pn
3.8.05

Nursing Ethics:
Irish Cases and Concerns

Dolores Dooley and Joan McCarthy

Gill & Macmillan

Gill & Macmillan
Hume Avenue
Park West
Dublin 12
with associated companies throughout the world

www.gillmacmillan.ie

0 7171 3576 4

Index compiled by Cover to Cover
Print origination in Ireland by Red Barn Publishing, Skeagh, Skibbereen

The paper used in this book is made from the wood pulp of managed forests. For every tree felled, at least one is planted, thereby renewing natural resources.

A catalogue record is available for this book from the British Library.

Contents

Section One: Patient-Nurse Relationship

Section Two: Living and Dying

Section Three: Resources, Justice and Accountability

Section Four: Nursing Ethically

Appendices

Foreword

This excellent text exploring ethical issues in nursing within the context of the Irish Health Service is both timely and welcome. While there are some very useful international texts now available to the Irish nurse, concerned with the ethical dimension of practice, one that acknowledges the culture and socialisation of Irish nursing and the Irish health service is long overdue. The authors, from a base of many years of experience teaching ethics to nursing and medical students, and to qualified practitioners, invite the reader to confront and examine, with new eyes, taken-for-granted elements of practice; or in the authors' words 'unquestioned and habituated practices'. Some graphic examples are cited, such as the taking of blood without consent or the sharing of clothes versus personal belongings for intellectually disabled residents. The authors also provide a broad range of clinically relevant topics in a clear and considered manner.

Much thought has been given to the experience and the educational needs of the primary audience for this text. The layout of the text takes the reader from the context of nursing practice and the nurse–patient relationship (the known), through the difficult moral issues surrounding living and dying, resource allocation and justice, to, for some practitioners and students, the largely unknown terrain of ethical theories. Each chapter is carefully introduced with chapter-focused learning objectives highlighted at its commencement. There are numerous scenarios, narratives and experiential learning activities included in the text. This will help the reader to engage at an emotional, as well as a cognitive, level, with the text – and with the issues raised. Material is well referenced throughout, with further reading also provided in end-of-chapter reading lists. Interesting concepts such as 'moral space' are introduced to the reader. The discussion of this concept deftly reminds the reader that we all practise within a context and organisational structures. Both the context and the organisational structures of the health service (or health-care institution) can have a significant impact on one's ability both to perceive the moral and to follow through on decision actions in relation to an identified moral issue. This surely is an area worthy of further attention by practitioners, regulatory bodies and those who lead and manage the health service.

Alongside the standard topics one has come to expect in this type of introductory nursing ethics text, the authors also explore ethical issues surrounding some more recent biotechnological developments that are fast becoming recognised as mainstream 'treatments'. Chapter 11, *Selecting for Sex*, is one such very pertinent example.

The tension between the focus in Western thinking on individual autonomy versus African and Asian focus on communalism and interdependence is articulated sensitively and clearly. Indeed, from discussion of this tension across a number of chapters, the reader is better equipped to deal with some of the disquiet expressed both by practitioners and in the more recent health-care ethics literature. This disquiet surrounds the potential weaknesses of an overriding focus on individual autonomy in thinking about ethical issues in health care, in relation to an individual rendered vulnerable by illness and disease; and/or by the power structures within which health care is often delivered. This, I suggest, is an important discussion. Elemental to it is an analysis of the required tensions between respecting the person of the patient, including the patient's right to decision making, and the requirements of professional responsibility on the one hand, with an acceptance of the interdependent nature of human beings, families and society, and the social dimension of illness and disease, on the other.

As Ireland moves forward to embrace the health reform agenda, issues of justice, decisions regarding what is appropriate resource allocation, and what a member of the general public can reasonably expect both from the health service, and from the practitioners who work within it, will become very salient and contentious issues. The authors helpfully draw out some of the key elements that require consideration, and provide some helpful analysis and lines of argument for the novice discussant. This is a complex and at times confusing terrain. The text provides some very useful signposts to guide the concerned practitioner and citizen in discussions that will often prove contentious. Nonetheless these are discussions which, as members of a society that cares about the quality of the health care provided to its citizens, we should not sidestep or leave only to the 'experts'.

Nurses are used to concerning themselves with the micro level of resource allocation; however, as Dooley and McCarthy suggest, this may not be enough. Nurses, as responsible practitioners and concerned citizens, may also need to engage with macro and meso allocation discussions. This section of the text allows the reader to confront both the uncertainty in this area, and the requirement to decide what the level of engagement of the nurse should be, given a particular set of circumstances, rather than simply accept unexamined tradition.

The authors then move on to introduce the reader to a number of theoretical perspectives that can be brought to bear to help ethical analysis, judgement development and decision making. The language of the different ethical theories enables different elements in a situation to gain salience. The final section in the text gives a more detailed description of a number of ethical theories, both contemporary and traditional, and highlights the main claims of each. Strengths and weaknesses of each of the frameworks are considered, as is the answer each theory proposes to the question of how one should behave to live a morally good life.

This text is a very welcome addition to the Irish health literature scene. It is timely in terms of the changes in Irish nursing education, to undergraduate degree-level studies for registration, and postgraduate master's level for specialist and advanced practice. It is also timely in terms of the Irish health service reform agenda, an agenda in which nurses will play an intimate part. I commend the authors for their substantive and stimulating contribution to thinking about the ethical dimension of nursing practice. Many nursing students, both undergraduate and postgraduate, will gain much from studying this text for years to come.

Professor P. Anne Scott

Acknowledgements

We are indebted to numerous people who have helped us in various ways to write this book. First and foremost, we would like to thank all of the nursing and midwifery students who have shared with us their experiences and worries about nursing and midwifery practice over the years of teaching nursing ethics. We are especially grateful for the contributions of Antoinette Woodman and Olive Long.

We would also like to express our appreciation of the support we have received from our colleagues in the Catherine McAuley School of Nursing and Midwifery, University College Cork. We applaud the Head of School, Professor Geraldine McCarthy, for recognising the important role that nursing ethics has to play in the education of nursing students and ensuring its inclusion in undergraduate and postgraduate nursing curricula. We would also like to thank Alice Coffey, Angela Flynn, Jill Murphy, Rhona O'Connell, Eileen Savage, John Sweeney, Teresa Tuohy, Mark Tyrrell and Teresa Wills who gave us invaluable feedback on individual chapters and cases in the text.

We are grateful too to Mary Donnelly and Deirdre Madden, Department of Law, University College Cork, whose expertise in legal and ethical questions in relation to health care have greatly enhanced the scope of the book. Friends, Clare Treacy and Sharon Murphy, have also given us the benefit of their critical and exacting perspectives on various cases and contexts.

Our gratitude also goes to the staff of Gill & Macmillan and, especially, to Regina Barrett, Marion O'Brien, Aoileann O'Donnell and Emer Ryan who hurried us along with the greatest of patience and speed.

We would especially like to thank Professor P. Anne Scott, Head of School of Nursing, Dublin City University, for agreeing to write the Foreword for *Nursing Ethics: Irish Cases and Concerns*. As Professor Scott is one of the pioneers of the development of nursing ethics in Ireland, we deeply appreciate her early encouragement and ongoing support for the book.

Finally, we would like to pay tribute to our partners and families, especially Desmond Clarke for his steady encouragement in the work of applying ethics, and Patricia O'Dwyer for her critical insights and careful reading of the whole of the text.

Of course, any mistakes or inaccuracies are our own.

Introduction

Nursing Ethics is a domain of inquiry that focuses on the moral problems and challenges that nurses face in the course of their work. It involves an exploration and analysis of the beliefs, values, attitudes, assumptions, arguments, emotions and relationships that underlie nursing ethical decisions.

In some ways, nursing ethics can be viewed as one area of health-care ethics alongside others such as medical ethics and dentistry ethics. Similar to these, nursing ethics focuses on ethical issues that arise in patient/professional relationships, such as autonomy, consent, veracity and confidentiality. It also considers obstacles to good care that health professionals must grapple with – scarce resources, social injustice and incompetent or immoral colleagues, for example. Most health professionals address these different issues and challenges at diverse levels (Holm 1997: 150–151).

Nursing ethics can also be understood as distinct from other fields in health-care ethics in important ways. Nursing ethics is connected with the unique history, goals and practices of nursing. In addition, many nurse ethicists pay particular attention to the quality of the relationship the nurse has with patients and their families (Fry 1989: 20). Moreover, the institutional and socio-cultural positions from which nurses make ethical decisions are considered to be significantly different from the positions of other professionals (Storch 2004: 1–16).

In the past twenty years, the field of health-care ethics in general has rapidly expanded to try to address the moral and metaphysical seismic shifts that have occurred as a result of technological advances at the beginning and end of life. Today, human beings can create life, modify life and prolong life in ways that make the wildest of science-fiction stories sound tame. Clinical ethics committees, research ethics committees and commissions are being instituted to attend to the moral uncertainty and moral challenges that go along with such rapid changes. Nursing ethics can be seen in a process of development that addresses these challenges and moral uncertainty.

While nursing ethics has also expanded rapidly in response to change, it is well to remember that it is not just a recent phenomenon, the 'Josephine come lately' or 'poor relation' of other fields in health-care ethics. In fact, according to Marsha Fowler's doctoral research, nursing ethics has a long and distinguished history which demonstrates that nurses have been profoundly and intimately concerned with good nursing practice and the welfare of society as a whole for decades (Fowler 1984). The first documented textbook, for example, was Isabel Robb's *Nursing Ethics: For Hospital and Private Use*, published in 1900 and reprinted several times. In addition, the first journal of nursing, *The Trained Nurse*, which began in 1888, published a six-part series of articles on ethics in nursing. Since its inception in 1900, *The American Journal of Nursing* (AJN) has published over 400 articles on ethical issues up to the 1980s (Fowler 1997: 31).

At the beginning of the twentieth century, the language of obedience, vocation and service predominated in the nursing ethics discourse. Today, in the twenty-first century, writers place emphasis on good judgement, autonomous decision making and professional and personal accountability. What is common to both early and recent discourse, however, is an understanding of the ethical life as one that is most deeply lived in relationship with others. To be ethically alive on this view is to be aware, attentive, and understanding of the ethical obligations and responsibilities we share with and for others. A Canadian nurse ethicist articulates this perspective in the following way:

> [N]ursing ethics is about being in relationship to persons in care. The enactment of nursing ethics is a constant readiness to engage one's moral agency. Almost every nursing action and situation involves ethics. To raise questions about ethics is to ask about the good in our practice. Are we doing the right thing for this patient? Are we listening to this person's need for pain relief? Are we respecting a family's grief over their dying child as they struggle to squeeze out a few extra days or hours for the child through alternative therapies? Are we ready to stand up for what we know to be right when we face a situation requiring us to perform a procedure that we are confident is not appropriate and that violates the dignity of another human being? Are we willing to find time to debrief after complex situations to determine how we could have done better, with a commitment to doing everything in our power to prevent similar situations from occurring in the future? (Storch 2004: 7)

We offer this nursing ethics text in recognition of the long-standing ethical engagement of Irish nurses and midwives in improving the lives of people in their care. In the following chapters, we explore and analyse situations drawn from the everyday practice of nurses in Ireland and elsewhere as well as some exceptional situations where life and death issues arise. This text does not view ethics solely as an academic or theoretical subject but rather as an engaging, challenging activity that demands the development of a range of skills and intelligences.

We use different moral frameworks to draw out different ethical features of each of these situations. While, for simplicity's sake, we pay most attention to traditional ethical frameworks such as principle-based approaches, we also draw on more contemporary perspectives such as narrative ethics, in order to bring to the foreground different ethical dimensions that may arise in health-care settings.

We believe that, given the international and multicultural nature of nursing practice, there should be a variety of moral frameworks to support ethical understanding and development. As with all other areas of inquiry, the development of nursing ethics has not occurred in a vacuum. History, culture, gender relations, political and economic forces, health-care policies and organisational hierarchies all contribute to the often vastly different roles and responsibilities that nurses assume locally and globally. We believe that, because Irish nurses work in very different kinds of health-care settings, they need to be able to draw on a variety of moral paradigms in order to expand their agency.

The text is the first of its kind for teaching nursing ethics in Ireland. It introduces the reader to the process of ethical reasoning and resolution through interactive learning, with the goal of engaging the reader through an exchange of cases, analysis and questions. Many of the cases are concrete narratives drawn from everyday experiences of nurses in Irish hospital wards, operating theatres, clinics and community health centres. Where relevant, we also include cases drawn from other countries. The narratives highlight a number of ethical questions and issues that are then explained and discussed in the text. In each chapter, a range of activities and suggestions is offered to encourage the reader to tease out the moral questions raised in the text. Each chapter offers Summary Learning Guides to facilitate a revision of concepts and definitions that aid in the project of developing greater ethical literacy for nurses in practice. Terms highlighted in bold are explained in the Glossary at the end of the text.

The overall aim of the book is to provide Irish nurses with a resource that will support and empower them in the challenging role they have in Irish health care. Specifically we intend this book to provide the critical, reflective and imaginative skills to enable them to become more informed and more confident decision makers.

Nursing Ethics: Irish Cases and Concerns is divided into four sections with a brief introduction to each section. The first three explore and analyse different case narratives as the basis for consideration of the patient–nurse relationship, decision making at the beginning and end of life, justice in resource allocation and strategies of accountability in practice. In considering these situations, our discussion draws on a range of different ethical frameworks that are more fully explained in the final section of the text.

Section One:
Patient–Nurse Relationship

This section focuses on moral values that are central to the patient–nurse relationship. These values are also key conditions of the empowerment of individuals to make important decisions in relation to their health care and wellbeing. These include autonomy, truth telling, confidentiality and informed consent.

The first two chapters explore and analyse the notion of patient autonomy. Chapter 1 defines autonomy as involving self-determination and self-authorship and explains why the freedom of individuals to make their own life choices is considered so important in many countries. Chapter 2 describes and analyses two cases which illustrate the different kinds of demands that the principle of respect for autonomy places on nurses working in different health-care settings: general hospital and community. It also discusses the notion of paternalism and the challenges that arise when respect for autonomy seems to conflict with the need to protect vulnerable patients from harm.

Chapter 3 tells the story of an autonomous patient who is lied to about her condition and a nurse whose conscience is clearly troubled because she is party to the deception. In analysing the case, this chapter explains and evaluates two different moral theories on truth telling and it enumerates the arguments for and against truthful conversation with patients. This chapter anticipates the later discussion of informed consent since understanding of and information on one's condition are a pre-requisite for patient consent. Truth telling is also one of the themes addressed in Chapter 4 which explains the relationship between conscience and integrity and introduces the notion of moral space as a means of supporting the nurse's moral agency and advocacy role.

Chapters 5 and 6 explore another moral issue that impacts on patient autonomy and the patient–nurse relationship: the obligation on nurses to respect patient confidentiality. Chapter 5 refers to professional codes of practice in determining the scope of confidentiality and it indicates those circumstances where an exception to confidentiality might be made. Chapter 6 extends the discussion of confidentiality through an analysis of two cases which raise the troubling tension between the duty to protect a patient and the duty to warn another. The chapter argues that, to be ethically engaged in the fullest sense is to be alive to the world of the patient from the patient's point of view, while acknowledging that there are others whose voices and interests must also be heard and served.

The final two chapters in this section assess the role of the requirement of informed consent in the patient–nurse relationship. Chapter 7 introduces and explains the various elements of informed consent and considers, especially, the role of nurses in enabling patients to participate fully in decision making regarding their medical treatment and nursing care. What the case in Chapter 7 illustrates is that informed consent is more a process of understanding and deliberation than a single act of assent or compliance. With this understanding of informed consent, we turn in Chapter 8 to the additional challenges that the requirement of informed consent poses to nurses who undertake research involving human participants. We highlight the controversial role of one public health nurse in the United States Tuskegee clinical trial and we also explore a second case narrative which illustrates some of the issues that arise in undertaking research with children.

– 1 –

Respecting Patient Autonomy

Objectives

At the end of this chapter, you should be able to:

- Define **autonomy** and describe the four elements of an autonomous decision;
- Distinguish between moral and nonmoral decisions;
- Explain why autonomous capacity is held in high regard;
- Consider two different views of why autonomy deserves respect;
- Explore different ways in which autonomy can be respected in health-care settings.

INTRODUCTION

The term autonomy derives from the Greek words, *autos* ('self') and *nomos* ('rule', 'law', 'governance') and originally referred to the self-rule of Greek independent city-states. Today, however, we associate autonomy not just with nations but also with persons, acts and decisions. In addition to meaning self-rule, it has acquired meanings such as self-governance, liberty, self-authorship, freedom of the will and self-determination.

An *autonomous person* is usually taken to be someone who is capable of making important decisions about their own lives on the basis of their own beliefs and values. While there is some disagreement among ethicists as to the exact features of an *autonomous decision*, we suggest that for any act to qualify as autonomous, it should be autonomous in each of the following four senses:

a) *Free or voluntary*: carried out in the light of an individual's own thoughts, feelings, desires or intentions.

b) *Intentional*: intended by the individual. The act is not committed in error or as a result of ignorance.

c) *Informed*: performed with an understanding of the situation, an awareness of the consequences and a knowledge of alternatives.

d) *Deliberative*: the result of a considered weighing of the likely consequences.

In order to tease out what these different senses of autonomy might demand of a decision maker, consider the following scenario.

Case 1.1: Deciding Where to Go

Mairéad is a forty-year-old woman who has been working as a care assistant in the local hospital for the past twenty years. She has made up her mind to return to education to become a nurse and she must now decide which college she will apply to in order to begin the undergraduate programme in nursing.

Before applying, Mairéad writes to the four institutions that teach nursing in the south west, for information about their programmes. She also makes an appointment with the coordinators in each.

Taking into consideration the content of the available programmes, the distances involved, and what she learns from visiting the coordinators, Mairéad decides to apply to the Clare Institute of Technology (CIT), the college that is nearest to her home.

Mairéad's decision to apply to CIT in this case could be considered autonomous in each of the four senses:

a) It is *free* or *voluntary* because, even though she might have been influenced by her meeting with the coordinator in CIT, it is unlikely that Mairéad was unduly influenced. All of our decisions are inevitably influenced, to some degree, by other people's views or desires. However, a decision is considered free when it is not *coerced* by other people. Similarly, a decision is considered free, when it is not made under the influence of drugs or a pathological condition.

b) Given Mairéad's travels to different institutions and her meetings with various coordinators, it could be said that she has decided to apply to CIT with some *purpose* – she *intends* to study in Clare rather than, for example, in Dublin or Wexford.

c) It is clear that Mairéad has taken the time to *inform* herself fully of the content of programmes, the institutions offering them and the demands on her time that undertaking an undergraduate programme involves.

d) Finally, given her preparation, it is probable that Mairéad has *considered* all the information that she has gathered and *weighed* the likely costs and benefits of her decision.

Activity

While the choice of a particular undergraduate programme in nursing is likely to be voluntary, intentional, informed and deliberative, our everyday decisions are not always autonomous in each of these four senses. Some may be wholly voluntary but not informed; others may be fully informed but ill-considered. Think of one decision that you have made in the past month – to date someone new, for example, or to go to the cinema. In which of the four senses, if any, would you say that your decision was autonomous?

Moral and Nonmoral Decisions

Notice that, while Mairéad's choice of programme is autonomous, it is a practical, rather than a moral decision. Mairéad's decision to go to CIT reflects the values that Mairéad places on things such as education (programme content), convenience (distance to travel), and efficiency (visit to the coordinator). Her decision expresses a personal preference rather than a moral position.

On the other hand, decisions that are moral in nature are decisions that concern significant moral interests such as human rights and liberty, justice and welfare. For example, while Mairéad's choice of college is a nonmoral choice, the earlier decision that she made – to return to college to become a nurse – is, in the main, a moral decision. This is illustrated in the following excerpt from Mairéad's story.

Case 1.2: Deciding What to Do

Mairéad wanted to become a nurse as far back as she could remember. As a child, she had been captivated by the stories told to her by her favourite aunt, who worked as a midwife in a local hospital. As a teenager, she had avidly followed the TV series, *Marcus Welby* and *Nurse*, the equivalent when she was growing up of shows such as *Flying Doctors* and *ER*.

However, because she was unsuccessful in securing a training place in an Irish hospital, and because the family finances couldn't support her training in the UK, Mairéad decided to take a job as care assistant and apply again for nursing at a later date. By the time she was ready to move on, however, Mairéad had met and married Tom. Her life of the last twenty years was a (happy) blur of supporting Tom on their farm and raising their family.

Now that the children were off pursuing their own careers, Mairéad was once again contemplating a career in nursing. One worry remained, however – the care of her father. Mairéad's mother had died ten years previously, and her father, now eighty-one and suffering from rheumatoid arthritis, was growing more feeble and immobile every day. Mairéad knew that even with the support of the public health nurse, with Tom's help and home help, her father would soon need full-time care.

Her choice seemed to be a stark one. If she stayed at home, she could look after her father. If she enrolled on a nursing programme, it was likely that her father would have to be hospitalised. On the one hand, even though she didn't have a very good relationship with her father, she felt obliged to look after him in his last days. On the other hand, she felt that she had a lot to offer the patients who might come under her care and the colleagues with whom she might work.

Activity

Read Cases 1.1 and 1.2 and consider: what makes Mairéad's decision in relation to becoming a nurse a moral decision and her decision about which college she attends a practical decision?

Mairéad's choice between caring for her father and training as a nurse is a moral one because it involves two competing moral obligations – the obligation to look after an ailing parent and the obligation to look after the ailing people in the larger community. While Mairéad doesn't have a very good personal relationship with her father, she, nevertheless, feels that she owes him a daughter's duty of care. Such a duty is informed by the value that Mairéad places on family relationships and respect for one's parents.

On the other hand, while Mairéad's desire to train as a nurse is personal – she has always wanted to become a nurse – her choice is also informed by the values that she places on the prevention of suffering and promotion of health (nursing care for patients) and fidelity (to colleagues in health care).

In sum, while Mairéad's choice of nursing programme is determined by the practical values she holds in relation to education, convenience and efficiency, her choice to become a nurse is determined by the moral values she holds in relation to doing good.

Activity

We have suggested that decisions can be considered autonomous in each of four senses: they can be free, intentional, informed and deliberative. We have, earlier, concluded that Mairéad's choice of college is autonomous in each of these ways. Now, re-read Case 1.2 and decide whether or not Mairéad's decision to become a nurse in the first place is, similarly, autonomous.

While our decisions (moral and nonmoral) may be described as autonomous in one or more of the four ways we have just described, we also talk about *degrees* or *levels* of autonomy. Different acts may be more or less free, more or less informed, more or less deliberate. For example, all of the decisions or acts that we carry out in our daily life do not require the same level of autonomy as a career-related choice. You may consider that the choice to sit or stand while reading this book, or the choice of what to wear this evening do not demand the level of freedom or the kind of purpose and consideration that a career choice might require. You might be happy for someone else to tell you what to wear to a social occasion, for example, but you might well baulk if they insisted that you train as a journalist rather than as a nurse.

The weightier the decision in an individual's life and the lives of others, the more important it is that the decision is significantly autonomous. This is particularly the case when it comes to decisions that people make in relation to their health and welfare which touch on features of human life that are deeply meaningful – bodily integrity, birth, death and dying.

Acknowledging that health-care decisions are profoundly important however, does not mean that only those health-care decisions that are *fully* voluntary, intended, informed and deliberate qualify as autonomous. If that were the case, most of the decisions that most of us make would not make the grade. Following Beauchamp and Childress (2001: 59), we would argue in favour of the ideal of *substantial* rather than *full* autonomy in relation to health-care decisions. So, for example, we allow that a person's decision counts as autonomous even if it is motivated by some controlling influences and even if that person is not fully but only reasonably informed of the consequences of their decision.

Describing a person as autonomous then does not mean that they are the single originating source of all of their decisions or that they are the single author of the story of their own lives. Nor does it imply that individuals have complete control over all of their desires, intentions and deliberations.

> To restrict adequate decision-making by patients and research subjects to the ideal of fully or completely autonomous decision-making strips their acts of any meaningful place in the practical world, where people's actions are rarely, if ever, fully autonomous. A person's appreciation of information and independence from controlling influences in the context of health care need not exceed, for example, a person's information and independence in making a financial investment, hiring a new employee, buying a house, or selecting a university. Such consequential decisions must be substantially autonomous, but not necessarily fully autonomous. (Beauchamp and Childress 2001: 59–60)

Setting a minimum standard of this kind for autonomy makes sense because it includes the decisions that most ordinary people make. The significance of setting such a standard will become even more clear in Chapter 7 when we examine the concept of **informed consent**.

Activity

a) Take another look at the list of decisions that Beauchamp and Childress have suggested require the same degree of **substantial autonomy** as health-care decisions. They included decisions about:
 • Financial investments
 • Hiring an employee
 • Buying a house
 • Selecting a university.

Do you agree with Beauchamp and Childress here? Can you add two other kinds of decisions that you think would require the same level of autonomy?

b) Can you think of two decisions that, in your view, should be made on the basis of *full* or *complete* (and not just substantial) autonomy? Give reasons as to why you think this should be so.

Summary Learning Guide 1.1

The concept of autonomy:

- Refers to such capacities as self-rule, self-governance, liberty, self-authorship, freedom of the will and self-determination;
- Refers to a person who is capable of making important decisions about their own lives on the basis of their own beliefs and values;
- Refers to decisions or actions that are free, intentional, informed and deliberative;
- Refers to a continuum of levels of autonomy from very little, to substantial, to full autonomy.

THE IMPORTANCE OF AUTONOMY

The capacity that human beings have to act autonomously is valued very highly in the western Judaeo-Christian tradition. This is so for a number of reasons which are summarised here and explained below. Autonomy is argued to be important because:

i)   It enables human beings to be accountable for their actions;
ii)   It is considered core to personal identity;
iii)   It is the basis of respect for human rights.

a)   The fact that human beings are the kinds of creatures who can act or refrain from acting on the basis of their own deliberative capacities enables them to take responsibility for and to account for their decisions in a way that has been recognised throughout human history. For example, religious stories might bemoan the decisions of Lucifer, Adam and Eve to turn away from God but their ability to make such a choice is nevertheless a central feature of the Christian belief system. In addition, classic plays and novels such as *Hamlet* and *Pride and Prejudice* focus on and appraise the choices and the subsequent lives of their main protagonists. Popular music also celebrates those who can say, 'I did it my way' or who 'can shout out, I am who I am'.

From the sublime to the ridiculous and from the traumatic to the trivial, the ability of human individuals to choose on the basis of their own ideas of what is the right thing to do has been lauded down the centuries by very many cultures across the world. Whether individuals choose to conform, to reform, to rebel or to refuse, individual creativity is everywhere honoured.

b)   The relationship between autonomy and personal identity is profound. Because human beings have a sense that they have an important role to play in decisions that affect their lives, autonomy is considered to be core to personal identity. For example, if computers or astrology charts could find a life partner for us with greater success than we can achieve by ourselves, would we hand over our futures to them? Perhaps. However, we generally don't because part of the pleasure of planning a romantic entanglement, a career or a garden is the knowledge that we ourselves are, to some degree, responsible for the outcome.

In making a decision, in choosing one particular path over another, individuals have a sense that they are participating in their own self-creation on the basis of their personal choices. In turn, the self that they help to create – the nurse, the parent, the politician, the lover – is the author of further self-creating choices.

Notice that this view does not insist that people are *completely independent* or the *sole* authors of their lives. While individuals exercise some autonomy in their self-creation, their personal identity is also dependent on their physicality and their relationships with others. In addition, it is made intelligible by the culture, history and circumstances out of which they emerge and from which they draw their self-understandings.

c) Historically the concept of autonomy has been used to champion the rights of various groups to equal treatment and opportunities and to challenge oppressive regimes and institutions on the basis that they deny or abuse it.

Political philosophers of the late twentieth century such as Isaiah Berlin (1969), John Rawls (1971) and Ronald Dworkin (1977) place autonomy as a central value of modern liberal societies and argue that the success of these societies can be measured by the extent to which they provide the conditions under which human beings can express their autonomy.

This way of approaching the social and political arrangements of a society as a whole might also be applied to specific social provisions such as health care and particular institutions. We might ask, for example, to what extent the Irish health-care system protects and promotes the autonomy of those who use it and those who work in it. Or, we might ask to what extent a hospital or health-centre protects or promotes the autonomy of patients under its care.

RESPECT FOR AUTONOMY

Because of the significance attached to autonomy, respect for autonomous choice is a core element of many different philosophical and political

Activity

In this section, we suggested three arguments as to why autonomy is considered important in Anglo-American cultures. In sum, autonomous capacity, makes human beings accountable, supports a sense of self and is the foundation of respect for human rights.

a) Reflect on each of these arguments again and see if you agree or disagree with any of them.

b) For some cultural groups in China, Japan and other parts of Southern Asia and Southern Europe, family and communal decision making is afforded a privileged position, and individuals are encouraged to place the interests of their family and community above their own. List any merits that you see in this approach to decision making.

theories. Two philosophers, the eighteenth-century German, Immanuel Kant (1724–1804), and the nineteenth-century Englishman, John Stuart Mill (1806–1873), have greatly influenced the way in which we understand what respect for autonomy involves.

Kantian Autonomy

Kant appealed to the **deontological** belief – that some things are intrinsically or inherently good, that each person is intrinsically valuable or has unconditional worth because they have the capacity to be autonomous. For Kant, human dignity resides in the fact that each person has a **free will** which they can follow independently of their passions or desires. In his view, human beings can be distinguished from many other sentient creatures because humans are not wholly determined by their own immediate desires.

Believing that human beings are able to act freely and independently of personal desires, loves and hates, Kant argued that they are capable of prescribing general moral rules or principles for themselves to follow. They can legislate for their own conduct. The neo-Kantian, Thomas Hill, takes this to mean that:

> [T]he autonomy of a moral legislator means that, in debating basic moral principles and values, a person ideally should not be moved by blind adherence to tradition or authority, by outside threats or bribes, by unreflective impulse, or unquestioned habits of thought . . . must try not to give special weight to his or her particular preferences and personal attachments . . . In other words, at the level of deliberation about basic principles, morality requires impartial regard for all persons. (Hill 1991: 45)

On the Kantian view, human beings have a capacity for free, **rational** and **impartial** decision making. This means that they are able to decide a course of action on the basis of careful reflection and in the absence of coercion from authority or custom. In addition, they can decide the best course of action independently of their own personal preferences or inclinations.

It is on the basis of this kind of autonomous capacity that each human being has a special status that deserves protection and respect for Kant. In his terms, disrespecting a person's autonomy would involve treating an individual merely as a means to another's ends and not in terms of their own ends:

> So act that you use humanity, whether in your own person or in the person of any other, always at the same time as an end, never merely as a means. (Kant 1997 [1785], 38)

Millian Autonomy

In his well-known thesis in *On Liberty* (1859), John Stuart Mill also promoted respect for individual autonomy (or liberty) but on different grounds from those of Kant. Mill viewed each person as worthy of respect, not because of their rationality or impartiality, but because of their unique individuality. He appealed to the **utilitarian** view – that an action is morally good if it gives rise to more good than evil – to support his position. For Mill, respecting individual autonomy gives rise to more good than evil – society ought to respect autonomy because, in the long term, society benefits from doing so:

> The worth of a State, in the long run, is the worth of the individuals composing it . . . a state which dwarfs its men in order that they may be more docile instruments in its hands even for beneficial purposes – will find that with small men no great thing can really be accomplished. (Mill 1981: 187)

In other words, on the Millian view, individual freedom is compatible with and contributes towards the good of society as a whole. It follows that a person ought be allowed to act according to their own life's plan, their own beliefs and values whether or not their actions are considered wise, or good or foolish by everyone else (One needs to read this text of Mill as referring to both genders when he uses the language of 'small men' etc.)

The only occasion, for Mill, when a state or an individual is justified in interfering in individual liberty is when a person's action causes harm to others. He distinguishes between public and private morality, between those of our actions which affect others in society – other-regarding actions – and those which affect only ourselves – self-regarding actions. This is a classic liberal position which holds that the freedom of the individual can be compromised only when it is in competition with the rights and freedoms of other individuals. Respect for autonomy requires, in this view, that we not interfere with the self-regarding acts and decisions that people make.

> [T]he only purpose for which power can be rightfully exercised over any member of a civilized community, against his will, is to prevent harm to others. His own good, either physical or moral, is not sufficient warrant. He cannot rightfully be compelled to do or forbear because it will be better for him to do so, because it will make him happier, because, in the opinions of others, to do so would be wise, or even right. These are good reasons for remonstrating with him, or persuading him, or entreating him, but not for compelling him, or visiting him with any evil in case he does otherwise. (Mill 1981: 68)

Respecting Autonomy in Health Care

Drawing on the insights of both Kant and Mill, some health-care ethicists have suggested a **principle** or **rule** of autonomy to guide all health

Activity

It could be argued that most human actions affect other people apart from the agent of the action.

a) Make a list of three actions that an individual might perform which would clearly affect other people.

b) Can you think of any actions that are exclusively self-regarding actions?

c) Consider whether or not it is a matter of degree, that some actions might be more self-regarding than others?

professionals in relation to their care of patients. Such a principle obliges health professionals to behave in certain ways toward patients. Tom Beauchamp and James Childress, for example, are two ethicists who have given an important role to the concept of autonomy in health care. They delineate the principle of autonomy in the following way:

> This principle [of autonomy] can be stated as a negative obligation and as a positive obligation. As a negative obligation: Autonomous actions should not be subjected to controlling constraints by others . . . As a positive obligation, this principle requires respectful treatment in disclosing information and fostering autonomous decision-making . . . Respect for autonomy obligates professionals in health care and research involving human subjects to disclose information, to probe for and ensure understanding and voluntariness, and to foster adequate decision-making. (2001: 64)

Negative autonomy refers to non-interference with others' choices. It simply means that health professionals are obliged not to interfere with or constrain a patient's autonomous decisions in relation to their health (as long as the exercise of their autonomy does not substantially infringe on the autonomy of others). Positive autonomy places more substantive obligations on health-care workers. It obliges health professionals to recognise, support and enable the unique values, priorities and individuality of patients.

CONCLUSION
This chapter has explained and defended the need to respect individual autonomy. Firstly we defined autonomous decisions as those that are substantially voluntary, intentional, informed and deliberative and we distinguished between decisions that are largely moral and those that are not. We suggested that very many of our decisions, moral and nonmoral, are

Activity

a) Can you think of any examples from your practice where you felt obliged to constrain the autonomous decision of a patient in your care?

b) Can you think of any examples from your practice where you supported and enabled the autonomy of a patient in your care?

c) Based on what you have learned about the concept of autonomy so far and on the definition of the principle of autonomy provided by Beauchamp and Childress, briefly define the principle of autonomy in your own words as a guide for your practice.

Summary Learning Guide 1.2

Autonomy is important because:

- It enables people to be accountable for their actions;
- It is core to personal identity;
- It is fundamental to the defence of human rights.

Autonomy deserves respect because:

- It is an expression of the rational and impartial nature of human beings (Kant);
- It contributes to the good of society as a whole (Mill).

The principle of autonomy obliges the nurse:

- To refrain from interfering or constraining the autonomy of patients (except where that autonomy might seriously limit or harm others);
- To enable and promote the autonomy of patients.

---

not autonomous in each of the four senses. In addition, we suggested that different acts may be considered autonomous to different degrees. Given that an individual's acts might be considered in terms of a continuum of autonomy, we argued that a person's health-care decisions need to be substantially (but not necessarily fully) autonomous to qualify for protection and promotion.

We also proposed, in this chapter, that individual autonomy is important because it is a prerequisite for personal accountability, personal identity and human rights. We further indicated two philosophical views of why autonomy deserves respect: Kant's argument that respect for autonomy recognises the human capacity for rational and impartial decision making, and Mill's argument that a society which respects individual autonomy is ultimately a better society than one that does not.

Finally, we briefly introduced the idea of a principle of autonomy that might serve to guide nurses in their practice. Chapter 2 will describe and analyse two cases which illustrate the different kinds of demands that the principle of respect for autonomy, in its negative and positive senses, places on nurses working in different health-care settings.

The following terms are explained in the glossary:

autonomy	principle
deontological theory	rational
free will	rule
impartiality	substantial autonomy
informed consent	utilitarian

– 2 –

Autonomy and Vulnerability

Objectives

At the end of this chapter, you should be able to:

- Distinguish between negative and positive obligations of autonomy;
- Define and discuss the principle of **beneficence**;
- Distinguish between **weak** and **strong** forms of **paternalism**;
- Discuss the challenges that arise when respect for autonomy seems to conflict with the need to protect vulnerable patients from harm.

INTRODUCTION

In Chapter 1, we defined the principle of autonomy as a rule which obliges health professionals to act in particular ways in relation to patients in their care. We suggested that the principle placed a negative obligation on the nurse – not to interfere with or constrain patients' autonomous decisions – and a positive obligation – to acknowledge, support and promote the decision-making capacity of patients.

The following case illustrates the kinds of demands that the principle of respect for autonomy, in its negative sense, places on a nurse who is working in a hospital setting. The case is concerned with the ways in which a patient's autonomy can be constrained.

Case 2.1: The Patient who Wants to Go Home

Sean is seventy-two years old and has been living alone since the death of his partner five years ago. He is in the early stages of Alzheimer's disease and is currently in the city general hospital recovering from a minor operation. Up until recently, he has lived a very active and independent life, devoting himself to charity work and to his beloved garden.

During the day, Sean is generally fine, good humoured and cooperative with staff and fellow patients. However, as the evenings draw on, Sean is inclined to become agitated and distressed. He insists to staff and other patients, often loudly and aggressively, that he wants to go home to tend to his flowers and vegetables. He has taken to wandering the corridors of the hospital, trying to leave; on a few occasions, he has managed to get as far as the hospital car park.

The staff have tried various strategies to reassure Sean. They have told him that his neighbour is caring for his garden and they have also tried some mild sedatives. However, even when asked during his most lucid periods in the day, Sean tells staff that he would prefer to go home, whatever the risk, and that he misses his house all the more when night draws on.

Most recently, Sean managed to leave the hospital altogether and was found by an off-duty hospital porter, wandering in a very busy shopping area looking for a bus to take him home. This has prompted the team to meet to decide on what can be done to ensure Sean's wellbeing and safety and the welfare of other residents on the ward. The resident doctor suggests that they give Sean a stronger sedative in the evening, while the ward manager suggests that they use an electronic tag so that staff are alerted and the door of the ward is closed when Sean tries to leave the hospital.

Sean's story will strike a chord with many nurses, health professionals and carers who look after people with varying degrees of dementia, and it illustrates some of the key ethical issues that arise in relation to their care, such as, for example:

- Whether or not Sean's attempts to return home should be considered autonomous acts;
- The obligations, if any, of the health-care team to respect Sean's wishes;
- The obligations of the team to ensure Sean's safety and wellbeing;
- The obligations of staff to respect Sean's autonomy and, at the same time, ensure the wellbeing of all the patients in their care.

You might think of other issues that are relevant here, but we will focus our discussion on respect for Sean's autonomy and concern for his welfare.

Through general conversation, or as a result of applying a relevant clinical assessment tool, it might be established that Sean's dementia is sufficiently advanced to cloud his judgement seriously. Staff might determine that Sean's stage of dementia is increasingly undermining his ability to make autonomous decisions and that he is all but non-autonomous. While he seems perfectly lucid during the day, his night disturbances on the ward and his escapades into a large and impersonal city are serious causes for concern.

On the other hand, staff might determine that Sean is only in the early stages of Alzheimer's and that he could well manage both to find his way home, and to look after himself there for some time to come. If Sean is acting freely, if his intentions are clear and not mistaken, if he is reasonably informed of the risks at stake and can weigh the reasons for and against his hospitalisation, then Sean's decision to go home can be considered to be substantially autonomous.

However, whether Sean is considered to have substantial autonomy or no autonomy, his safety and welfare are an issue. Concern for his safety might lead the team to appeal to a second principle, that of beneficence, in order to help them in deciding what to do. We will briefly explain this principle before considering its application to Sean's situation.

THE PRINCIPLE OF BENEFICENCE

Since the time of Hippocrates (460–377 BC), health-care professionals have been advised to act for the benefit of their patients. This advice is often conceived in terms of the principle of beneficence which minimally requires that health professionals avoid harming patients and ideally requires them to promote patient health and wellbeing. (The twin tasks of avoiding harm and promoting good are often cast as two principles in the ethics literature: **nonmaleficence** – do no harm – and beneficence – do good – but for the purposes of this chapter, we take the principle of beneficence to incorporate both meanings.)

The parable of the Good Samaritan in the New Testament, Luke 10:34, is a good example of the *ideal* form of beneficence (Beauchamp and Childress 2001: 167). In that story, a man travelling from Jerusalem to Jericho is beaten and robbed and left for dead. His plight is ignored by two other travellers but he is eventually found by a stranger who, moved to pity, pours oil and wine on the man's wounds, bandages them and brings him to the nearest inn to care for him there.

Activity

a) Write a list of three acts of kindness in ordinary life that might be considered *ideal* acts of beneficence.

b) Write a list of three acts a nurse might perform in the course of her work that might be considered *ideal* acts of beneficence.

c) Do you think that it is possible for nurses to live up to the ideal of beneficence in all aspects of their professional lives?

Many ethicists and many ethical codes accept a less than ideal notion of beneficence as a requirement of professional conduct. Even so, while health professionals are not expected to be extremely altruistic and self-sacrificing, nevertheless, they are required to prevent and remove the conditions that cause harm and to promote good. Many Professional Codes of Conduct for Nurses implicitly appeal to the principle of beneficence to guide the professional conduct of nurses. For example, An Bord Altranais, the Irish Nursing Board's Code of Conduct states:

> The aim of the nursing profession is to give the highest standard of care possible to patients. Any circumstance which could place patients/clients in jeopardy or which militate against safe standards of practice should be made known to appropriate persons or authorities. (An Bord Altranais 2000a)

And according to the American Nurses Association (ANA):

> The nurse's primary commitment is to the health, welfare, and safety of the client. (ANA 1985: sec.3.1, p.6)

Because the patient in Case 2.1 is at risk of harm if he leaves the hospital, the health-care team has an obligation under the principle of beneficence to take this into consideration. The issue that arises for the team is one of balancing its obligations both to respect Sean's autonomy and, at the same time, to protect him from harm. This might mean that the team will have to make what is called a **paternalistic** decision in relation to Sean. The concept of paternalism and its implications for Sean's care are discussed in the following section.

PATERNALISM

As the term itself indicates, to act paternally towards a person is to act in a fatherly way towards them. Drawing on the traditional role of the father in a family, this conjures up the idea of someone who makes most of the decisions for his children and who is motivated in doing so by his conception of what is in their best interests.

For Beauchamp and Childress, the analogy of the responsible father translates easily to reflect the role of the health professional:

> A professional has superior training, knowledge and insight and is thus in an authoritative position to determine the patient's best interests. From this perspective, a health care professional is like a loving parent with dependent often ignorant and fearful children. (Beauchamp and Childress 2001: 178)

However, the traditional notion of the role of the father in relation to his children has been challenged in different ways:

- As an inadequate conceptualisation of family relationships – the heterosexual nuclear family is only one model of family life;
- As unjust – as unnecessarily authoritarian and undemocratic, for example;
- As counterproductive – children are happiest when their views are treated with respect.

Activity

a) Can you think of analogous examples where paternalistic practices in health care might be considered inadequate, unjust and counterproductive?

b) If we conclude that the term 'paternalism' is an unhelpful way of capturing some of the decisions that health professionals have to make on behalf of their patients, can you thing of another term? Would 'maternalism' be more useful? Or do you think we might run into similar difficulties with this term?

c) Many public health nurses, midwives and other nurses describe the people they care for in the community or other health-care settings as *clients* rather than *patients*. However, for the purposes of this text, we have decided to retain the more traditional word, patient. Take a few moments to reflect on what these different terms conjure up for you. Do you think that labelling someone in a particular way changes our behaviour toward them?

Weak Paternalism

Not all acts of paternalism are considered to be morally unacceptable. **Weak paternalism** limits the freedom of substantially *non-autonomous* individuals – those whose capacity to decide is compromised because they are unconscious, ignorant, careless, fearful, depressed or severely emotionally stressed.

On this understanding of paternalism, which is accepted as obligatory by ethicists and health professionals generally, the object is to protect individuals from self-inflicted harm.

> Intervention in the life of a substantially non-autonomous dependent became and remains the most widely accepted model of justified paternalism. That is, the paradigmatic form of justified paternalism starts with incompetent children in need of parental supervision and extends to other incompetents in need of care analogous to beneficent parental guidance. (Beauchamp and Childress 2001: 177)

Examples of weak acts of paternalism are:

- Raising the rails of the bed of a post-operative patient;
- Preventing a patient from removing their IV tube while they are asleep or unconscious;
- Performing the Heimlich manoeuvre in an emergency without permission.

Looking at the case study of Sean in the light of this discussion of weak paternalism, we can see that if the health-care team concludes that Sean is substantially non-autonomous, then its decision to intervene, albeit paternalistic, would be morally acceptable. In this situation, Sean's freedom of movement could, justifiably, be restricted, because his decision to go home would not be considered to be an autonomous one.

In short, constraining Sean does not disrespect his autonomy. He is not exercising autonomy in this instance. However, one might say more positively that the health-care workers are respecting Sean in his substantially non-autonomous state. The task that would then remain for the team would be a practical one of deciding what is the most appropriate, least restrictive and effective course of action to take in order to ensure Sean's safety.

Strong Paternalism

On the other hand, the team could determine that Sean has only a mild degree of cognitive impairment and could thus conclude that his desire and decision to return home are substantially autonomous. If, in spite of this conclusion, they decide to restrict Sean's freedom for what they perceive to be his own good, their interference needs a stronger justification than was required for **weak** paternalism.

The terminology of **strong** and **weak** paternalism can be confusing. It helps to think of the terms as referring to the justification required in each: weak paternalism, because it acts to protect non-autonomous individuals, calls for less rigorous defence or justification. Any act described as **strong**

paternalism is far more controversial. Strong paternalism demands considerably more stringent justification precisely because the patient is substantially autonomous. Strong paternalism limits the freedom of substantially autonomous individuals out of concern for their (supposed) 'good' or 'wellbeing'. In effect, strong paternalism elevates the principle of beneficence over the principle of autonomy when the two are in conflict.

Viewed in this way, paternalism is dis-empowering and typically involves one or more of the following: lying, deception, manipulation, coercion, non-disclosure of information. Examples of acts of strong paternalism are:

- Using patronising language such as 'Aren't we looking well today?' or 'There's no need to be worrying your head about that';
- Behaving in ways such as keeping patients waiting, turning one's back on patients;
- Ignoring patients, speaking about them (but not to them) when they are in the room;
- Making decisions without informing or involving autonomous patients.

Many contemporary ethicists argue that acts of strong paternalism are morally unacceptable because they interfere with autonomous choice. For example, Isaiah Berlin (1992) draws on the liberal philosophy of John Stuart Mill, outlined in Chapter 1, to reject paternalistic interventions in cases of substantial autonomy. For him, the authority to make decisions resides in the individual.

> I wish to be an instrument of my own, not other men's acts of will. I wish to be a subject, not an object . . . deciding, not being decided for, self-directed and not acted upon by external nature or by other men as if I were a thing, or an animal, or a slave incapable of playing a human role, that is, of conceiving goals and policies of my own and realising them. (Berlin 1992: 131)

This position also finds support in the arguments of the Irish legal medical expert, Mary Donnelly, who suggests that it is patients who are the most appropriate people to make health-care decisions because they are the ones who are immediately and directly affected by the consequences of any decision made:

> This in no way denies the importance of the doctor's [and nurse's] expertise but it acknowledges that the patient is an expert too in relation to how she lives her life and the consequences and risks she is prepared to make. (Donnelly 2002: 17)

For Donnelly, patients and health professionals do not necessarily have the same values concerning what constitutes benefit or harm to them. Unless there are exceptional circumstances where they might be self-deceived or ignorant, Donnelly argues in favour of assuming that people are best placed to know their own desires, values and beliefs.

If we applied this rejection of strong paternalism to the case of Sean, we would have to conclude that if the health-care team considers that Sean's decision to go home is substantially autonomous, the team would not be justified in interfering with it. The team may disagree with it, may consider that it is imprudent and foolish and may advise Sean that, in going home, he is putting his health and welfare at serious risk. However, respect for Sean's autonomy requires that the team not interfere with his choice.

Activity

So far, in analysing Sean's situation, we have suggested only two possibilities – that Sean's decision to go home is either non-autonomous or substantially autonomous. However, there is at least one other alternative.

Staff might determine that Sean's decision to go home is *partially* autonomous. For example, they might agree that it is un-coerced, purposeful and adequately informed but they might also consider that Sean has not sufficiently thought through the risks at stake in going home. The challenge here is one of determining the degree to which the health-care team might be justified in interfering with the autonomy that Sean does have.

If this were the case, how would you suggest that the health-care team might proceed? Notice that this situation calls for a response that invokes 'somewhere in-between' weak and strong paternalism.

Summary Learning Guide 2.1

The Principle of Beneficence:

- Obliges the nurse to protect patients from harm (nonmaleficence) and to promote their health and welfare;
- Is explicitly stated in many professional codes of conduct.

Paternalism:

- Describes actions that are carried out for the good of patients;
- Can be weak: intended to prevent harm or promote the good of patients who are non-autonomous e.g. unconscious, demented, fearful.
- Can be strong: intended to prevent harm or promote the good of patients who are autonomous. Strong paternalism privileges the principle of beneficence over the principle of autonomy when the two come into conflict.

PROMOTING AUTONOMY

As was indicated in the first half of this chapter, the principle of autonomy has negative and positive implications for nurses. So far, we have been exploring the negative obligation that the principle places on nurses – not to interfere with or constrain patients' substantially autonomous decisions in relation to their health.

The following section explores the different ways in which nurses might promote and enable the autonomy of patients in their care. This positive obligation on the part of the nurse is underlined by the Irish Nursing Board, An Bord Altranais, in its recent document, *The Scope of Nursing and Midwifery Practice Framework*, which states that:

> Nursing care should be delivered in a way that respects the uniqueness and dignity of each patient/client regardless of culture or religion. (An Bord Altranais 2000b: 3)

The document also lays stress on the duty of the nurse to promote the 'active involvement' of an individual and their family, friends and community in all aspects of their health care and to encourage 'self-reliance' and self-determination'. It goes on to cite values that underpin the delivery of nursing care:

> Fundamental to nursing practice is the therapeutic relationship between the nurse and the patient/client that is based on trust, understanding, compassion, support and serves to empower the patient/client to make life choices. (An Bord Altranais 2000b: 3)

The following case study, which looks at the challenges faced by a public health nurse in relation to a family in her care, will help us to tease out some of the issues involved in promoting patient autonomy.

Case 2.2: The Patient, the Carer and the Public Health Nurse

Eileen is the local public health nurse for a small rural community in the west of Ireland. As part of her caseload, she regularly visits Mr William Murphy who is at the end stages of lung cancer and is expected to die within the next three months. During her visits, Eileen has developed a friendly relationship with William's daughter, Anne.

Anne, who is now fifty-two, had a job in the local post office until the death of her mother two years ago. At that stage, she took unpaid leave from work in order to stay at home and care for her father. On one of Eileen's recent visits to the Murphy home, Anne told her about a painful sore that she had on the nipple of her left breast. She seemed very embarrassed to show Eileen her breast but when she did, Eileen became immediately concerned. She thought that the sore might well be a simple reaction to some skin product or detergent or some form of dermatitis. However, she was also concerned that it might be a rare form of breast cancer that affects one breast and usually starts out as a rash that develops into a painful lesion.

Ann confided in Eileen that she had been to her local GP two months previously and had been given an antibiotic cream. However, the condition had not cleared up and, on her second visit, the GP had suggested that she go to the regional hospital for a mammogram. Anne told Eileen that she had refused point blank to do this for a number of reasons: she did not want to leave her father at this crucial time; she did not think that she could cope with the idea that she herself might be ill; and she felt that she would not be able to hide any bad news from her father. In short, while she was worried about her own situation, she did not want to know. She had left the doctor's surgery and had made no further appointment. She reckoned that she might be able to address the situation after her father had passed on.

Eileen did not want to alarm Anne any further, but she knew that if Anne did indeed have some form of cancer, time was of the essence. She wondered how much information the doctor had given her about her condition and if he had actually told Anne that she might have a form of cancer. She wondered how she might best help Anne to make the right decision.

The case of Anne and William is an example of a situation where there is conflict and uncertainty. It would seem that Anne must decide whether to delay treatment for a possible serious condition in order to spend more time with her father, or have treatment and risk missing out on his last few weeks with her.

The case raises a number of ethical issues such as the right of the nurse to interfere with Anne's apparently autonomous decision not to know her condition, and the scope of the public health nurse's duty to carers and their families as well as to patients. However, because we want to explore the positive requirements of the principle of autonomy, we will try to answer one specific question in this section: How best might Eileen understand her obligation to promote Anne's autonomy in this situation?

Promoting Autonomy
In this case, Eileen could decide that her moral obligations to Anne are fulfilled if she provides her with more information about her possible condition. This approach casts the relationship between the nurse and the patient as a contractual one, where there is a provider and a consumer, or an expert and a lay person. In this view, the task of the nurse is to make sure that patients are informed of the nature of their illness, the risks and benefits of any proposed treatment and any alternative procedures. On this **contractual model**, both nurse and patient are perceived as distinct parties with distinct tasks and obligations. To promote autonomy, on this model of the nurse–patient relationship, is to inform patients fully and allow them to make their decision. The nurse is the informer or the one who ensures that information is provided and the patient is the decision maker.

However, it could be suggested that this understanding of the nurse–patient relationship does not fully capture what goes on in situations where a person is often extremely vulnerable and does not at all fit the picture of someone capable of making substantially autonomous decisions. When people are ill, their values, beliefs and desires are often unclear and there is far more uncertainty as to how these might be realised. Importantly people very often want to revise or modify their preferences in the light of their illness. The situation of Anne and William is certainly one where illness contributes to vulnerability and uncertainty as to what to do, and this reality needs to be addressed.

We want to suggest an alternative more **narrative** and contextual approach to the promotion of autonomy to the contractual model. This approach recognises that decision making can involve both *independence* and *interdependence*. It acknowledges both the vulnerability of the patient and the dynamic nature of decision making (McCarthy 2003; Parker 2001: 304–11; MacKenzie and Stoljar 2000).

Where there is this kind of vulnerability, we suggest that the role of the nurse expands. Her task is not simply to provide information to enable decision making, but also to support patients in identifying and articulating their values and intentions so that they are better able to choose whatever treatment (or non-treatment) might be consistent with their core desires and values. According to this view, patients may not yet know what they want, or may want different, even conflicting things.

The emphasis here is not on confirming the separateness of nurse and patient – one informs and one decides – but on acknowledging the interdependence of patient and nurse. In our case study, Anne is dependent on Eileen to help her to consider her options in the light of her concerns about her father and her own health, and in relation to her overall goals, beliefs and values. In order to fulfil her obligations to both William and Anne, Eileen is dependent on her relationship with Anne. This view of autonomy sees information as shared information, something that runs in both directions. It sees decision making as a mutual process where the emphasis is on communication as dialogue, listening and attention to body language, not only communication as information provision.

This understanding of the obligation to promote patient autonomy is also consistent with the role of the nurse as patient **advocate**. Specifically, Fry and Johnstone describe the nurse's advocacy role as one that emphasises communication skills and support in a way that is similar to the narrative approach. Their account of advocacy

> views the nurse as the person who helps the patient discuss his or her needs, interests, and choices consistent with the patient's values and lifestyle. (Fry and Johnstone 2002: 38)

For a more detailed account of advocacy, see Chapter 4 of this text. For a more detailed account of narrative, see Chapter 19 of this text.

Activity

Take a few moments to reflect on the challenge that faces Eileen in relation to her obligations to William and Anne. How do you think Eileen might proceed?

An emphasis on good communication is particularly pertinent to the situation facing the public health nurse in Case 2.2. Effective nursing care in community situations such as this one is dependent on a partnership existing between the nurse (Eileen) and patient (William) and carer (Anne). Unlike nurses working in acute-care settings, for example, it is likely that public health or community nurses will have long-term relationships with individuals and families that last over a number of years.

At the outset, both Anne and Eileen need to gather more information. For example, is there a family history of such lesions/carcinoma on the breast? Anne's age is also a consideration. Eileen will also need to establish what, for Anne, is the most difficult aspect of the situation as it currently stands. Telling her father, perhaps? At present, there is insufficient evidence of anything sinister to tell William and thereby worry him unnecessarily. Eileen may reflect with Anne as to what might be the worst-case scenario – that indeed she has a malignant lesion/lump in her breast – and they may consider the alternative – that this is a benign lesion. Either way, through a process of elimination, Eileen could empower Anne to give consideration to a possible course of action that would not necessitate her being away from her father for any length of time. Anne might make an appointment for a mammogram in the knowledge of a 4- to 6-week waiting period. In the interim, she has the opportunity to cancel the appointment and has time to reflect on and become more familiar with the situation. Anne might also request the GP to take a swab of the lesion and send it for analysis to test the appropriateness of the antibiotics used in the first instance. Eileen might offer to accompany Anne for the mammogram and suggest that a relative visit William to be with him while Anne attends her appointments.

In guiding and supporting Anne, Eileen is able to take a more contextual or situation-based perspective that makes links between Anne's health status and William's health status and the goals and values of all concerned. Moreover, Eileen's approach acknowledges that, for Anne, her relationship with her father and his ill-health are central to her decision making in relation to her own condition. Neither William nor Anne can be viewed as isolated individuals who are simply choosing for themselves. They are deeply involved with each other, and the question of their wellbeing extends far beyond their own immediate state of health. The contemporary ethicist, Thomas Hill, expresses a similar approach to respecting autonomy in the following passage:

> Respecting people's autonomy requires resisting the temptation to 'take charge' of their lives without their consent, but it does not deny anyone the choice to share with others, to acknowledge one's dependency, to accept advice, or even to sacrifice for the interests of others. The right of autonomy allows people some room to make their own choices; it does not dictate what those choices should be. (Hill 1991: 49)

Activity

The approach to decision making, as we have just outlined it, seems very attractive and practical. However, can you think of any difficulties or concerns that might arise when a nurse adopts it in relation to a vulnerable patient?

One difficulty with this approach is that the nurse may not have time or the skill for this kind of dialogue. No doubt, Eileen is a hard-pressed public health nurse with a heavy caseload and many demands on her time; she may feel that Anne's situation is an additional drain on her resources which distracts her from her professional obligations to William.

In addition, given the long tradition of paternalistic practices in the Irish health-care services generally, Eileen may well mistake her own values for those of Anne. She may, unwittingly and with the finest of intentions to empathise, impose her own values on Anne. One understanding of empathy is useful here and is articulated by the ethicist, Howard Brody:

> In a culture that prizes autonomy and independence, we may fondly imagine that most people are whole and intact, unlike those who suffer from disease . . . Charity tends to assume that I start off whole and remain whole while I offer aid to the suffering. Empathy and testimony require a full awareness of my own vulnerability and radical incompleteness; to be with the suffering as a cohuman presence will require that I change . . . Today I listen to the testimony of someone's suffering; tomorrow that person (or someone else) will be listening to my testimony of my own. Today I help to heal the sufferer by listening to and validating her story; tomorrow that sufferer will have helped to heal me, as her testimony becomes a model I can use to better make sense of and deal with my own suffering. (Brody 1987: 21–2)

In Brody's analysis, the demand of empathy does not require us to 'step into another's shoes' in order to understand their pain. It does not presuppose that it is ever possible to understand another's pain fully. The other person is always 'other' to us; their difference persists, resisting assimilation under the umbrella of mutual understanding. Instead, empathy demands that we bear witness to our own vulnerability and lack so that we stand, not as whole to part, or healthy to ill, but as a 'cohuman presence'. In this view, nurses cannot offer patients the reassurance that they know and understand them – only the acknowledgement that they have listened and heard. In this view, too, no nurse is untouched by a patient's pain and vulnerability; there is professional engagement, not detachment.

Different situations demand different responses. Autonomy and its protection and promotion demand different responses. Sometimes patients may explicitly ask for information and support; sometimes they may need the nurse to decide with them or for them. Sometimes they may need only time to reflect. Sometimes, and this can often be the hardest thing of all to provide, they may need a 'cohuman presence', a person who is strong enough in their own vulnerability, to be able to recognise and bear witness to a patient's pain (McCarthy 2004:65–71).

Activity

a) Apply the **narrative** approach to the first case of this Chapter, Case 2.1. How might it change the way in which the health-care team approaches Sean's requests and attempts to go home?

Following Brody, the team might take the time to listen to and validate Sean's own story: the staff might try to explore with Sean what it is about home that he particularly misses. Might his love of gardening find an outlet in the hospital setting? Might his worries about home mask other concerns? They might begin by acknowledging and making space for Sean's wishes, whether or not they determine that it is appropriate to fulfil them.

Summary Learning Guide 2.2

The contractual approach to promoting autonomy involves:

- Recognising the patient as an independent decision maker;
- Conceiving the nurse as a provider and the patient as a consumer of a health sevice;
- Informing patients of the nature of their illness and the risks and benefits of proposed treatments;
- Professional detachment.

The narrative approach to promoting autonomy involves:

- Recognising the vulnerability of the patient as a decision maker;
- Conceiving the patient as an interdependent decision maker;
- Viewing information-giving as shared communication;
- Professional engagement.

CONCLUSION

This chapter has explained and defended the importance of the principle of respect for autonomy and it has suggested ways in which it might be realised by nurses. In addition, a related principle, beneficence, has been defined and the tensions between autonomy and beneficence explored. Finally the chapter has suggested two different ways in which the task of promoting autonomy can be conceived.

Now that we have come to the end of our discussion, it is important to acknowledge that not everyone would agree with privileging autonomy over other human values. There are many who believe that personal autonomy, and, in turn, individual rights, have been afforded far too much weight in western democracies and that the lives of vulnerable groups and of communities as a whole have suffered as a result (See Chapter 19 of this text for some further discussion of this position). You might remember that we touched on this issue in the first case study where we pointed to a tension between supporting the wishes of an individual patient, Sean, and caring for the welfare of all the patients on his ward whose evenings were disturbed by his activities.

The ethicist, Donna Dickenson (2001), herself a strong advocate of patient autonomy, points out that while the US and European ethics literature and laws are dominated by what she calls a 'liberal, rights-based' approach, where the patient is seen as having the right to override medical opinion, this is not universally the case. Citing Ireland and some southern European countries such as Italy and Spain as exceptions, she suggests that the prevailing view in Ireland is one where:

> The patient has a positive duty to follow the doctor's instructions and to maximize his or her own health and well-being. . . . (Dickenson 2001: 285)

Activity

Take a moment to reflect on Dickenson's perspective on the patient's position in Ireland. Do you think that she captures the real situation for patients (such as Sean) in Irish hospitals and other health-care settings? Is talk of patient autonomy merely aspirational, the preoccupation of idealistic academics (such as ourselves) or is it a realistic possibility?

The following chapters continue to discuss autonomy and its scope in health-care decision making. Specifically, respect for autonomy requires the health professional to tell the truth (Chapters 3 and 4); respect patient confidentiality (Chapters 5 and 6); and ensure the informed consent of patients to accept or refuse treatment (Chapters 7 and 8).

The following terms are explained in the glossary:

advocacy
beneficence
contractual model
impartiality
non-maleficence

paternalism
strong paternalism
weak paternalism

– 3 –

Truthful Conversations

Objectives

At the end of this chapter, you should be able to:

- Compare and contrast two different moral theories on truth telling;
- Discuss how the practice of truth telling supports patient autonomy;
- Give reasons for a general principle of truth telling;
- Define **justification** and its contribution to moral agency;
- Evaluate the use of **therapeutic privilege** in withholding the truth of a diagnosis.

INTRODUCTION

The experience of being lied to by someone who we normally expect to be truthful can generate a complex set of emotions: anger, confusion, sadness, distrust and suspicion. These feelings reveal a great deal about the role of trust in supporting relationships that are important in our lives. Interactions with nurses require the firm establishment and maintenance of trust. Once trust is lost or undermined, a sense of security and confidence in health-care professionals is correspondingly threatened. A decision of an individual nurse or doctor to deceive patients is not simply a matter affecting their own conscience. It is also a decision that could have serious social and professional repercussions.

Truthful communication of diagnoses in health care is often defended by reference to respect for the autonomy of patients. As outlined in Chapter 1, autonomy emphasises the importance of patient self-determination: patients are entitled to choose how they wish to lead their lives. Knowledge of one's state of health or information about illness seem, in general, conditions for choices about the future.

The value of respect for personal autonomy and the implications for truthful communications in health care are based on a long tradition of philosophy. Here we look at two traditional moral theories where truthful communication and respect for individual autonomy are seen as central to human relationships.

KANT AND DEONTOLOGY: FOCUS ON DUTY

The rigorous **deontological** philosophy of the eighteenth-century German philosopher, Immanuel Kant, recommends a strict observance of truth telling. The term **deontological** is from two Greek terms: *deon* = duty and *logos* = knowledge of. In a **deontological theory**, actions are judged right or wrong on the basis of what we should know to be our 'duty'. We know the rightness or wrongness of an act by our reason, inner conscience or moral intuition or God's commands. Kant's view depends critically on the concept of rationality. He argues that, as human beings, we are born with a reasoning power or capacity that enables us to know what is right or wrong. This same power informs us of the requirements of the moral law.

According to Kantian deontology, some actions are simply wrong. They are 'intrinsically wrong'. In claiming that some actions are intrinsically wrong, deontologists mean that no anticipated good outcome can give moral warrant or **justification** for carrying out these actions. To use an example, let us say that torturing innocent human beings is intrinsically wrong. This means that no number of anticipated positive results or good outcomes from torture (such as getting valuable information) can make such torture 'right'. Likewise, to say that lying cannot be morally defended means that no number of seemingly good outcomes, for the liar or the one lied to, can justify lying.

Staying with these examples, why is it that good consequences would never warrant torture of the innocent or the act of lying? In the *Metaphysical Principles of Virtue* (1797), Kant explains the relationship between truthfulness and the dignity of humanity in a person. Right actions promote or foster human dignity and respect for human beings. Wrong actions undermine dignity and respect, of the one lying and the person lied to.

> The greatest violation of man's duty to himself considered only as a moral being is the opposite of veracity: lying. Dishonour, which goes with lying, accompanies the liar, like his shadow. Lying is the throwing away and, as it were, the obliteration of one's dignity as a human being. Lying, as intentional untruth in general, does not need to be harmful to others in order to be blameworthy. Even a really good end may be intended by lying. Yet to lie even for these reasons is through its mere form a crime of man against his own person and a baseness which must make a man contemptible in his own eyes. (Kant 1968: 90–91)

Notice that from this rigorous deontological perspective, lying, even for reasons of supposed kindness or benevolence is still wrong because it debases the one lying. Moreover, Kant believes that lying also treats the person we lie to with disrespect for their autonomy: we are using the other person as a *means for our own ends* – perhaps to make the job easier or because we cannot bring ourselves to share bad news. Kant puts it this way: 'Lying is a crime of man [woman] against his [her] own person.' He asks: 'Should I lie to extricate myself from a difficult situation?' No, is the categorical response! No matter the motivation, in Kant's philosophy, expected good consequences do not make the lying right. Consequences are irrelevant to the moral evaluation of actions.

This strong and unqualified denunciation of some actions is what Kant means by the **categorical imperative**. We know what our duty asks of us if we ponder a simple question: Would I wish everyone to behave as I am now proposing to do in these circumstances? If we cannot answer yes to this question, we should stop and ask why. Is there something wrong about everyone choosing to perform this action?

Activity

a) Do you agree with Kant's claim that lying is *always* wrong? Can you envisage any circumstances that would justify lying?

b) Do you think that Kant is overstating his case by saying that lying is a serious violation of oneself as a human being? A violation of others?

c) Reflect on any situation in your life where someone you trust has lied to you and you subsequently found out. Discuss how you felt about being deceived. Does this reflection help give you insight into what is wrong with lying?

UTILITARIANISM: FOCUS ON CONSEQUENCES

The deontological theory is strikingly different from other ethical theories such as **utilitarianism**. Whereas deontology argues that some actions are simply wrong regardless of the good consequences, utilitarianism is a **consequentialist** theory. This indicates the centrality of consequences of actions when we are morally evaluating an action. Acts are not right or wrong in themselves. Utilitarians stress that the rightness or wrongness of an act is determined by looking to what follows from the choices of individuals. If we maximise human wellbeing or happiness, it is a moral action. If human suffering and degradation occur, the action is immoral. The challenges of utilitarianism become clear: human beings take great responsibility for anticipating the outcomes of choices. While utilitarianism is a very prevalent moral position in the world of health economics, politics and social policy-making, we will, in Chapter 18, study some of the difficulties in living according to a utilitarian ethic.

JOHN STUART MILL: RESPONDING TO KANTIAN ETHICS

The famous nineteenth-century utilitarian philosopher, John Stuart Mill, knew Kant's theory very well. This is illustrated in his famous essay, *Utilitarianism*. Rather than argue, as Kant did, that consequences are irrelevant to the moral quality of actions, Mill took the maxim of utilitarianism to be: 'Do what has the best effects over-all'. Unlike Kantian ethics, Mill's argument is that it might be necessary to lie if doing so would likely, and in a particular situation, protect individuals from harm. Mill asks: What if lying would serve to achieve the greater happiness and welfare of individuals and society? Utilitarians see their great strength in emphasising what is good or bad for people based on the preferences of people. What matters in terms of the goal of morality are specific consequences for happiness and human wellbeing affecting persons' lives. This is in contrast with the beliefs of deontologists who stress the importance of abstract rules, divine commands or intuitions that are supposed to define what is moral. Notice that the utilitarians have a daunting task of trying to gauge accurately what consequences are likely to follow from any chosen action. Sometimes, as in the case study in this chapter, predicting likely consequences can be a serious challenge.

Summary Learning Guide 3.1

If you approach truth telling as a **Kantian deontologist**, you will believe:
- That lying is intrinsically wrong;
- That lying is against the moral law;
- That, by lying to others, we treat both them and ourselves with disrespect;
- That no anticipated good consequences from lying will make it right.

If you approach truth telling as a **consequentialist** or **utilitarian**, you will believe:
- That no actions are intrinsically and always wrong;
- That the rightness or wrongness of lying depends on the consequences of lying;
- That the consequences must foster wellbeing and minimise suffering;
- That the judgement of likely consequences is rigorously demanding and requires that you know the patient and context thoroughly.

Against this background of deontology and utilitarianism, consider the following case study. The clinician in charge decides not to communicate the truth to a patient with a brain tumour. While reading the case, jot down your first, unanalysed response to the decisions taken.

Case 3.1: Following Orders to 'Lie'?

Sarah was a forty-year-old married woman who had two children aged fourteen and eight. Clinical tests confirmed that Sarah had an inoperable brain tumour with a prognosis of less than a year to live. Her husband, Paul, had been informed of the diagnosis but Sarah had not. Paul requested that Sarah's doctor not tell his wife of the medical findings. With some reluctance, the doctor complied with the husband's wishes. The nurses were told of this decision. The family, doctor, nurses and ancillary staff on the floor knew of Sarah's diagnosis but no one informed her. Nursing her proved very difficult as she regularly stated, 'I know something serious is wrong with me' or asked: 'What's wrong with me?' She could not understand why the test results weren't being discussed with her. Paul didn't have anything to tell Sarah either and tried to be comforting and reassuring. He didn't seem as anxious as Sarah about not getting the test results.

As one of the nurses on the floor, I had little contact with the patient, fearing that she would also ask me directly about the situation. When I did have to see her, I was very efficient and cheerful, but certainly brisk. I knew I was avoiding contact because, when you're a nurse, it's almost impossible to say nothing, especially if the patient asks. I felt very distressed about the guilty feelings I had from my involvement in this deception. It was more difficult when Sarah's children came to see her and asked me: 'Will my mum be home and well again soon?' I worried that I would let something slip as I was never too sure exactly what the doctor had told her or her husband, Paul. I deeply believed that she had a right to the truth about her own life and felt caught in a painful conflict of conscience.

EVIDENCE-BASED ETHICS: ATTENTION TO THE HUMAN STORIES

Evidence-based nursing is much emphasised in the literature on nursing practice. There, 'evidence' is determined on the basis of systematically structured research studies that are aimed at making recommendations for improved nursing care. Similarly evidence-based ethics deploys the concept of 'evidence'. Here, 'evidence' means the data gathered from careful, systematic patient observations, listening to patients and colleagues, and recording such data in order to argue for a certain ethical practice. In the case above, Sarah is providing evidence to the nurses, the clinicians and the family that she desires communication and understanding about her condition.

The following quote from Sissela Bok considers truthful conversation in relation to terminally ill patients:

> It has always been especially easy to keep knowledge from terminally ill patients. They are most vulnerable, least able to take action to learn what they need to know, or to protect their autonomy. The very fact of being so ill greatly increases the likelihood of control by others. And the fear of being helpless in the face of such control is growing . . . the possibility of prolonged pain, increasing weakness, the uncertainty, the loss of power and chance of senility, the sense of being a burden. (Bok 1978: 244–5)

Bok's quote might resonate with Sarah's case because, what one first notices in this narrative is that there is considerable fear, anxiety, annoyance and apprehension on the part of the patient. Sarah is baffled and anxious about the silence of the doctors and nursing staff when she asks questions. She simply cannot understand why no one is discussing test results with her. Sarah also would surely notice the change in manner of the nurse who seems to be avoiding conversations and spends little time in the room.

Activity

Reflect back on the particulars of this case.

We explained above that gauging consequences is difficult but very important if one is reasoning as a utilitarian. A good utilitarian has to ask: Were there good reasons for obstructions to Sarah's liberty? How would you answer the following questions?

a) Are the consequences of *not* informing Sarah more conducive to maximising the good (for whom?) than the results of informing her?

b) How would you gauge the likely consequences of telling or not telling Sarah the truth of her condition?

c) From a Kantian point of view, withholding the truth is wrong. By refusing her understanding, you are objectifying Sarah and treating her as a *means to other people's ends and not as a valued end in herself*. Consider: What other people's ends might be displacing concern for Sarah?

STRONG PATERNALISM – A BARRIER TO RATIONAL CHOICE

In this case, both the doctor and the husband adopt the stance of **strong paternalism**. Recall that **strong paternalism** refers to actions that obstruct the exercise of choice by *a competent and autonomous person*. The motive for strong paternalism here may well be beneficence but, when you notice paternalism in action, a pertinent question is always: Is this decision truly being taken for the wellbeing of the patient or are other motives dominant such as self-interest or self-protection? Thomas Hill links the idea of a 'right of autonomy' and the idea of a 'rational decision maker', offering some insight into the case at hand:

> The right of autonomy is only a right to make one's choices free from certain interferences by others. Among these interferences are illegitimate threats, manipulations, and blocking or distorting the perception of options. A rational decision maker wants not only to have a clear head and ability to respond wisely to the problems present to him; he wants also to see the problems and the important facts that bear on them realistically and in perspective. Thus one can also manipulate a person by feeding him information selectively, by covering up pertinent evidence, and by planting false clues in order to give a distorted picture of the problem situation. (Hill 1991: 32–3)

VERACITY: ADHERING TO THE PRINCIPLE OF TRUTH TELLING

Avoiding manipulation of the patient requires a conscientious adherence to a **general principle of veracity** or truth telling. This principle states the broad sweep of obligations to tell the truth to patients. The following formulation of the general principle of truth telling incorporates several elements for practice:

The health professional should:

1. tell patients the truth about their diagnoses,
2. in a measured manner,
3. in language the patient can understand,
4. unless there are good reasons to believe that a degree of harm,
5. more serious than a temporary emotional depression, would follow as a result of telling the diagnosis.

a) Would you add anything further to these points on truthful communication?

b) Would you challenge anything in this statement?

c) On your reading of Case 3.1, do you think it likely that Sarah would suffer a serious depression from the communication of her diagnosis?

Arguments against Truthful Communication

In the literature on truthful communication, there are standard arguments for concealment of the truth. As you read the following, ask whether they are valid or evidence-based arguments–where 'evidence' means the result of your systematic observations and reflections from your nursing experience.

1. **Argument from ignorance**: the patient is not capable of understanding the truth.
2. **Argument based on patient request**: the patient does not wish to know and has made this clear.
3. **Argument from beneficence**: the truth would be harmful to the patient. (Higgs 1999: 511)

Take time to consider these standard arguments for a moment. On *argument 1*, if we set the standard for understanding one's illness too high, no patient except the clinicians themselves would qualify for hearing of their diagnosis. If we recall the general principle of truth telling, the obligation stated there as a value is to explain an illness to the patient in language they can understand. The case of Sarah gives no evidence that she could not understand what the doctors would tell her about her brain tumour. So, in the case of Sarah, the first argument above clearly does not apply.

On *argument 2*, the staff get repeated requests from Sarah for information about her illness. No patient likes the tragic news of serious illness. Sadness is painfully normal. Anticipating that another will be distressed at bad news should not be confused with evidence that they do not wish to know. Should the nurse or doctor second-guess Sarah's sincerity in asking the questions? The second argument would not apply in this case. (In the following chapter, we meet Michael who clearly does not wish to know!)

Finally, on *argument 3*, in claiming the truth is harmful to the patient, one needs to reflect honestly on the evidence for anticipated harm. On reflection, evidence may be more difficult than realised. Is concern about Sarah's wellbeing central in this decision? The nurse's conscience is very uneasy. Is that because she sees no evidence for deception?

a) Give reasons for your choice from the following options regarding how best to serve Sarah's wellbeing and show respect for her and the family:

- Avoid encounters with Sarah.

- Seek a case consultation with the staff on the ward.
- Explicitly lie about the test results.
- Disclose the test results with reassurances of care.

b) Consider the nurse's situation. She is involved in deceiving Sarah, yet she had no input into the original decision to deceive. In effect, her moral agency is being curtailed. Does the nurse have any room to manoeuvre in this situation? As a nurse in the unit, how would you try to negotiate and resolve your conscience dilemma?

Moral Principles and Exceptions

In many situations of health care, you may be asked to explain how you would justify or defend your views about, for example, consent, truth telling, confidentiality, or constraints on autonomy. Being prepared to give reasons means that we are willing to continue in growth as moral agents. **Justification** involves giving reasons for adherence to truth telling in general. But, justification is also about giving reasons why an **exception** to truthfulness is necessary in a particular situation. For example, the doctor in the case may generally agree with the practice of truth telling but judge now, in the concrete circumstances, that it is not appropriate. If this is so, then the doctor is clearly choosing to make an exception to the general principle of truth telling. This path requires justification.

The nature of the general ethical principle stated above is precisely that: it expresses a basic value or set of values that we wish to protect. We can, with consistency, strongly affirm the general principle and yet recognise that there might be circumstances where we must set aside the general presumption because other competing values are deemed more important at this time. So the rule in the general principle operates 'most of the time' and functions as a 'rule of thumb' for most situations.

Exceptions and Dangers of Self-deception

If we find ourselves appealing to the exceptions much more than the general principle, we are probably beginning to doubt seriously the value contained in the general rule or principle. On the other hand, we might verbally endorse the value of being truthful but through repeated exceptions reveal a lack of sincerity or **weakness of will** in our conviction about the value of truthfulness. Accepting general principles is one way of endorsing the cumulative experience of human valuing. When we endorse the moral importance of certain values, we are agreeing to the general acceptability of what is called an 'ethical norm'. The norm of 'telling the truth as a general rule' is defended by appeal to the moral value of respect for the autonomy of individuals whose condition of health is primarily their business, their concern and an area of profound meaning in their life.

As with all exceptions to ethical principles, if we put aside the general rule in a particular case, reflection is required regarding the concrete patient and specific clinical realities that are known. Taking the full range of human, patient, personal and health realities into account, we must then consider the reasons for thinking that a particular case is an exception and that a deceptive communication or non-communication of information is called for.

Recall that Immanuel Kant was not in favour of exceptions for lying. The **categorical imperative** against lying means just that: there can be no exceptions! Kant held this very stringent view because he deeply believed that as human beings we are always in danger of self-deception. Some contemporary deontologists do argue for reasoned exceptions but this is a revision of Kantian thought, a revision that would probably cause Kant to stir in his tomb.

Arguments for a General Rule of Truthful Communication

Four standard arguments are commonly given to support a general principle of truthful conversation with patients (Higgs 1999: 507–12). Consider these and see whether you would endorse them as good working arguments for truth telling.

1. Moral argument: The patient as a human being has a right or entitlement to know what is discovered about their health and what options are available for treatment. Being kept in ignorance shows a lack of respect for a person's desire to have some 'control' in their life. So, the moral argument focuses on the wrongfulness and harm to the person and their freedom of choice in concealing the reality of illness from them.

2. Clinical argument: Treatment and or emotional adjustments are considerably facilitated if the patient knows what they are being treated for, what therapeutic options they could choose and why doctors or nurses might recommend certain treatments over others. This clinical benefit of truth telling assumes that the patient has also been given a chance to ask questions about other alternative treatments to those suggested by the doctor or nurse.

3. Psychological argument: Knowing and understanding diagnoses that are communicated with hope helps to provide psychological support against isolation in illness. Such conversation with hope that everything will be done to help the patient can minimise the worst imaginings and fears about the disease process. Knowing that therapies and pain control are available for an illness enables the patient to seek help from medical staff, nurses and family members. Deception and concealment hinder such positive benefits.

4. Practical argument: The patient will find out the diagnosis whether they are told by a health professional or not. The patient finds out the diagnosis by intelligent guessing. A charade of pretence is usually unsuccessful in protecting the patient from the truth. Sarah in Case 3.1, for example, is aware, reflective and most likely alert to all clues of nurse activity, tests she has been given and plans being made for treatment. Guessing one's diagnosis rather than being treated with respect as a competent adult affects trust and openness with the health professionals involved in the deception.

Therapeutic Privilege

Often, health professionals appeal to the obligation to look out for the wellbeing of patients to justify their decisions. This is part of the basis for the doctor's decision not to communicate truthfully with Sarah. In this decision, the doctor appeals to what is known as **therapeutic privilege**. Therapeutic privilege assumes that the doctor or health professional knows best what is in the interests of the patient. In granting this, we see a subtle move from medical expertise to moral expertise. The 'privilege' idea in **therapeutic privilege** is an entitlement for the health-care professional to withhold information *if* they think the information given to the patient would run the risk of seriously harming the patient. Notice how this privilege was incorporated in the general principle of truth telling above.

Beauchamp and Childress believe that use of the therapeutic privilege is very controversial because it can be over-used in order to avoid difficult challenges in communication with patients. What is required is *a sound medical judgment that to divulge the information would be potentially harmful to a depressed, emotionally drained or unstable person* (Beauchamp and Childress 1989: 91).

Is an appeal to **therapeutic privilege** in this context a beneficent decision? Sarah is not unstable or depressed, though she is indeed worried. Communication to Sarah of the fact that she has a brain tumour clearly is likely to cause considerable distress, tears and fear. But fear and distress are the state that Sarah is in while not knowing. The application of the therapeutic privilege in this case seems totally unjustified. Non-communication in this case prevents Sarah from beginning the human process of internalising the very difficult news of her illness. One could argue that the practice of nursing and medicine precisely involves nurses and clinicians in learning the art of compassion, listening and creativity in helping patients in distress after receiving bad news. If this process is considered tangential to health-care practice, a reassessment of the goals of health-care provision might be warranted.

Summary Learning Guide 3.2

Truthful conversation (truth telling):

- Is defended as a fundamental moral value in health-care practices;
- Is founded on respect for personal autonomy;
- Can be expressed in the form of a general principle;
- Requires skilful communication and listening to foster hope for coping with one's illness.

The principle of truth telling is not absolute but it:

- Allows for exceptions in certain specific situations;
- Requires that any exceptions be justified or defended by evidence from the concrete realities of a case;
- Considers therapeutic privilege as one such exception but one that requires caution in its use.

The medical doctor and ethics writer, Jay Katz, proposes a new model of trust in the health-care context, a model that endorses the fundamental importance of communication to achievement of good medical practice and respectful patient care.

> Both parties need to relate to one another as equals and unequals. Their equalities and inequalities complement one another. [Health professionals] know more about the disease. Patients know more about their own needs. Neither knows at the outset what each can do for the other. This trust cannot be earned through deeds alone. It requires words as well. It relies not only on [health professionals'] technical competence but also on their willingness to share the burden of decision making with patients and on their verbal competence to do so. It is a trust that requires professionals to trust themselves in order to trust their patients, for to trust patients, [they] first must learn to trust themselves to face up to and acknowledge the tragic limitations of their own professional knowledge. (Katz 2002: 102)

In his work, Katz emphasises the 'tragic' limitations of communication in health care. An escalation of efforts at communication by both the doctors and nurses with Paul and Sarah would greatly assist the health-care team in comprehending the fears and hopes of the couple. It would reveal the values and plans that are central in the life stories of this couple and their children. Notice how different the focus is if one approaches the family as a **narrative unit**, a group of people bound together by stories that tie them: the focus turns on the family as an integral whole, needing help and listening. The focus might become how to help this family absorb and negotiate the illness of a loved one. The zoom lens then moves away from the health professionals' concerns about how to avoid Sarah, how to communicate, how to follow up the diagnostic news, and so on. The **narrative approach** is only hinted at here. As a contemporary moral theory, it is examined more fully in Chapter 19.

Activity

If Sarah does not understand her illness because she has not been taken seriously as a questioning patient, the possibility of achieving consent to treatment is undermined.

a) What if the doctor decides to administer steroids in an effort to remove pressure from the brain tumour? Sarah may well ask you as the nurse, 'What is the medication? Will it help?' What would you tell her?

b) If Sarah gets severe headaches as her tumour progresses, what then would you tell her?

CONCLUSION

A patient's compliance with therapies is normally facilitated in proportion as they understand their illness and know why a therapy is given. Ignorance, on the other hand, fosters detachment from such involvement in therapies. The doctor in the case here engages in a convoluted deception to Sarah. Her questions encourage him and the nurses to construct additional misleading answers precisely in order to maintain the charade of deception begun by conceding to Paul's request. The health professionals have capitulated to the insistent needs of the patient's husband. This is questionable in displacing the attention to the fundamental respect owed to Sarah as the ill patient.

In this chapter, we explained two traditional moral theories – deontology and utilitarianism. We enumerated the arguments for and against truthful conversation with patients. The general principle of truth telling was defined. It was argued that, if exceptions to truthful conversations become the rule, the general value of truthfulness is correspondingly destroyed. To avoid this, the need for evidence-based justification in making exceptions was explained.

In a subsequent chapter that discusses informed consent, the impact of this case becomes clear. Consent relies on accurate understanding of one's illness and the options proposed for treatment. This is a general point to be stressed about honest communication of illness: it is a necessary condition for informed consent. So, if one takes a decision not to divulge information, the next decision is what to do about achieving a process of informed consent. If informed consent is set aside, there is always the impending challenge not only of moral turpitude but also a real possibility of litigation should anything serious transpire in the treatment of a patient.

The following terms are explained in the glossary:

autonomy
beneficence
categorical imperative
consequentialism
deontological theory
evidence-based ethics
justification

narrative model of ethics
principle of truth telling
strong paternalism
therapeutic privilege
utilitarianism
veracity
weakness of will

– 4 –

Advocacy and Integrity

Objectives

At the end of this chapter, you should be able to:

- Explain how **conscience** and **integrity** are related;
- Assess the role of nurse **advocacy**;
- Evaluate the meaning and possibilities for **moral space**;
- Explore the role of family members in decision making;
- Discuss how cultural differences influence the practice of truth telling;
- Enumerate the moral consequences of *how* one tells the truth.

INTRODUCTION

Chapter 3 raised ethical challenges that arise from the hierarchies of health-care institutions and management. Working in an institutional structure that retains a hierarchy of authorities, the nurse in Case 3.1 seems morally compromised in a deception with which she does not agree. Her **conscience** is clearly troubled and her sense of **integrity** may well be undermined. In such circumstances, if the nurse assumes the role of patient **advocate**, she may want to argue for Sarah's right to know but feel restricted by the accepted lines of authority for discussing diagnoses and prognoses with patients.

This chapter explores how the realities of conscience and integrity come into play in advocacy. The role of advocacy – speaking on behalf of patients' needs, preferences and moral values – can be a controversial one. Exercising it may challenge one's own beliefs and one's sense of integrity, causing conflicts and moral distress. Even while trying to represent patients' values and needs, advocacy may bring nurses into conflict with colleagues and institutional expectations of authority demarcations.

INTEGRITY AND MORAL CHARACTER

To be known as a person of integrity is considered a positive endorsement of the individual's moral character. **Integrity** means 'soundness, reliability, wholeness and integration of moral character' (Beauchamp and Childress 2001: 36). According to ancient and more recent sources in the moral traditions, the idea of **moral integrity** means fidelity in adhering to moral norms.

The virtue of integrity represents two aspects of a person's character:

1. The first is a coherent integration of aspects of the self: emotions, aspirations, knowledge etc. so that each complements and does not frustrate the other.

2. The second is the character trait of being faithful to moral values and standing up in their defence when necessary. (Beauchamp and Childress 2001)

The notions of moral agency and moral autonomy are inherent in the idea of integrity. Becoming a moral agent requires authorship of one's own moral life. When we begin to reflect on who we are as young adults, we find that we have already been instilled with a range of values, principles and moral beliefs. Influences that have shaped our young moral life are extensive: family, church, educational system and friends. But if we are to become 'author' of our own moral lives, more seems required. Yeo and Ford explain this requirement of adopting a reflective stance about our inherited beliefs:

> As we question what we inherited and the external authorities to which we are subject, we reject some things and accept and deepen others. We shape our own moral code or make the code we inherited more fully our own by assuming responsibility for it. In doing so, we become more fully autonomous, directing our own moral life rather than being guided solely by others. Our sense of integrity develops as we assume greater control over and accountability for our moral lives. (in Yeo and Moorhouse 1996: 268)

Persons can be said to lack moral integrity if a number of deficits in their character become consistent: self-deception, insincerity, bad faith, and hypocrisy. These character deficits represent a severing in the connections between a person's emotions, actions and moral convictions. Perhaps the most common deficiency is the lack of sincerely held, fundamental moral convictions, but no less important is the failure to act on professed moral beliefs.

Beauchamp and Childress give this analysis:

> Their [nurses] moral commitments may create morally difficult situations in which they must either compromise on their fundamental commitments or withdraw from the care of the patient in question. Yet, compromise seems, by definition, what a person of integrity cannot do; such a person must not sacrifice his or her deep moral commitments. Does this mean that action involving compromise is inconsistent with maintaining integrity? Will it turn out on close inspection that moral integrity in modern health care is little more than a dogmatic insistence that one's cherished values are higher than others' values? (Beauchamp and Childress 2001: 36)

The authors here explain that situations that compromise integrity can often be avoided if participants:

1.   recognise the fallibility of their own moral views, and
2.   respect others' perspectives.

But participants in a dispute can also use mechanisms to nurture conscientious decisions such as: consultative institutional processes – regular on-site case conferences, for example, or hospital ethics committees.

> A moral climate of mutual respect together with channels of reasoned recourse in institutions can usually prevent people from feeling that their integrity has been compromised. (Beauchamp and Childress 2001: 37)

FAMILY ROLE IN HEALTH-CARE DECISIONS

One area that challenges a nurse's convictions may arise when a family member insists on a decision that goes contrary to the patient's own preferences. By all accounts, the case of Sarah illustrated in Chapter 3 is not infrequent in health care. Families believe that they have a privileged role in advising clinicians and nurses about what their loved one should be told. In turn, the nurse's desire to be advocate for the patient may seriously conflict with family expectations and demands.

Case 4.1: When the Patient Doesn't Want to Know

Michael is forty years old, single and living on his own. He has been suffering from abdominal paint that has grown increasingly more severe. He is beginning to experience a great deal of constipation and nausea. When he is persuaded to go to the doctor, he makes it clear to his mother and later to his doctor that if he has any serious illness, he simply doesn't wish to be told. 'I'm just one of those people who thinks that ignorance is bliss and I've always trusted that doctors will do whatever they can to help me.' When he sees his family doctor, he restates his wish not to know and insists that he does not wish his mother to be told either. He is referred to a consultant, Dr Wilkins, and confirms his wish not to know his diagnosis. Michael also mentions this desire not to know to the general practice nurse in the family doctor's office and to the nurse specialist in the consultant's rooms. In subsequent meetings with Michael, Dr Wilkins does not approach the issue of test results even though they indicate a diagnosis of colon cancer with some metastasis to lymph nodes. This could respond quite well with surgery and follow-up chemotherapy. He advises Michael that he has arranged a bed for him at the local regional hospital.

In hospital, the nurse, David Jennings, is in the ward and Dr Wilkins explains the test results to him as the nurse in charge, but explains that he plans to respect Michael's request not to be informed. He believes that to do otherwise would be disrespectful to Michael. He reassures Michael that he is in good hands and has every reason to feel hopeful of recovery. David Jennings feels uncomfortable about this easy acceptance of Michael's request but then explains that Michael's mother is already in hospital. She insists that she has a right to know what is wrong with Michael and what is being done in relation to his treatment and care. Contrary to Michael's request not to tell his mother, Dr Wilkins decides to discuss Michael's diagnosis with her. He asks Nurse Jennings to respect the decision.

Dr Wilkins is convinced on ethical grounds that cooperating in Michael's request is both:

1.   the way to respect this particular patient's autonomy, and
2.   the way to foster his wellbeing and show benevolence.

Dr Wilkins endorses one argument given for non-communication of the truth: *the patient does not wish to know.*

Activity

a) While not planning to disregard Michael's request not to know, would you try to understand Michael's story further? What do you think motivates him to choose to remain ignorant of his situation?

b) Why, do you think, did Michael make a point of telling the nurses of his wishes?

c) What reasons can you offer for Dr Wilkins' decision to tell Michael's mother of his condition? Would you come to a different conclusion? Try to give reasons for your answer.

Because a patient asks not to be told of a diagnosis does not mean that communication with the patient ceases. In this case, there may be a more significant story to be learned from ongoing conversations with Michael. This may be especially important if the request not to know is buttressed by deeper fears, intimations of mortality or concern at losing control in a lengthy illness. In brief, a request not to have truthful communication may, paradoxically, be an invitation for conversation.

Paternalism with Permission

Michael's plea to remain ignorant of his illness offers a **waiver** of consent to information for both the doctor and the nurses. The waiver gives moral consent to the doctor's nondisclosure. This waiver proves awkward in this case because Dr Wilkins is hopeful that treatment will bring Michael to reasonable recovery. But the decision to accept the waiver from Michael has consequences that might prove difficult to deal with later. Michael's waiver has implications for any informed consent that may be needed for invasive procedures and most certainly any proposed surgery that is recommended.

Sometimes when a patient offers such a waiver, they delegate decisional authority to another person such as a family member. This is not the case here. Michael's request is an explicit agreement to allow the doctor and nurse to practise **paternalism with permission**. They are here authorised to proceed with decisions without consent from Michael and also without discussing therapeutic options available to Michael.

However, when a patient gives such permission for ongoing paternalism, it may be advisable not to make any decisions in stone! Continued conversations and further test results may mean that it will be necessary to revisit Michael's decision not to know.

Yeo and Moorhouse argue that, from the standpoint of autonomy, the challenge is to determine what the patient really wishes. Michael seems to have waived his right to know. To insist on telling him would be to confuse a right to be informed with an obligation to be informed (Yeo and Moorhouse 1996: 164). Respect for autonomy does not go so far as forcing people to live up to what we happen to think are their obligations.

Summary Learning Guide 4.1

The concept of 'paternalism with permission' refers to:

- An autonomous decision by a patient to accept decisions taken by medical and nursing staff;
- A form of patient consent to forego the right to be informed of diagnosis, prognosis and therapeutic options;
- An exercise of the patient's right not to know.

'Paternalism with Permission' causes difficulties:

- If medical interventions (diagnostic or therapeutic) are required that would normally require explicit consent;
- If understanding is necessary to achieve patient compliance with treatment;
- If it is not revisited and reviewed by health-care staff.

Respecting Cultural Differences

Family requests to be involved in decision making about competent relatives poses challenges especially if one is nursing in western culture or more typically North American culture. For the past twenty years, western health-care ethics has emphasised the centrality of patient autonomy and the individual's right to self-determination. However, other cultures have not uncritically accepted this emphasis. As a result, health-care staff cannot assume that the dominantly western desire for truthful communication with the individual patient is the rule to follow, especially if they are nursing patients from non-western cultural backgrounds.

Following an exclusively western practice may be disrespectful of a particular patient whose cultural meanings are other than western and even at odds with western values and practices. Some ethnic groups and cultures expect that communication from doctors and nurses would be with the family first, before the patient, and sometimes instead of the patient. In many parts of the world, such as Africa, Pakistan and Eastern cultures, as well as in North America, there has been a subtle move to reaffirm greater decision authority for families especially in areas of dispute about terminal illness. A narrow focus on patient autonomy has been criticised,

> as being non-contextual and based on an abstract concept that the individual is isolated and disconnected from the many relationships within which he or she actually exists. (Moazam 2000: 34)

But while respecting cultural differences, allowing an authoritarian family to be decisive in the decision-making process has its own dangers too. Patients seeking their own communication with health professionals may be eclipsed in the caring and solicitude of the family and may, privately, not agree with the family prioritising their own cultural upbringing. A nurse or doctor who is too facile in generalising in the domain of cultural practice is likely to make errors of judgement. More importantly facile generalisations moving from cultural practice to patient preferences may result in disrespect for the unique individuality of the patient in favour of the generalised cultural practice. *'The [health professional] must use discrimination, judging encounters with each patient and family on their own merit'* (Moazam 2000: 35).

A similar challenge to the hegemony of western ethical views on autonomy comes from Peter Kasenene speaking about African values:

> In African traditional ethics, autonomy, the ability to think and act independently and freely, is limited by the emphasis put on communalism. African societies emphasize interdependence and an individual's obligations to the community. An individual who disregards the family or the community and does what he or she thinks to be right, is regarded as anti-social. Thus, excessive individual autonomy is regarded as being a denial of one's corporate existence. (Kasenene 2000: 351)

As Ireland becomes an increasingly multicultural society, health-care professionals will require informed awareness of moral differences in cultural practices that would influence decisions taken about communication concerning diagnoses, prognoses, treatment options, and so on. This is not a simple matter since the need to achieve patient participation in decision making may confer legal obligations on health-care professionals.

ADVOCACY: A CONTROVERSIAL OBLIGATION

One definition of **advocacy** states:

> Advocacy is concerned with promoting and safeguarding the well-being and interests of patients and clients. It is not concerned with conflict for its own sake . . . advocate means, 'one who pleads the cause of another' or 'one who recommends or urges something'. This indicates that advocacy is a positive, constructive activity. (UKCC, United Kingdom Central Council for Nurses, Midwives and Health Visitors' Code of Conduct, 1992)

In the same vein, Graham Rumbold understands the role of nurse advocate as part of the duties that a nurse takes on in joining the profession of nursing. One of the main duties or functions undertaken by nurses is to ensure that patients' rights are recognised and respected. Patients have the right to expect, with the assistance of nurses' advocacy, that, whatever is done to or for them will be in their best interests (Rumbold 1999: 251).

Along similar lines, the Irish Nursing Board, An Bord Altranais, proposes that nurses should aim to provide high standards of care and to protect patients from harm.

> The aim of the nursing profession is to give the highest standard of care possible to patients. Any circumstance which could place patients/clients in jeopardy or which militates against safe standards of practice should be made known to appropriate persons or authorities. (An Bord Altranais 2000)

Activity

Pause and consider the positions stated above.

a) On the understanding of 'advocacy', propounded by the UKCC, by Rumbold and by An Bord Altranais, where do nurses stand with respect to their power as advocate if they feel that patients are being mistreated or otherwise not having their rights respected?

b) Do nurses have the authority or freedom to speak out on behalf of patients who, perhaps for complicated reasons, are unable to do so themselves?

These questions ask you to connect the apparent duty of advocacy with the larger institutional and professional context of nursing. Is advocacy a realistic ideal serviced and encouraged within health-care institutions?

Moral Space for Advocacy

There is frequently a gap between aspirations and moral hopes and expectations. Within the health professions, it seems increasingly recognised that the duties of nurses, especially advocacy expectations, require some institutional recognition. With this joint tension and requirement in mind, we introduce the idea of **moral space**. Moral space is a concept that functions as an umbrella term. It embraces many elements within the health-care context. The concept is elaborated here but will come into play in subsequent chapters as well.

The many dimensions that make up moral space are put in place to create and sustain an atmosphere that facilitates the exercise of advocacy and respects diversity of conscience among professionals. The following elements are included in moral space.

> This 'space' is not an identifiable physical place (like a room) but rather refers to:
> • an institutional health-care context,
> • where a philosophy of respect for professional and patient moral autonomy is fundamental,
> • where mechanisms are available for communication of conscientious objections,
> • where these communications are facilitated by designated nurse personnel,

- where discussion and non-intimidating recognition of conscience differences regarding work practice are made possible,
- where discussion of moral differences is facilitated through an informal forum,
- where such a forum becomes a professionally expected mechanism for review of cases that bring ethical challenges to the fore.

Professionals who criticise the idea of advocacy often argue that the institutional hierarchies, organisational structures and authority powers tend to obstruct rather than encourage the nurse's role of giving voice with patients in relation to their rights. The concept of moral space, fleshed out as it is above, is meant to argue for such provisions that would make advocacy and diversity of conscience more visible and respected realities in health care.

Advocacy as a Contested Ideal

The literature in nursing ethics shows that advocacy is strongly commended by some authors and recommended with caution by others. There is considerable uncertainty and there are multiple interpretations about what this 'advocacy' requires. It is argued that because of the lack of clarity in operationalising the concept of advocacy, it is a potentially risky role to adopt (Mallik 1997; Kuhse 1997).

Some authors urge that, because it is unclear and because of the unrealistic demands within the structure of health-care systems, the advocate role neither can nor should impose such fraught obligations on nurses (Willard 1996). Others prefer to think of advocacy as 'power transferral' from the professional back to the patient. According to this view, advocacy is defined as 'involving, informing, supporting and protecting clients so that they can make their own health-care decision' (Bartter 1996: 223).

Many authors link the meaning of advocacy with the role of facilitating the exercise of autonomy for patients. It might be helpful for readers to review the distinctions between the contractual and dialogical models for facilitating autonomy, laid out in Chapter 2. More active roles for the nurse in facilitating patient autonomy build on more robust conceptions of autonomy. In the facilitating interpretation of advocacy, the nurse's role is to assist patients in assuming a sense of control or authority in a situation where, for many reasons, they might feel much out of control.

Joan Liaschenko argues that advocacy can be understood as clearly having a moral sense. It emphasises speaking to someone on behalf of a patient. Advocacy is also viewed as doing work that connects patient and services for the purposes of influencing some patient outcome. But Liaschenko also believes that advocacy requires knowing something about the goods of human life as well as how they relate to the best interests of a particular patient. By 'the goods of human life' she means 'those values in living that seem to be recognised universally as fundamentally important or essential to human and humane living' (Liaschenko 1998: 12).

Gadow chooses a form of 'existential advocacy' as a concept that incorporates respect for autonomy in very active terms. In this model of advocacy, individuals are assisted by nurses to exercise their self-determination authentically. In Gadow's model, the role of nurse advocate involves more than simply ensuring that the patient's wishes are considered and respected.

Existential advocacy refers to:

> the effort to help persons *become clear about what they want to do*, by helping them discern and clarify their values in the situation, and on the basis of that self-examination, to reach decisions that express their reaffirmed, perhaps recreated, complex of values. (Gadow 1989: 85)

Gadow offers a very demanding model of advocacy that could not be equally attained with all patients and, in some cases, is not possible at all. This would especially be the case with 'silent patients', such as non-conscious patients, who are unable to express their preferences.

ADVOCACY AS A POLITICAL STANCE

If nurses could be more actively involved in structuring mechanisms for conference consultations, decision reviews and team meetings, encouraging the advocacy role might be better warranted. Verena Tschudin would not agree to relinquish the obligation of nurses to act as advocate but rather sees adoption of the advocacy role as part of nurses' reclaiming of their professional identity. She claims that the notion of advocacy is a political stance and increasingly is seen as having the conviction or courage to stand up for a person against a system that is often unjust.

> On occasions, we have to be sure that we say *no*, especially to exploitation and misuse. Being treated unfairly and unjustly is never acceptable. When clients and patients in our care are at risk, we have to use the advocacy role and challenge the people concerned. This is not simply an ethical duty, but also a political act. (Tschudin 1999: 152–3)

Helga Kuhse is more worried about endorsing the advocacy role for nurses in the context of many institutional settings where autonomy for nurses is not promoted. Kuhse challenges the implicit assumption that nurses must carry out decisions of doctors regardless of their own moral point of view. She questions the reality of nursing life at present by asking: Are nurses regarded as autonomous health-care professionals and moral agents or are they seen as *dependent functionaries whose role it is to do the moral bidding of others?* (Kuhse 1997: 200).

Kuhse concludes that, in spite of the challenges facing the role of advocacy, it would be a mistake for nurses to reject the metaphor of the nurse as patient advocate.

> The central value of the metaphor lies in its power to shape actions. It focuses attention firmly on the proper primary 'object' of nursing care – the individual patient or client – and highlights such positive qualities as courage and assertiveness. These qualities – traditionally strongly discouraged in nurses and women – are sorely needed if nurses are to

fulfil their professional and moral responsibilities to patients. (Kuhse 1997: 206)

Activity

a) Consider Kuhse's understanding of advocacy, its pitfalls and strengths. Are there institutional barriers to the practice of nurse advocacy? Consider the following text from Yarling and McElmurry and discuss whether this represents your experience of the institutional reality of nursing in Ireland:

> The nurse *is often not free to be moral*, that is, a nurse is often not free to honor the commitment to the patient, whether the commitment takes the form of responding to the patient's request for no further treatment, of keeping the patient free from unnecessary suffering, or of performing whatever functions may be required by professional standards of nursing and by excellence in nursing practice. (cited in Kuhse 1997: 200)

b) Does the notion of moral space in all its concrete recommendations help or hinder the possibilities here?

c) Would you agree with Tschudin that advocacy is an ethical and political duty for nurse practice?

CONSCIENCE AND MORAL SPACE

When conscience conflicts arise because of disagreements with a decision taken by a clinician on a case, such as that of Sarah in Case 3.1, nurses are often confronted with difficult moral choices especially if they accept Tschudin's injunction to take advocacy as an ethical duty. But if there is going to be an endorsement of the challenge of advocacy, the idea of **moral space** needs to be discussed more broadly in professional contexts. The concept of moral space emphasises the need for closer harmonisation between nurse theory and practice, between institutional structures and ethically sensitive delivery of health care.

The ideas of Yarling and McElmurry speak of a kind of dissonance between education and nurse practice that resonates with the idea of 'moral space',

> A gap between what nurses are taught about how they should act and how in reality they are expected to act. There surfaces 'a profound moral dissonance' between nursing education and nursing practice which extends to the core of professional identity and leaves nurses essentially morally unintegrated professionals who are not self-determining, moral agents. (Yarling and McElmurry 1986: 67)

The Nursing Code of Conduct from An Bord Altranais (2000) writes about the importance of patient understanding:

> It is necessary for patients to have appropriate information for making an informed judgment. Every effort should be made to ensure that a

patient understands the nature and purpose of their care and treatment. In certain circumstances there may be a doubt whether certain information should be given to a patient and special care should be taken in such cases. (An Bord Altranais 2000)

Activity

a) On the basis of this statement, do you think that the Irish Nursing Board is recommending that the nurse participate in the process of communicating information to the patient? Does your professional experience confirm this interpretation?

b) Do you think that nurses can mobilise support within the profession to be more involved in the communication process with patients about diagnoses or prognoses? Think of some reasons why nurses should not have responsibilities of this kind.

The Irish Charter of Patients' Rights is one document that seems to assume rights such as:

1) Patients should be given access to details of their medical condition and treatment, including the results of tests and examinations.

2) It is a patient's right, on discharge, to be informed of the nature of their medical condition and follow-on treatment by their General Practitioner. (Department of Health 1990)

The case of Sarah, 3.1, would pose serious conflicts with both sets of guidelines cited here.

Summary Learning Guide 4.2

Nurse advocacy:

- Is a controversial concept that is strongly endorsed by some writers and presented with caution by others;
- Calls for a nurse to represent patient values and preferences;
- May cause conflict when patient preferences conflict with a nurse's professional or moral beliefs;
- Can be understood as an ethical duty and political act;
- Is a metaphor that focuses on positive qualities such as courage and assertiveness;
- Needs to be promoted and facilitated by institutional moral space.

COMMUNICATING THE TRUTH WITH RESPECT
The manner of truthful communication may be thought incidental to the moral obligation to be truthful as a general rule. But this is not the case.

The manner of communication can make the difference between a patient quaking with anxiety or experiencing relief and trust in what is to come. So, in addition to the important decision about *whether to tell a patient* about a clinically determined diagnosis/prognosis, two elements in the art and practice of truthful communication are essential to consider:

1. How much to tell, and
2. How to tell.

The following distinctions range from the important moral differences between overt lying and subtle, gradual and limited disclosure.

In Michael's case, the health-care team could consider gradual but subtle communication of what Michael will be undergoing (tests, surgery, chemotherapy). This can be done at the same time as the health-care team respects Michael's request not to know. Sharing with Michael where he is going now and why does not implicate nurse or doctor in a charade of deception or lying. Dr Wilkins has not lied to Michael and does not ask the nurses to lie. Dr Wilkins is also not deceiving Michael. He is simply not telling him what he and the health-care team know about Michael's illness. However, as we saw, the moral challenge in Dr Wilkins' approach is his decision to disclose Michael's details to his mother without getting permission from Michael.

Obligations of veracity are difficult to determine outside specific patients' contexts, but the following generalisations may be considered about types of disclosure and non-disclosure.

*   **Respect for a patient's request not to be told** the truth of a diagnosis cannot be interpreted as a permission or justification to the health-care team to lie.

*   **Explicit lying** is telling a person something that you know to be untrue with the intention of having them believe that it is true. Such lying to a recognised autonomous patient is profoundly difficult to justify morally, even if one invokes the therapeutic privilege.

*   **Therapeutic privilege** (see Case 3.1) endorses the withholding of information from patients because one judges it will be extremely harmful. The 'privilege' does not endorse lying to the patient.

*   **Deception that does not involve lying:** This approach is often considered easier to justify than lying. Arguments are not convincing. Consider: If a nurse tells a 60-year-old terminally ill patient that he will be 'right as rain in no time'. How do you construe this? It certainly is an effort to cheer up the patient but is it being deceptive? Does it threaten the relationship of trust between nurse and patient?

*   **Non-disclosure or minimal disclosure**: These methods are usually less difficult to justify than overt lying. This is especially the case if health professionals know of special cultural practices or customs in a family that are approved by the patient as well as family members.

- **Cautious disclosure**: In terms of amount of information to be given, a paced disclosure that is attentive to a patient's questions for more understanding is a prudent approach to consider. Cautious disclosure stresses accuracy and empathy. Cautious disclosure avoids what is called 'truth dumping' and 'terminal candour' (Beauchamp and Childress 2001: 286). Dispensing information gradually means greater accuracy as test results are offered to the health-care team. Gradual disclosure also builds on levels of indeterminacy and ambiguity that are constant features of clinical diagnoses.

The Art of Communicating

Finally there are the sensitive skills of how to tell, how to engage in a truthful communication. This skill is a pre-requisite for patient respect. It is a skill that can be learned well. In addition to the art of making honest judgements, communicating illness calls for skills in speaking without technical jargon. It also necessitates a listening that is sensitive to subtle signals and body language. These skills can make the difference in one's efforts to provide helpful, compassionate and hope-giving assistance to the patient. For example, because a patient is almost certainly moving into stages of dying does not mean that hope is no longer applicable. Hope refers again to the dimension of trustful expectation that all care and communication will be provided to respond to the needs of the whole person.

CONCLUSION

In the two chapters just completed, we have explored two case narratives with ethical challenges:

Case 3.1: Sarah is a woman who is clearly autonomous and requests information about her condition. However, the doctor decides not to tell her about her illness, primarily (it seems) because her husband requests him not to do so. The nurse, in the case, does not agree with the doctor's decision and experiences considerable moral distress of conscience. She believes that she lacks the moral space to discuss her serious reservations about this decision. A question we were left with is: should the nurse have done more?

Case 4.1: Michael is a man who has explicitly asked not to be told of his illness and adds that he does not wish his mother to be informed of his diagnosis. The doctor agrees to Michael's request not to tell him but does inform Michael's mother. The nurse is left wondering why the mother was told contrary to Michael's explicit request.

The concept of integrity and a steadfast conscience was discussed and shown to rely on a person's development of moral agency and the expansion of moral space within which to exercise it. The role of advocacy for nurses was also reviewed and seen to be a controversial concept but one that writers are slow to abandon. Advocacy encourages active commitment to represent and respect patient preferences. The role of advocate may, at times, come into serious conflict with institutional role expectations and the nurse's moral beliefs. When these conflicts occur, further reflection is needed to decide on moral priorities – professional and personal.

The following terms are explained in the glossary:

advocacy

conscience

holism

integrity

moral distress

moral space

paternalism with permission

sexism

waiver

– 5 –

Respecting Patient Confidentiality

Objectives

At the end of this chapter, you should be able to:

- Explain the principle of confidentiality and its importance;
- Refer to professional codes of practice and legal precedents that offer guidelines in making judgements about confidentiality;
- Discuss circumstances where it might be justifiable to qualify the principle of confidentiality.

INTRODUCTION

In Chapter 1 of this text, we described the principle of autonomy as a rule that obliges nurses to relate with patients in a particular way, namely to respect the health-related decisions that patients make. The principle of confidentiality is another such rule that places an obligation on nurses, namely to respect the confidences that patients share with them. By extension, this means that a nurse is also obliged to keep confidential patient information that she might gain from sources other than the patient in her care (Mills 2002: 45).

Confidential information is usually understood to be private information that a person shares with another on the understanding that it will not be disclosed to third parties. Keeping patient confidentiality is considered important because of its role in building patient trust and protecting patient autonomy and **privacy**. It is also considered important because the consequences of respecting patient confidentiality are generally seen as positive.

Confidentiality is a core element of all human relationships; thus it is basic to building trust and confidence between patient and nurse. Keeping confidences is a form of keeping a promise or bond. In effect, the nurse promises the patient to keep a bond of trust – the patient trusts the nurse to keep confidence and the nurse trusts the patient to tell the truth.

Keeping confidentiality expresses respect for autonomy and privacy. Firstly, it enables patients to be open about personal issues, concerns and questions, and enhances their capacity to make decisions about their health care. It also acknowledges that it is the patient who must live with the consequences of the decision (not the nurse). Secondly, respecting a patient's choice to keep certain information about them confidential – deciding not to tell a family member about their illness, for example – recognises the patient's right to privacy.

The philosopher, Sissela Bok, emphasises the importance of individual rights to privacy and, linking them with autonomy, argues that conflicts about concealing or revealing personal information should be understood as conflicts of power. She claims:

> Conflicts over secrecy – between state and citizen . . . or parent and child, [or between nurse and patient] or in journalism or business or law – are conflicts over power: the power that comes through controlling the flow of information. To be able to hold back some information about oneself or to channel it and thus influence how one is seen by others gives power; so does the capacity to penetrate similar defenses and strategies when used by others . . . To have no capacity for secrecy is to be out of control over how others see one; it leaves one open to coercion. To have no insight into what others conceal is to lack power as well. (Bok 1989: 19)

Finally, not only is the keeping of confidentiality considered worthwhile because it is viewed as an implicit part of the nurse–patient relationship, but it is also seen as a means of ensuring other important benefits. For example, the trust engendered through confidentiality:

- Creates an open and supportive environment that encourages patients to disclose more of their symptoms and worries, fears and phobias;
- Ensures a better diagnosis and a higher quality of care;
- Secures greater agreement and compliance with procedures and treatment;
- Encourages individuals – in particular, vulnerable individuals – to seek help and increases their contact with the health services.

In sum, the keeping of patient confidentiality is considered important because it is basic to a relationship built on trust and respect. It is important also because the consequences of keeping confidentiality are generally beneficial to patients in ensuring better outcomes for them.

Activity

a) Give one example from your professional experience of an occasion where the breaching of a patient's confidentiality undermined their trust in the health professions.

b) Re-read Bok's argument that conflicts about disclosing or not disclosing personal information are about power. Can you think of any example from your professional experience that might support Bok's view?

Summary Learning Guide 5.1

Confidential information:

- Is private information that a person shares with another on the understanding that it will not be disclosed to third parties.

Keeping patient confidentiality is important because it:

- Builds patient trust;
- Protects patient autonomy and privacy;
- Contributes to good treatment and care outcomes.

PROFESSIONAL AND LEGAL ACCOUNTABILITY

Professional Codes

Because it has long been held as an honoured bond between health professionals and patients, the keeping of confidentiality has been enshrined in both professional and legal codes. It was first articulated in the Hippocratic Oath (c. fifth century BCE):

> What I may see or hear in the course of the treatment or even outside of the treatment in regard to the life of men, which on no account one must spread abroad, I will keep to myself, holding such things shameful to be spoken about. (Translated by Ludwig Edelstein, 1943)

Florence Nightingale also set high standards for the nurse–patient relationship in relation to confidentiality. In 1859, she advised nurses in the following terms:

> And remember every nurse should be one who is to be depended upon, in other words, capable of being a 'confidential' nurse. She does not know how soon she may find herself placed in such a situation; she must be no gossip, no vain talker, she should never answer questions about her sick except to those who have a right to ask them. (Nightingale 1859, 1992, 70)

While the ancient oath points to shamefulness on the part of the health professional for breaking confidence, Nightingale draws attention to breaches of confidentiality that can happen through gossip and self-aggrandizement. She also indicates that anyone who asks for information about a patient must have a **right** to do so.

Modern codes of professional conduct for health professionals echo both Hippocrates' and Nightingale's stress on the professional–patient relationship and they also place emphasis on the notion of a presumed right on the patient's part to confidentiality. For example, the Irish Medical Council describes confidentiality as a 'time-honoured principle of medical ethics. It extends after death and is fundamental to the doctor/patient relationship. . . .' (Irish Medical Council 2004: 16.1)

However, where contemporary codes differ from earlier ones is in the acknowledgement they make that some circumstances may give rise to the need for the principle of confidentiality to be qualified in some way. Such circumstances include situations where the rights of those *other* than the patient may be at risk. These codes are discussed in detail in the following sections.

Activity

a) Nightingale suggests that confidentiality may be breached through 'gossip' and 'vain talk'. Can you think of contemporary examples where such breaches might arise?

b) Can you think of any other circumstances where, in the process of ordinary, everyday routine activities in a clinic or hospital, patient confidentiality might be breached?

Legislation

In addition to being protected by professional codes, confidentiality is also protected by law, on the basis of court decisions and also on appeal to such mechanisms as the Irish Constitution and the European Convention on Human Rights.

The Irish Courts, for example, recognise a right to privacy (and, by implication, a right to confidentiality) which is loosely derived from the Irish Constitution:

> Though not specifically guaranteed by the Constitution, the right to privacy is one of the fundamental personal rights of the citizen which flow from the Christian and democratic nature of the State . . . The nature of the right to privacy must be such as to ensure the dignity and freedom of an individual in the type of society envisaged by the Constitution, namely, a sovereign, independent and democratic society. (Hamilton P in *Kennedy and Arnold v Ireland* [1987] cited in Madden 2002)

The European Convention on Human Rights also protects privacy under Article 8:

> Everyone has the right to respect for his private and family life, his home and his correspondence.

However, just as professional codes consider exceptional circumstances where the principle of confidentiality might be qualified, so, also, legal rights to privacy are not considered absolute. The European Convention, for example, also stipulates under Article 8 that:

> There shall be no interference by a public authority with the exercise of this right except such as is in accordance with the law and is necessary in a democratic society in the interests of national security, public safety or the economic well-being of the country, for the prevention of

disorder or crime, for the protection of health or morals, or for the protection of the rights and freedoms of others.

What is at the heart of qualification of the right to privacy in Article 8 is a concern for the interests of others and the public interest generally.

Qualifying the Principle of Confidentiality
While the principle of confidentiality holds an honoured place in professional codes and laws, serious extenuating circumstances occasionally call for the principle to be qualified in some way.

The challenge for a nurse who is faced with such circumstances is to consider them carefully, to examine the implications of relevant codes and laws and to decide a course of action that she thinks best fulfils her various obligations as a carer, a professional and a citizen.

Disclosing with Permission
The least controversial circumstance that might arise is one where confidential information is shared between health professionals working in a multidisciplinary team. However, while many might presume that it is acceptable for members of a team to disclose to each other confidential information about a patient, even in this instance, care needs to be taken. The Code of Professional Conduct of An Bord Altranais, for example, advises nurses to use their professional judgement in relation to such disclosure:

> Information regarding a patient's history, treatment and state of health is privileged and confidential. It is accepted nursing practice that nursing care is communicated and recorded as part of the patient's care and treatment. Professional judgement and responsibility should be exercised in the sharing of such information with professional colleagues. (An Bord Altranais 2000)

While the Irish Medical Council does not address this point, the UK General Medical Council advises doctors to ensure that patients are aware that information might be shared:

> You should make sure that patients are aware that personal information about them will be shared within the health care team, unless they object, and of the reasons for this. (General Medical Council 2000: 8)

Disclosing Without Permission
While these situations might be more contentious and troubling, there is considerable international consensus on what might be deemed grounds for qualifying the principle of confidentiality *without* the permission of a patient. Generally codes delineate four circumstances where a health professional might justifiably share confidential information with people other than the patient or the multidisciplinary team. These circumstances relate to the interests of: the law, the patient, society, and other individuals. An Bord

Altranais addresses only one of these, but all four are explicitly detailed in the Irish Medical Council Guide 2004 as follows:

> There are four circumstances where exception may be made in the absence of permission from the patient:
>
> • When ordered by a Judge in a Court of Law, or by a Tribunal established by an Act of Oireachtas.
>
> • When necessary to protect the interest of the patient.
>
> • When necessary to protect the welfare of Society.
>
> • When necessary to safeguard the welfare of another individual or patient. (Irish Medical Council 2004: 16.3)

We will examine each of these circumstances in turn and will focus on the fourth concerning the interests of third parties, in order to identify and tease out some of the knottier problems that arise in relation to confidentiality.

1. When Obliged under the Law

Circumstances where the law can require a health professional to disclose confidential information include criminal investigations where the records of a suspected individual in a crime (e.g. road traffic offence, shooting offence) may be sought, and legal actions where a professional might be asked to testify in a court or tribunal. They may also relate to Infectious Diseases Regulations which place an obligation on doctors and other health professionals to disclose information about 'notifiable' diseases to the public health authorities.

The Guidelines of An Bord Altranais advise nurses to seek legal and professional advice should they be required to disclose information to a court of law.

> In certain circumstances, the nurse may be required by a court of law to divulge information held. A nurse called to give evidence in court should seek in advance legal and/or professional advice as to the response to be made if required by the court to divulge confidential information. (An Bord Altranais 2000)

2. To Protect the Interests of the Patient

In many situations, patients are likely to agree that the protection of their interests requires disclosure to a third party – where insanity is a defence in a criminal action, for example, or for insurance purposes. However, ethical problems arise if the health professional and the patient disagree as to what is in their best interests.

On such an occasion, a nurse might be torn between maintaining a patient's trust, on the one hand, and exercising the duty to protect a patient from harm, on the other. Circumstances where such conflicts arise might involve patients who share information with a nurse in relation to abuse, neglect or suicidal intentions. In cases of abuse or neglect, the patient – young or old – may feel so dependent or fearful that they refuse to permit the nurse to disclose the abuse. In cases of threatened suicide, a patient may be so severely depressed that they cannot rationally decide where their best interests lie.

3. To Protect the Interests of Society

As we concluded in Chapter 1, the right of an individual to exercise autonomy is limited by the similar rights of others to live autonomously. So, also, in the case of confidentiality, the interest of a patient in having confidences protected is limited by the legitimate interests of others. Those interests may be deemed to outweigh an individual's right to confidentiality in circumstances where nondisclosure threatens the wellbeing and welfare of others. For example, a nurse might be justifiably concerned to learn that an airline pilot or bus driver suffers from epilepsy, or that a patient has murderous intentions and seems capable of carrying them out. In these circumstances, the health and even lives of members of the public are at risk if the nurse does not disclose this information to other relevant parties.

4. To Protect the Interests of Another Individual or Patient

The fourth set of circumstances is similar to the third, just outlined, in that it concerns the interests of persons other than the patient. However, these circumstances concern not the public at large or society as a whole, but particular identifiable individuals who are at serious risk of harm which disclosure of information might avert or minimise. The widely reported court case which first stipulated that health professionals had a legal obligation to breach confidentiality in circumstances where identifiable third parties were at risk is the United States case of *Tarasoff v. the Regents of the University of California* (1976).

In that case, the California Supreme Court imposed on a psychotherapist a limited duty to warn a presumed intended victim of a patient's aggression. The case came about when the parents of a murdered student, Tatiana Tarasoff, sued the University of California and the professionals involved for their failure to notify them that their daughter was in grave danger. Her killer, Prosenjit Poddar, had been undergoing outpatient psychotherapy with the student health services, during which he had admitted to having violent fantasies in relation to Tarasoff. The therapist, who learned from Poddar's friend that he had purchased a gun, took steps to hospitalise him for further evaluation – against his will, if necessary. However, Californian law makes involuntary hospitalisation difficult and, while Poddar was still at large, he shot and killed Tarasoff and was subsequently convicted of second-degree homicide.

The parents claimed that the defendant (University of California, therapist and campus police) failed to notify them or their daughter that she was in danger. The providers involved claimed that they could not warn Tatiana Tarasoff because it would violate patient confidentiality. The case was initially dismissed but, after several appeals, the California Supreme Court overturned the dismissal. In 1976, it stated:

> [O]nce a therapist does, in fact, determine, or under the applicable professional standards reasonably should have determined, that a patient poses a serious danger of violence to others, he bears a duty to exercise reasonable care to protect the foreseeable victim of that danger. (*Tarasoff* v. *the Regents of the University of California* [1976])

The court noted that the duty to protect might be fulfilled in different ways, such as issuing a warning to the presumed intended victim or others likely to tell the potential victim of the danger, notifying the police, or initiating steps reasonably necessary under the circumstances.

This duty or obligation on the part of health professionals to warn an identifiable person who is at risk of serious harm, which was articulated by the Californian Supreme Court in the Tarasoff case, has also been expressed in many contemporary codes. In particular, many codes explicitly place a duty to warn on professionals in relation to serious communicable diseases. The Irish Medical Council, for example, puts it in the following way:

> Where others may be at serious risk if not aware that a patient has a communicable infection, a doctor should do his/her best to obtain permission from the patient to tell them, so that appropriate safeguards can be put in place. If the patient refuses to consent to disclosure, those who might be at risk of infection should be informed of the risk to themselves. (Irish Medical Council 2004: 16.9)

The position of the Medical Council in relation to disclosure in these circumstances is supported by the Irish Data Protection Acts 1988 and 2003 and the EU Data Protection Directive 1995. Specifically the Irish Acts permit disclosure of otherwise confidential information where 'required urgently to prevent injury or other damage to the health of a person' (Data Protection Acts 1988 and 2003: Section 8(d)).

Summary Learning Guide 5.2

Professional Codes and Laws

- Professional codes stipulate that patients have a right to confidentiality.
- Confidentiality is also protected by law: court decisions, the Irish Constitution and the European Convention on Human Rights.

Qualifying the Principle of Confidentiality

The principle of confidentiality is not considered absolute. Exceptional circumstances where the principle may be qualified include:

- When obliged under the law;
- To protect the interests of the patient;
- To protect the interests of society;
- To protect the interests of another individual or patient.

A Duty to Warn: Whom? What? When? How?

While the law (legislation and court decisions) and professional regulations clearly stipulate a duty on the part of health professionals to warn those at risk, there remains some uncertainty in relation to the precise circumstances that would prompt the disclosure of information (who to warn about what) and also in relation to the process of carrying out such a duty (when and how to warn). However, some guidelines exist.

1. *In relation to whom to warn about what:*
   - The Californian Supreme Court stipulates that the person at risk must be *identifiable*, and that the risk to them must be one of a *serious danger of violence*.
   - The Data Protection Directive 1995 permits disclosure in *urgent* circumstances to *prevent injury or other damage*.
   - The Irish Medical Council cites *serious risk* as a condition of disclosure.

2. *In relation to when and how:*
   - The Californian Supreme Court advised taking steps that were *reasonably necessary under the circumstances*.
   - The Irish Medical Council directs a doctor to *do his/her best to obtain [the] permission* of patients to disclose any information.

What these provisos indicate is a general concern that confidentiality is not breached lightly: that the decision to disclose is not made in haste without due care and consideration of all concerned in the situation.

The following case which relates to the duty to warn will help to illustrate some of the complex ethical tensions that arise when a nurse must contemplate breaching confidentiality in these circumstances.

Case 5.1: Married with HIV

Mr Murphy, a successful forty-two-year-old businessman, reported to the Health Adviser/Counsellor in the Genitourinary Medicine (GUM) Clinic of a large regional hospital after being confidentially informed that his blood test was positive for antibodies to the Human Immune Deficiency Virus (HIV). The patient had no symptoms.

The Health Adviser, Norma Flynn, informed Mr Murphy that although he did not have AIDS, there was between a 5 and 35 per cent probability that he would develop the disease within the next five years. He was also told that he could probably infect others through sexual contact, by sharing needles, or by donating blood and blood products. He was counselled not to donate blood, and to engage in 'safe sex' – that is, sex that did not involve the exchange of bodily fluids such as semen.

Mr Murphy then revealed that he was bisexual, and that he believed that he had contracted the infection during one of his homosexual encounters. He also said that he was married with four children. Norma advised Mr Murphy to inform his wife of his diagnosis. But Mr Murphy refused to do so, saying that his wife did not know anything about his bisexuality and that telling her would ruin his marriage and his life.

Activity

Consider this case in relation to what you have read about confidentiality so far. How do you think Norma might resolve the situation?

In the case of Mr Murphy, Norma Flynn must decide whether she should inform Mrs Murphy about Mr Murphy's condition or whether she should protect the confidentiality of the therapeutic relationship. It seems that she must choose between two competing moral obligations – the obligation to keep patient confidentiality and the obligation to protect another person whose life may be at risk if she fails to disclose. To help her in making the decision, she must ask herself the following questions about the situation:

1. What values are protected by the principle of confidentiality and are they relevant in this case?
2. Does she have an obligation to protect a third party who is not her patient?
3. If there are both a duty to a patient and a duty to a third party, which is the most compelling duty?
4. If Norma Flynn is considering telling Mrs Murphy, how much should be told?

1. As we indicated earlier, the principle of confidentiality is basic to all human relationships, is essential to the promotion of trust between nurse and patient, and is an expression of respect for patient autonomy and privacy. The positive consequences to the patient of keeping confidentiality are also considered important.

In the case of Mr Murphy, the patient is adamant that his wife should not be told. He believes that if she were to find out, his marriage and family, and his life as a whole, would be irreparably damaged. There is much at stake for him. In considering his situation, Norma is obliged to maintain his trust in her as much as possible; she is also obliged to respect his autonomy – that is, the decisions he makes in relation to his own life.

In addition to these duties, Norma must also consider the consequences of disclosure – what Mr Murphy might do if his relationship with her, with the Clinic and with his family breaks down. Should he lose the support that he might receive there, Mr Murphy might well be in a far more dangerous position, to himself and to others, than he is now.

Norma's concern about the long-term consequences of breaking Mr Murphy's trust are echoed by utilitarian ethicists such as Helga Kuhse who is concerned that allowing exceptions to the rule of confidentiality with the intention of protecting third-party interests will not achieve their intended effect in the long term (Kuhse 1999: 493–6). Kuhse's basic concern is that a more relaxed confidentiality requirement on the part of health professionals will inhibit people who are most in need of health services from availing of them:

> The point is that if known breaches of confidentiality are likely to prevent individuals from seeking treatment or to hinder them from seeking treatment in a timely fashion, then a rule requiring disclosure is likely to do more harm than good. (Kuhse 1999: 495)

The cost of breaches of confidentiality is the loss of patient trust and the subsequent inability to support patients to modify behaviour that is harmful to others. In brief, in Kuhse's view, while harm might be prevented on some occasions, in the longer term, the overall harm to society will not be reduced.

2. On the other hand, even though Mrs Murphy is not her patient, it could be argued that Norma also has a moral obligation to protect her. Not just the autonomy of Mr Murphy, but also that of his wife is very much at risk in this situation. While the consequences of disclosure might be serious for Mr Murphy, the consequences of nondisclosure are also serious for Mrs Murphy. The most compelling argument for disclosure is a health-related one, based on general agreement that early access to anti-retroviral therapy and health-care management are likely to prolong the health and welfare of individuals with HIV (Woodman 2003: 7).

Norma might also consult relevant professional and legal regulations. For example, the guidelines of the Irish Department of Health and Children (2001) and the UK Society of Sexual Health Advisers (SSHA) (2004) acknowledge that sexual health advisers have a professional duty to protect third parties, and an important function of GUM clinics in Ireland and elsewhere is the process of **partner notification**. Partner notification, or contact tracing, describes the process whereby individuals who may have been in contact with a sexually transmitted infection (STI) are contacted (by the partner or by the health professional) in order to prevent the spread of the infection.

From a legal point of view, the Tarasoff case and other legislation indicate that there is a duty to warn an identifiable third party of serious danger. In this case, the third party is both identifiable and in serious danger: either Mrs Murphy is already HIV positive and is in need of treatment, or she is in danger of contracting HIV and needs to take precautions against it.

3. The ethical dilemma that Norma is faced with then is very real – she has a duty to the patient, Mr Murphy, and she has a duty to his wife, Mrs Murphy. It seems that she cannot fulfil both duties at once – if she fulfils her duty to Mr Murphy, she must neglect her duty to Mrs Murphy and vice versa.

On the one hand, seeing that Mr Murphy is her patient, Norma might be inclined to privilege her duty to him over her duty to Mrs Murphy. On the other hand, she might think that while the therapeutic relationship may suffer and Mr Murphy's autonomy be undermined, the implications of nondisclosure are far more serious for Mrs Murphy. In which case, Norma might conclude that the duty to warn is the more compelling duty.

Accepting that she has a compelling duty to warn Mrs Murphy, Norma must next decide how to proceed. Again, she can draw on available guidelines. For example, the Irish Medical Council, as outlined, directs doctors to *do their best* to seek the permission of patients to disclose and that, having failed to secure permission, they should then disclose only where the risk is serious. It would seem that even when it is accepted that one duty (to disclose) outweighs another (not to disclose), there remains an obligation to continue to try to meet both obligations at the same time.

As a first step, then, Norma must make every effort to secure Mr Murphy's permission to disclose. Were she able to persuade Mr Murphy that he should tell his wife, or were she to secure his permission for her to disclose his HIV status, Norma would be able to fulfil both of her obligations – she would maintain Mr Murphy's trust and she would protect Mrs Murphy.

But what if Mr Murphy could not be persuaded? What then? It would seem that Norma would have to take what she sees as the least harmful course of action – breach confidentiality and inform Mrs Murphy.

4. If Norma decides she should tell Mrs Murphy, what should be told? This fourth question is based on a working principle, the minimalist principle of disclosure. We formulate the principle this way: 'Tell a relevant third party only the minimum that is necessary to achieve the end of disclosure.' This can afford protection of patient confidence as much as possible, while recognising an obligation to disclose pertinent information to achieve the legal requirement or to protect a third party from danger. So the question Norma can ask if she is pondering whether or not to tell Mrs Murphy of her husband's situation is: what information is essential for Mrs Murphy to know to achieve protection for her and perhaps encourage her to come into the clinic for testing herself?

Norma is looking at a clinical situation where Mr Murphy is diagnosed HIV positive and her primary concern is how she can protect relevant third parties, specifically his wife. But she is aware that Mr Murphy is seriously worried that, if he does tell his wife or allow her to be told, she may also find out that he is bisexual. This might be a worse outcome than telling her that he is HIV positive. Since it is not true that HIV is contracted only through sexual experience, that Mr Murphy is bisexual seems not relevant information to tell Mrs Murphy. Norma might think Mrs Murphy should know her husband's sexual orientation. But why?

Knowing details of her husband's sexuality seems extraneous to the objective of due care to protect Mrs Murphy from infection with HIV. Perhaps Mr Murphy's sexual orientation is information that should be left entirely to conversation between Mr and Mrs Murphy. Perhaps too, if Norma made it clear to Mr Murphy that she has no intention of telling his wife about his sexuality, it would persuade him to undertake the conversation with his wife. Alternatively Norma could offer to discuss the diagnosis together with both Mr and Mrs Murphy. If Mrs Murphy asks Norma how her husband contracted HIV, or if Mrs Murphy comes near to the sexuality issue, Norma can explain that, on these questions, she thinks a conversation between them is more fruitful and respectful.

Activity

If Mr Murphy refuses to tell his wife, the case seems, inevitably, to evolve into a 'win–lose' situation, where Mr Murphy wins and Mrs Murphy loses or vice versa. Consider what you have read about this case so far. Can you think of any other way that Norma might address her dilemma?

CONCLUSION

This chapter has focused on the ethical challenges that keeping patient confidentiality affords to nurses. While we have considered the important role that confidentiality plays in the nurse–patient relationship, we have also explored the kinds of circumstances where breaching confidentiality seems ethically warranted.

We have ended this chapter with a troubling conclusion: that in some ethical dilemmas, someone must win and someone must lose. In order to determine whether or not this is an inevitable outcome of the process of ethical reasoning, we will examine a second case on confidentiality in the following chapter. This case also concerns a set of circumstances where the duty of confidentiality seems to conflict with the duty to warn, but the situation in this case is far more complex.

The following terms are explained in the glossary:

confidential information
partner notification
privacy

public interest
right

The Confidentiality Process

Objectives

At the end of this chapter, you should have:

- A deeper understanding of the process of respecting patient confidentiality;
- An increased awareness of the various dimensions of moral engagement;
- Additional skills in interpreting and analysing ethical situations.

INTRODUCTION

In Chapter 5, we explained and explored the principle of confidentiality and considered what a nurse might do in a case where she has both a duty to her patient and a competing duty to a third party. We suggested at the end of the chapter that, in the case of Mr Murphy, there were compelling reasons why confidentiality should be breached. However, we left open the question of how a nurse might proceed once she had arrived at such a position. One of the tasks of this chapter is to address this question.

To do so, we will first examine a second set of circumstances where the duty of confidentiality seems to conflict with the duty to warn. This case, 6.1: Living in fear with HIV, is even more morally complex than our first confidentiality case, 5.1: Married with HIV. Such complexity will make clear the kinds of moral expertise that a nurse (or midwife) needs to have in order to address such situations adequately.

Case 6.1: Living in Fear with HIV

When Chi Chi was three months pregnant, she came for a check-up to the ante-natal clinic at the Rotunda maternity hospital where I work. Her admission form revealed that Chi Chi was thirty years old, was originally from Somalia, and had been living in Dublin for two years. She was married and had two children – a boy of ten and a girl of six. As I was the midwife assigned to look after Chi Chi, I told her about the blood screening and HIV screening that we generally carried out for pregnant women in the clinic. It seemed to me that she had fairly good English and she agreed to all the tests.

At her next appointment, I was present when the Registrar told Chi Chi that her HIV test was positive. After the Registrar left, I tried to comfort Chi Chi but she was very distressed and fearful. I explained the test results and talked to her about some further tests that needed to be carried out to determine the progress of the HIV virus.

I also advised her about taking precautions in relation to sexual contact with her husband, and urged her to visit the clinic again in a few days.

On her return visit, Chi Chi immediately agreed to go on an anti-retroviral therapy drug-treatment programme aimed at controlling the HIV virus and minimising the risk of its transmission to her unborn child. However, she got very distressed and agitated when the discussion turned to her husband, Charles. I talked to Chi Chi about safe sex practices and the need for Charles to come to the hospital himself for counselling and testing.

However, Chi Chi was horrified at the thought of telling Charles. She said that they rarely talked of such matters. She told me that since they had escaped from their war-torn country, Charles had become very despondent and increasingly violent towards her. In tears, she said that she was afraid for her life and for the lives of her children most of the time. She was terrified that telling Charles about her HIV status would be the death of her.

Like the case of Mr Murphy, the case of Chi Chi also involves a duty of confidentiality (to Chi Chi) and a seeming conflicting duty to a third party (Charles).

If, in this case, the midwife, Margaret Murphy, were to apply the guidelines and follow the reasoning of the health adviser we met in Case 5.1, she might conclude that Charles ought to be informed that he was at risk.

Activity

Consider what you have read about this case so far. How do you think the midwife might address the situation? As you reflect, re-read Chapter 5 and list the reasons why the principle of confidentiality might, justifiably, be breached in this instance. List reasons why the principle of confidentiality should not be breached in this case.

The Ethical Context

As you considered Case 6.1, it might have struck you that the situation of Chi Chi and Charles is far more complex than any case we have discussed so far in the text. As such, we suggest that it calls for a far more sophisticated approach than a simple weighing of arguments for and against disclosure. To view Chi Chi's situation through the lens of confidentiality alone would be an oversimplification of the ethical issues that arise. These include not just confidentiality, but also the possibly abusive situation in which Chi Chi is living, the relationship between the midwife, Margaret, and Chi Chi, the threat of violence toward her, and the vulnerability of both Chi Chi and Charles as African asylum seekers living in Ireland.

Some questions that the midwife needs to consider are:

1.   What does she know of Chi Chi's living situation?
2.   Are there obstacles that might prevent the building of trust between Chi Chi and herself and constrain Chi Chi's ability to make decisions in relation to her health?

3.	How serious is the threat of violence toward Chi Chi?
4.	Does Charles need help?

1. What does Margaret know about Chi Chi's current living situation and background? Chi Chi has already mentioned that her husband has become abusive since they arrived in Dublin. Margaret needs to know more about the level of violence or abuse that Chi Chi and her children are living with. Perhaps Chi Chi is in far more immediate danger from that than she is from her HIV status. Perhaps Chi Chi's children are in danger.

While the midwife may feel confident in her knowledge about attitudes towards HIV/AIDs in Ireland, she must find out whether or not Chi Chi's Somali culture and community have views on HIV/AIDs that are relevant here.

2. Margaret must also consider how she might build trust with Chi Chi in order to support her in her situation. To do so, she must take into account the fact that differences between them – citizenship, ethnic origin, income, professional status, health – might be obstacles to building trust and rapport. In this situation, she is an Irish citizen, a white woman with professional status and expertise. Chi Chi, on the other hand, is a black woman living with a life-threatening stigmatising condition, in a home and a city that is, often, overtly hostile and racist towards her. Margaret needs to find out, for example, if Chi Chi's grasp of English is an obstacle to her understanding and decision making. Can Chi Chi afford the bus fare to get to the clinic? Or the medicines she will need? Margaret must also consider whether Chi Chi has had previous experiences with western health professionals that might impact on their relationship and on Chi Chi's ability to make informed decisions about her health care.

3. Chi Chi has told Margaret that she is afraid that her husband, Charles, will kill her if she tells him that she is HIV positive. Margaret needs to consider the threat of violence that Charles presents if he is informed – by Chi Chi herself, or by a health professional in the hospital. The likelihood of serious violence might well justify not telling him, at least for a period of time.

4. Margaret must also consider Charles. Firstly, it is possible that Charles is already HIV positive and that he may well have communicated the virus to Chi Chi himself. If so, he too is in need of treatment and care.

Secondly, Charles may need other kinds of help. Perhaps he, like many survivors of war, is suffering from post-traumatic stress or some other illness. The midwife might conclude that both Chi Chi and Charles are in need of support from a range of agencies, in addition to the maternity hospital services, in order for them to be enabled and empowered to come to terms with Chi Chi's diagnosis of HIV.

Ethical Expertise
In considering Chi Chi's situation, it is evident that complex situations make complex moral demands on the health professionals at the centre of them.

Activity

a) We have suggested that the midwife in Case 6.1 should address four concerns arising out of Chi Chi's situation. List any additional issues that you think might be important here.

b) How do you think a midwife should approach a case similar to that of Chi Chi but one in which the woman at risk of violence is white, Irish and middle-class? Do you think that she should take the same approach as Margaret does to Chi Chi or do you think that she should take a different approach? Give reasons for your answer. (See Fry and Veatch 2000: 282–4, for their account of such a case.)

These complex situations underline the need for nurses and midwives to develop different kinds of ethical expertise. Not only must they be aware of ethical principles and professional and legal obligations, but they must also be sensitive to the wider context in which the patient is trying to make decisions, and recognise that the relationship between professional and patient might itself be a source of moral concern.

Summary Learning Guide 6.1

Ethically complex situations demand the following moral capacities:

- Sensitivity to the patient's situation;
- Awareness of the need to understand and learn more;
- Consciousness of the variety of obstacles to building trust and empowering patients;
- Recognition that the patient may not be the only person in a situation in need of support.

Activity

Make a list of any other skills/expertise that you think Margaret might need in order to support Chi Chi.

CASE 5.1 FROM ANOTHER PERSPECTIVE

Given what we have learned from Case 6.1 about the demands of moral engagement, let's take a second look at Case 5.1. Recall that in the case of 'Married with HIV', in Chapter 5, we suggested that the health advisor, Norma Flynn, had a duty both to the patient, Mr Murphy, and to his wife, Mrs Murphy. We also argued that, on balance, Norma's duty to Mrs Murphy was more compelling because she was at risk of serious harm which disclosure might avert. We finished the chapter pondering what steps the health advisor might take next. The following case sheds some light on the course of action that Norma decided upon.

Case 6.2: Excerpt from the Journal of Bill Murphy

Since last month, I have been living in hell. I don't really know what to do. My four children, Mary, my workmates and friends in Skibbereen – what is going to happen when they find out? And if the Clinic has its way, they will, at least Mary will. But how can I possibly tell her?

It must have been Tom, I suppose. He's the only one I ever had 'real sex' with. That was three years ago when he came down to work in the Castle Hotel. I remember I could hardly believe it was happening. I never expected that I could ever have a loving relationship with another man . . . but I think I was able to love Tom.

And now, here I am. I wonder how he is. He must be qualified by now, doing his accounting somewhere. I wonder is he sick. Does he know what he has? Is he dead? Will I die? And Mary? . . .

As this case indicates, after his initial refusal to tell his wife, Norma decided to give Mr Murphy (Bill) more time to come to terms with his own situation before he (or she) would tell his wife about his HIV status. In addition, Bill agreed not to engage in any practice that might endanger anyone else, to attend counselling sessions with Norma and to keep a journal from which the above excerpt is drawn.

Activity

Critically evaluate the course of action that the health adviser has taken. Make a list of arguments in favour of her course of action. Make a list of arguments against her course of action.

The fact that Norma decides to take the time to support Bill to come to terms with his situation indicates that she is sensitive to his worries and fears and that she recognises the role that her relationship with him might play in empowering him in his health care and life decisions. But if Norma decides to promise Bill that she will not discuss his sexuality with his wife if she comes for testing, this too can help Bill experience a nonjudgemental attitude about bisexuality. This respect for sexual difference can also help empower Bill to agree to discuss his HIV diagnosis with his wife. A decision to discuss his sexuality with his wife might take more time.

The significance of the therapeutic relationship in these situations is recognised by many working in the area of sexually transmitted infection, such as the UK Society of Sexual Health Advisers (SSHA) whose guidelines lay particular stress on the obligations of the health adviser in this regard (2004). In addition, Antoinette Woodman's recent research on the practices of Irish Genitourinary Medicine clinics in relation to partner notification would, likely, support Norma's course of action (2003). In her thesis, Woodman argues that health professionals working with people who may have communicable sexually transmitted infections need to have a broad set of skills in order to deal with the understandable confusion, anger and hostility that they sometimes meet with in the course of their work. One health adviser whom Woodman interviewed as a part of her research goes to the heart of what is at stake in relation to disclosure:

> People can be very upset and even angry by the process of partner notification – they can see it as interference in their personal lives and it is – so one needs to be sensitive and non-judgemental. (Woodman 2003: 80)

In short, the impact that disclosure can have on individuals' lives cannot be underestimated and those whose task it might be to secure that disclosure must tread with great caution and care. In doing so, they, like Norma and Margaret, are challenged to do more than consult available moral, professional or legal guides. Such guides give direction and indicate boundaries but they do not (and cannot) provide individual solutions for specific situations. The process of finding individual solutions is one that, in addition to understanding and applying relevant rules, requires a range of interpretive skills on the part of health professionals. Some of these are identified in the following section.

Activity

Take a few moments to reread the three cases on confidentiality that we have examined in this chapter and in Chapter 5: 5.1 Married with HIV; 6.1 Living in Fear with HIV; and 6.1 Excerpt from the Journal of Bill Murphy. Compare the quantity and quality of information that is presented in each case.

INTERPRETING ETHICAL SITUATIONS

It is clear from the three cases on confidentiality that the way in which a nurse understands and approaches an ethically challenging situation has an impact on the therapeutic relationship between nurse and patient and makes a difference to the eventual outcome of the case.

For example, in Case 5.1, if Norma, the health adviser, were to focus on the fact that Mr Murphy was a successful businessman and unfaithful husband and not on his expressed worries about his wife and friends, she might be more likely to ignore the personal journey that has brought him to his present predicament. Norma's request that Mr Murphy, or Bill, keep a personal journal indicates that she recognises that the patient's own account of his situation is morally relevant. Indeed, as the journal tells the story of Bill's relationship with Tom, Bill becomes more of a person beset with his own demons and it seems likelier that Norma will be able to support him and his family.

Equally, if Margaret, the midwife, were to pay sole attention to Chi Chi's refusal to tell Charles about her HIV status, she would overlook what might well be the far more imminent danger facing Chi Chi and her children. Instead, when Margaret recognises the various ways in which Chi Chi's situation might constrain her ability to make good health-care decisions for herself and her family, she is in a better place to support and empower her.

In short, the way in which a nurse or midwife understands what is ethically relevant or important in a situation has an impact on her approach to it. Moreover, it might equally be argued that the way in which ethical cases are presented in books, such as this one, affects the way in which they are read and understood. For example, notice that Case 5.1 is reported in the third person; we read about Norma's dilemma with Mr Murphy as if it were a neutral account of observable facts. Take a few moments to read the case again, and consider what is told and what is not told – what is included in the account and what is left out of consideration. Do you think that this makes a difference?

Activity

Take a case from any one of the earlier chapters in this text and rewrite it from the patient's point of view. Do you think that viewing the situation from the patient's point of view might influence the way in which you understand the moral issues that arise therein?

CONCLUSION

While situations such as those of Bill and Chi Chi are, fortunately, rare enough, they enable us to achieve a better understanding of the complex nature of ethical decision making and engagement.

Focusing on the patient's own story and its context, as the health adviser and midwife have especially tried to do in Cases 6.1 and 6.2, makes clear that ethical decision making need not necessarily involve a win–lose situation – Mr Murphy loses, Mrs Murphy wins; Chi Chi wins, Charles loses; Bill wins, Mrs Murphy loses. Rather, ethical decision making is better viewed as a process of ethical engagement that is aimed at avoiding harm and benefiting *all* of those concerned in the difficult situations that arise.

Negotiating difficult moral terrain demands a range of competencies on the part of the health professionals involved – knowledge of ethical principles, codes and laws, as well as moral sensitivity and skills of interpretation and communication. In short, to be ethically engaged, in the fullest sense, is to be alive to the world of the patient from the patient's point of view, while acknowledging that there are others whose voices and interests must also be heard and served. In recent years, two ethical frameworks which place the patient at the centre of the ethical decision-making process have emerged. These are the *ethic of care* and *narrative ethics* and we explain and explore these approaches in Chapter 19.

The following terms are explained in the glossary:

ethic of care   narrative model ethics

Informed Consent to Nursing and Medical Procedures

Objectives

At the end of this chapter, you should be able to:

- Outline the moral and legal basis of informed consent;
- Consider the role of the nurse in relation to informed consent;
- Explain the modes of informed consent: explicit, implicit, tacit;
- Define informed consent;
- Explain and discuss three key elements of informed consent: competence, information and authorisation.

INTRODUCTION

With few exceptions, an individual's **consent** to undergo any health-care procedure – nursing or medical – or to participate in health-care research is viewed as an absolute ethical and legal prerequisite. In the past thirty years, it has been generally accepted that the process of gaining a patient's or research participant's consent centrally involves communicating with them about the nature of any proposed treatment or research. Therefore, what has become known as the principle or rule of **informed consent** is now widely used by ethical and legal theorists as well as health practitioners and researchers to convey the idea that a person should (a) be informed about and (b) freely consent to, any health-care treatment that they receive or any health-care research in which they participate.

The requirement of the informed consent of human participants in *research* has long been viewed as a process which protects their welfare and rights, and this is dealt with in greater detail in Chapter 8. The requirement for the informed consent of a person for *nursing or medical procedures and care*, however, is a relatively new phenomenon. It derives from a number of principles: nonmaleficence, beneficence and autonomy.

Firstly, it is viewed as a means of respecting a patient's privacy and dignity and protecting them from bodily invasion, assault, deception or coercion (nonmaleficence). Failure to obtain informed consent is viewed as undermining the relationship between the health professional and the patient. In some cases, it can lead to civil action (trespass, assault, battery) or criminal proceedings for common, aggravated or indecent assault.

Informed consent is also understood as a beneficent process, a means of promoting the health and wellbeing of the patient. The assumption is that patient involvement in decision making and treatment has therapeutic benefits:

- It encourages patient compliance with treatment and care procedures – for example, if a patient knows *why* there is a need to exercise, they are likelier to follow an exercise programme.
- It contributes to a better diagnosis, prognosis and quality of care – a patient who is involved in the decision-making process is likelier to provide more information about their condition and communicate their needs more readily.
- It enables individuals to communicate a more complete picture of the whole of their concerns in relation to a proposed treatment – for example, a man with terminal cancer may inform his consultant that he is more anxious to attend his son's wedding than he is to receive his weekly chemotherapy treatment.

The conception of informed consent as a nonmaleficent and beneficent procedure has long been the more generally accepted view in Ireland (Parker and Dickenson 2001: 285). More recently, however, the principle of informed consent has also been viewed as a requirement that protects and promotes the autonomy of individuals in health-care decision making. The idea is that a patient needs to be informed about the potential advantages and disadvantages of any proposed treatment and alternatives to treatment in order for them to reflect and deliberate on whether or not to accept or refuse the treatment that is offered. When an individual consents to the treatment that a health professional plans for them, they make the aims and objectives of the health professional part of their own. This means that the individual is not merely instrumental to another's ends, but, in fact, they take ownership of these ends.

A number of legal decisions in the last century have contributed to the understanding of informed consent as a principle that promotes autonomy. For example, in the landmark legal case from the United States, *Schloendoff* v. *Society of New York Hospital* (1914), Justice Cordozo stated:

> Every human being of adult years and sound mind has a right to determine what shall be done with his own body; and a surgeon who performs an operation without his patient's consent, commits an assault, for which he is liable in damages. ([1914] 211 NY 125)

In addition to determining that the absence of the consent of a competent patient to surgery amounts to assault, Justice Cordozo, emphasises here the 'right' of a competent adult 'to determine what shall be done with his own body'. A similar emphasis on autonomy as a basis for the legal requirement of informed consent can be found in the case law of many jurisdictions and in the more recent decisions of the Irish courts. In one Supreme Court case, for example, Justice Hamilton held that people who were incompetent retained their Constitutional rights including 'the right to life, the right to bodily integrity, the right to privacy, including self-determination, and the right to refuse medical care or treatment.' Referring to competent individuals, a second judge in the case, Justice O'Flaherty, concluded that 'there is an absolute right in a competent person to refuse medical treatment even if it leads to death' (*Re a Ward of Court* (1995) 2 ILRM 401, 431).(See Chapter 13 to learn more about the Ward of Court case.)

Activity

Consider Justice O'Flaherty's statement. He asserts that competent patients have a right to refuse treatment even if such refusal is not in the patient's best medical interest – in fact, it may lead to their death. Acknowledging such a right, O'Flaherty privileges the principle of autonomy over the principle of beneficence where competent patients are concerned. What is your response to O'Flaherty's judgement?

Codes of Professional Conduct usually oblige health professionals to secure the informed consent of patients to treatment. The Irish Code of Professional Conduct for each Nurse and Midwife, April 2000, for example, does not specifically use the terms autonomy or informed consent, but suggests that information is a condition of making an 'informed judgement':

> It is necessary for patients to have appropriate information for making an informed judgement. Every effort should be made to ensure that a patient understands the nature and purpose of their care and treatment. In certain circumstances there may be a doubt whether certain information should be given to a patient and special care should be taken in such cases. (An Bord Altranais 2000)

Activity

a) Compare what the Irish Code advises on informed consent with Provision 1.4 of the American Nurses Association (2001) *Code of Ethics with Interpretive Statements*. Consider the way in which the AMA Code links the requirement of informed consent with the principle of patient self-determination.

b) If you are sitting in class while you read this chapter, reach over and touch the person sitting on your right.

   i)   Consider how comfortable you were while you were doing this? Were you conscious of the need to respect the personal space of your fellow student? Did you hesitate and consider how you might touch them appropriately?

   ii) Reflect on your own response to being touched. Did it make you feel shy, self-conscious, vulnerable?

   iii) In the light of your response to this activity, take a few moments to consider what it must be like for people who are ill and in pain. Would you say that the routine of clinic or hospital ward desensitises nurses to the sometimes invasive nature of examination, treatment and care?

Summary Learning Guide 7.1

The requirement of informed consent derives from:

- The principle of nonmaleficence – avoiding harm to the patient; informed consent protects against assault, battery, deception, coercion;
- The principle of beneficence – doing good for the patient; informed consent improves therapeutic outcomes;
- The principle of autonomy – respecting autonomous choice; informed consent protects and promotes autonomy.

NURSING PRACTICE AND INFORMED CONSENT

For a long time, nurses worldwide have been concerned with the challenge of promoting patients' autonomy in the context of securing their informed consent to medical and nursing procedures. This challenge is made all the more complex because the precise role of the nurse in relation to the informed consent process is not always clear. For example, consultant doctors are often responsible for securing the informed consent of patients to various kinds of surgery or for issuing treatment instructions such as regimes of medicine or CPR/DNR (Cardiopulmonary Resuscitation/Do not Resuscitate) orders. However, while nurses do not, themselves, issue these orders, they are often the ones who are responsible for carrying them out. In addition, because of their level of contact with patients and families, they are the ones who witness the sometimes positive, sometimes negative, outcomes of decisions made.

Finally, as well as being involved in decision making for medical procedures, there are many procedures and care tasks for which nurses are directly responsible in their own right, such as wound care, taking blood, giving injections and vaccinations. Nurses are also responsible for providing patients with relevant information, offering advice, and exploring different options for treatment and care.

One well-known case, which draws attention to the tensions inherent in the role of the nurse in promoting the autonomous decision making of patients, is that of *Tuma* v. *Board of Nursing* (1979). This case, which will help us to reflect on the issues at stake, concerns a nurse, Jolene Tuma, who gave information about alternative treatments to a patient suffering from leukaemia.

Case 7.1: Informing the Patient about Alternative Treatment

In 1976, Jolene Tuma was a clinical instructor of nursing who was employed to provide nursing services while supervising students in the Twin Falls Clinic and Hospital, Idaho. Because of her interest in the special needs of dying patients, Nurse Tuma asked to be assigned to the care of a woman diagnosed with myeogenous leukaemia, Grace Wahlstrom. The patient had been informed by her doctor that her condition was terminal and that a course of chemotherapy was her best chance of survival. The doctor also informed the patient that the treatment was itself life threatening with undesirable side effects which reduced the body's defence

---

mechanisms and made the patient susceptible to infection. However, the doctor reassured her that treatment to prevent infection was also available.

While caring for her on 3 March, Nurse Tuma learned that the patient had been battling her cancer for twelve years and that she attributed her success thus far to the strength of her religious faith. Patient and nurse also discussed the side effects of chemotherapy and some non-traditional treatments for cancer, such as a diet programme and herbal medicines, which were being offered in another hospital. The patient indicated to Nurse Tuma that she would prefer to have her illness treated naturally and pleaded with the nurse to discuss some of these alternative treatments with her family that evening. Nurse Tuma agreed to do this.

When Mrs Wahlstrom told her family of the planned meeting, they contacted her doctor about the situation. Following on this, the doctor did not interfere with the arrangements. However, in the light of the patient's change of heart, he postponed the chemotherapy treatment scheduled for eight o'clock that evening.

When the nurse met with the patient and her family that evening, she told them about the prescribed treatment, its side effects and alternatives available. She also made them aware of the fact that Mrs Wahlstrom would have difficulty getting treatment, especially blood transfusions, if she left the hospital. In the light of the discussion, the patient and family decided that she should remain in hospital and continue chemotherapy. During the next two weeks, Mrs Wahlstrom did experience adverse side effects of the chemotherapy and was in a coma for much of the time. She died on 18 March 1976.

Later that month, the Board of Nursing of the State of Idaho received a complaint that Nurse Tuma had interfered with the doctor–patient relationship and that her action, in doing so, constituted unprofessional conduct. After a subsequent hearing which concluded that Nurse Tuma had acted unprofessionally, her licence was suspended by the Nursing Board and, later, by the District Court. However, these decisions were reversed when Nurse Tuma appealed to the Supreme Court of Idaho. That court concluded that there was *nothing in the statutory definition of 'unprofessional conduct'* which can be said to have adequately warned Tuma of the possibility that her licence would be suspended'. (*Tuma* v. *Board of Nursing*, [1979] 100 Idaho 74, 593 P.2d 711 n.66)

This case raises concerns about the nurse's obligations in relation to the requirement of the informed consent of Mrs Wahlstrom to her chemotherapy treatment. On this occasion, it seems that the patient did not fully understand what was involved in chemotherapy treatment, nor was she informed of any available alternatives to chemotherapy. The challenge for the nurse here is how she should respond in this situation. There are many issues at stake but we will address the following questions:

- What is required of health professionals in securing patient consent to treatment?
- How important is it that Mrs Wahlstrom be enabled to give informed consent to her treatment?
- Are there any reasons why the requirement of informed consent might not apply in this case?

- If her informed consent is required, how much information about her treatment should Mrs Wahlstrom be entitled to have?

Modes of Consent

If asked to think about consent, what might immediately spring to mind is the notion of **express** consent, consent that is made explicit, verbally or in writing. In the outline of the case concerning Grace Wahlstrom, for example, while it is unclear whether the patient signed a form or verbalised her consent, it is clear that her consent was explicit in nature.

But consent may also be **tacit** (silent or passive). Take the example of a group of nursing students who are asked to remain in class for the duration of a lecture. If, knowing what is involved in doing so, the students do not respond in any way – they neither nod nor shake their heads, they neither speak a word nor stand to leave – their informed passivity constitutes tacit consent. In such a case, a lecturer could not be blamed for assuming the ongoing cooperation of the students and continuing with the class.

Consent may also be implicit or **implied** by a person's actions. For example, a patient may hold out their arm in order that their blood pressure be taken. Or, in consenting to one procedure, such as giving blood, a patient may imply consent to another – having pressure placed on their arm in order to raise a vein from which to draw the blood, for example.

Of the three kinds of kinds of consent possible, express, tacit or implied, studies which explore the nurse's role in relation to consent generally find that patient consent to nursing care is often implied rather than expressed. Implied consent presents a particular challenge to health professionals generally because circumstances where a person implies that they consent to a procedure can easily be confused with circumstances where a person is merely complying with the request or wishes or instructions of the health professional. One study carried out in the UK by Helen Aveyard (2002), for example, points to such confusion between implied consent and compliance. The qualitative study examined the ways in which nurses obtained consent prior to nursing care procedures. To achieve this, it used six focus groups and in-depth interviews with thirty individual nurses in two UK teaching hospitals to gather information. In her analysis of the study's findings, Aveyard concluded that some nurses ignored the informational element of informed consent and that, as a result, many patients only complied with nursing procedures – followed nurses' requests – rather than actually gave informed consent. The nurses assumed that implied consent had been given for nursing care, when, in fact, the patient was merely complying with the procedure. For example, one of the study's participants, a nurse, observed:

> Some long-term patients, on heart tablets say, you assume they know what they are for . . . but then you ask them a question about it and you realize they haven't got the remotest idea what they are taking . . . they have a blind trust. Very odd. A lot of patients, you go up to them and they have been in hospital for about a week. You say to them,

Where would you like it and do you know what it's for' and they say 'I don't know what it's for, I had it stabbed in my arm yesterday and it bled a lot'. So I don't think people gain consent for every injection. (Interview 2) (Aveyard 2002: 204)

Aveyard concludes that because patient compliance can 'mimic' implied consent, nurses find it difficult to distinguish between them in practice, and she suggests an example of three different patients who present for vaccination.

Patient X holds her arm out from mere compliance, without information and possibly under duress. She is silent and the nurse misreads this act of compliance as implied consent and administers the vaccination. The patient is neither informed nor willing to have the vaccination. Meanwhile, Patient Y holds out her arm. She has had information but does not really want the vaccination.

Again she is silent and again the nurse misreads compliance for implied consent and administers the vaccination. A third patient, Z, holds out her arm. She has been well informed and actively wants the vaccination. Only patient Z can be said to have given implied consent to the vaccination, yet all three patients presented to the nurse in a similar way. (Aveyard 2002: 205)

While recognising that implied consent has a role to play in nursing care, Aveyard argues that it is essential that nurses are familiar with the meaning of implied consent, that they should consider carefully before assuming that a patient has implicitly consented to a particular nursing care procedure.

Given Aveyard's concerns in relation to implied consent and our concern to tease out the implications for Jolene Tuma in relation to the consent of Grace Wahlstrom, it is opportune to reflect on the meaning of informed consent generally.

Defining Informed Consent

Ethical and legal theorists might disagree about the precise number of elements involved or the way in which they are expressed (e.g. explicitly or implicitly), but they all agree that three elements are central to the meaning of informed consent:

1. Competence – the patient has the capacity to consent;
2. Information – the patient is informed of the nature, risks and benefits of the procedure;
3. Authorisation – the patient authorises a health professional to carry out a procedure.

The following definition of consent includes all three elements.

Informed consent takes place when a competent and informed person understands the risks and benefits at stake and authorises a health professional to treat them.

Activity

Write a brief definition of informed consent, in your own words. You can return to it later when you have completed your reading of this chapter.

Competence to Consent

Competence to consent to or refuse health-care treatment is a term used in relation to health-care decision making which reflects some of the features of autonomy that we have already explored in Chapter 1, namely, voluntariness, intentionality and deliberation. However, because the term competence, rather than the term autonomy, is often used in legal contexts to distinguish between those who are legally deemed fit to make decisions and those who are not, it is important to tease out what its specific role in health-care decision making is.

Competence is determined in both general and specific ways. Firstly, an individual might be considered competent or incompetent on the basis of their categorisation as a member of a particular group. For example, the general assumption is that all adults are competent to make decisions in relation to their medical treatment unless there is reason to think otherwise. Alternatively, from a legal point of view, children do not have decision-making power in relation to treatment until they are at least sixteen. (For a further discussion on the informed consent of children, see Chapter 8 of this text.)

Secondly, competence can be determined by referring to the specific health-care decision that is being made. In this context, competence is defined as 'the ability to perform a task' and the criteria which determine whether someone is competent or not vary according to whatever task is demanded (Beauchamp and Childress 2001: 70). Particular decision-making tasks are deemed to require particular competencies – for example, an individual may be considered competent enough to decide what to eat or how to dress, but not competent enough to decide on a course of medical treatment. In relation to health-care treatment, an individual may be deemed competent to consent to some treatments but not others. In addition, their capacity for making any given decision may fluctuate over time. Usually, the more complex the decision, or the more grave the procedure, the greater the capacity required on the part of the individual making it.

In relation to the determination of competence, Irish medical legal expert Deirdre Madden puts the following question:

> [D]oes the categorisation of an individual within a certain class or group determine his competence for all future decisions, or should the individual's competence be investigated in relation to each separate decision that may have to be made? (Madden 2002: 397)

Madden points to the danger of taking a general approach to determining competence. For example, she argues that classifying all those with chronic schizophrenia or all those with a learning disability as incompetent is likely to preclude many individuals from making decisions that they are, in fact, capable of making (Madden 2002: 397–8).

Whether in health-care situations or in criminal or civil law, **specific competence** is usually determined on the basis of an individual's ability to understand and use information and to weigh the consequences of their decision. Beauchamp and Childress define competence in the following way:

> Patients or subjects are competent to make a decision if they have the capacity to understand the material information, to make a judgment about the information in light of their values, to intend a certain outcome, and to communicate freely their wishes to care givers or investigators. (Beauchamp and Childress 2001: 71)

According to this view, a person is considered competent if they are able to understand a therapeutic procedure, can deliberate on its benefits and risks and freely decide in the light of this deliberation. This widely used standard of competence becomes a *clinical* assessment of competence when it is put into operation in empirical tests such as dementia rating scales, mental status examinations or tests for time-and-place orientation.

Outside the Mental Health Act 2001 there is no stated *legal* assessment in Ireland for determining competence (Donnelly 2002: 50). The 2001 Act, which applies to people suffering from a mental disorder, requires patient consent to treatment, provided that they have the capacity to:

- understand the nature of the treatment,
- its purpose, and
- likely effects.

While Irish courts have said little on how the competence of individuals is to be determined, one recent UK court case outlined some criteria for determining competence from a legal point of view. The *Re C* (1994) case was the first in the UK to recognise the right to refuse treatment. The case concerned a sixty-eight-year-old man who was diagnosed with paranoid schizophrenia and whose delusions included the belief that he was himself a surgeon. Nevertheless, the court decided that he was sufficiently competent to reject the treatment offered by his surgeon. The suggested treatment was intended to save the man's life and involved the amputation of a gangrenous leg. In making its decision, the court was satisfied that despite the man's mental illness and self-acknowledged delusions, he was nevertheless, competent: he

- understood the information,
- retained it and believed it,
- weighed the information, and
- made a choice in the knowledge that his decision might lead to his own death.

Donnelly advises that, in the absence of judicial discussion of criteria of competence, the test in *Re C* offers a useful reference point for health professionals working in Ireland. She argues that:

The test has advantages over the test set down in the Mental Health Act 2001 because, as well as looking at the patient's capacity to understand the proposed treatment, it also looks at the patient's capacity to believe the information and to apply it to his individual situation. It recognizes, for example, that a person suffering from a compulsive disorder such as anorexia nervosa might be entirely able to comprehend intellectually that death is the inevitable consequence of not eating, but he might not be able to accept that this information relates to his own situation. (Donnelly 2002: 51–2)

Activity

Consider Donnelly's view that the test in *Re C* is more comprehensive than the test for determining competence outlined in the Mental Health Act 2001. Briefly explain her reason for this. Do you agree that the test in *Re C* is a more useful means of considering the competence of people with anorexia nervosa? Can you think of any other illnesses where the test of *Re C* might usefully apply?

The case of *Re C* highlights a further concern in relation to the determination of competence. *Re C* refers to an individual whose life is at risk and who makes a seemingly strange decision that is at odds with the views of his surgical team. Disagreements of this kind between professionals and patients might often encourage the former to challenge the competence of the latter. However, in the case of *Re C*, the patient is deemed to be competent in spite of the disagreement about what is best for him.

The decision made by the court in this case indicates that care must be taken to distinguish between those decisions that are so bizarre as to raise concerns about a person's mental ability and those decisions that are based on reasons that others might not agree with and might even consider to be imprudent or irresponsible. In this regard, Donnelly makes the point that there is no 'inherent connection between the rationality of a patient's decision and the patient's competence' (Donnelly 2002: 47). Madden gives weight to this view by advising health professionals to make a distinction between the decision-making process and the result of the decision. Her rule of thumb is:

What is crucial is that the decision is not overridden on the basis of instinctive beliefs that no one in their right mind would have made such a decision, and that therefore the patient must be incompetent. (Madden 2002: 400)

Activity

a) Compare the case of a patient with paranoid schizophrenia with the case of a patient with anorexia nervosa. Why might the competence of the second patient be challenged but not the competence of the first?

b) In our case study, the patient, Grace Wahlstrom's committed faith and interest in alternative treatments for cancer might be considered strange by some health professionals. If Mrs Wahlstrom had decided, on the basis of her beliefs, to refuse chemotherapy indefinitely, do you think that her decision should have been overridden?

If we were to follow the arguments of Donnelly and Madden, Mrs Wahlstrom's wishes should be respected, because, however unusual or unorthodox, her views are not so bizarre as to raise questions about her competence, which is never in doubt. Indeed, in the light of what happened subsequently to Mrs Wahlstrom, it seems her concerns about chemotherapy had some merit.

Information

If an individual, such as Grace Wahlstrom in our case study, is considered competent to make decisions in relation to a possible medical treatment, and if it is accepted that they should be given information in relation to it, a further question arises. How much information should she be given? How much should an individual be told about the nature of a procedure, the risks of accepting or refusing treatment and any alternatives to the treatment? On the one hand, giving someone too little information about their treatment might seem patronising and pointless. On the other hand, giving someone too much information might prove unnecessary and counterproductive. The challenge is to establish some way of determining how much information is appropriate in any given situation.

The kind and level of information that a health professional gives to a patient will be directly influenced by the way in which they view the requirement of informed consent. If they see informed consent, primarily, as a requirement which ensures patient welfare, they are likely to discuss with a patient safety risks and side effects of a treatment. This is the approach that the doctor in our case study took in relation to Mrs Wahlstrom. On the other hand, if a health professional views informed consent as a process that protects and promotes patient autonomy, they are likely to view the provision of information in a much broader way. Indeed, they may well consider that information is more of an exchange and a dialogue than a disclosure and a monologue.

Three different standards of disclosure have emerged in health-care practice and some court decisions in various jurisdictions have added legal weight to them. These standards are the **professional standard**, the **reasonable person standard** and the **subjective standard**.

The Professional Standard or Standard Medical Practice

According to this standard, the level of information provided to a patient should accord with a practice accepted as proper by a responsible body of professional opinion. It is a level of information that a reasonably competent professional in the appropriate area of speciality would provide. This standard is often referred to as the 'Bolam test' from the case of *Bolam* v. *Friern Hospital Management Committee* (1957), which concerned the administration, without an anaesthetic, of electro-convulsive therapy (ECT) to a mentally ill patient to whom the risk of fracture was not explained. On that occasion, the court held that the doctor's non-disclosure of the risks involved in ECT was justified in the light of the patient's condition.

Reasonable Person Standard or Individual Material Risk Standard

The second standard of disclosure shifts the focus away from the views of the clinician and their profession and emphasises, instead, the perspective of the patient. This standard requires that whatever risks are considered important or material to the decision (whether or not to forego treatment) of a reasonable person should be disclosed. This is the newer and less accepted standard and was first explicitly stated in the case of *Canterbury* v. *Spence* (1972). In that case, a 19-year-old young man had suffered paralysis after undergoing surgery for a suspected ruptured disc. Justifying his nondisclosure at the trial, the doctor argued that informing the patient of a minute risk such as a 1 per cent risk of paralysis was not sound medical practice because it might deter patients from undergoing necessary medical procedures. However, the court rejected the sufficiency of the professional standard and recommended that a doctor must disclose those risks that a reasonable person would want to know about.

The Subjective Standard

While the reasonable person standard addresses the gap between what a professional might want to tell (perhaps out of concern for patient welfare) and what a patient might want to know (perhaps, in order to make an autonomous decision), a further problem is addressed by the subjective standard of disclosure. One difficulty that is inherent in the reasonable person standard is that not all persons are the same, nor is agreement easily reached as to what constitutes reasonableness. Fry and Veatch (2000: 338–9) define the subjective standard in the following way:

> [The subjective standard] requires disclosure of what a reasonable person would want to know modified by the unique needs and desires of the patient insofar as the practitioner knows them or ought to know them. This might require, for example, asking the patient if he or she has any special concerns. It might require the practitioner to add information based on his or her particular knowledge about the patient or on what the practitioner could reasonably be expected to know about the patient.

The focus of the subjective standard of disclosure is on providing information to promote and deepen understanding. It recasts the requirement of informed consent as a process that involves listening as much as telling and obliges the professional to engage with the individuality of patients rather than simply calculate what the reasonable patient might want to know. This approach focuses on asking patients questions to find out how much information they already have, how much information they might want to have and what their unique concerns are.

One example where the subjective standard might be used regularly is in midwifery. Heather Draper gives her understanding of special relationships that can develop between midwife and pregnant women when there has been continuity in care and preparation for birth over many months of pregnancy.

> The process of gaining consent prior to labour should be a process of counselling and an exchange of information, rather than a contract. The aim should be to facilitate discussion of what can reasonably be expected to happen under a variety of circumstances. This process of understanding and negotiation should be, and probably is, the norm in modern midwifery practice . . . It is not uncommon in midwifery for women to make birth plans prior to their confinements, in effect consenting or refusing consent, in writing, prior to the [birth] event. (Draper 1996: 27; see also Lewison 1996)

The birth plan is similar to an 'advance directive' that is, however, subject to change in conditions stipulated (e.g. whether an epidural is requested) before birth if the woman should decide. Where there is continuity of care between midwife and the pregnant woman, the consent process is very much ongoing, conversational and informing over many months for the midwife and pregnant woman.

The Situation in Ireland in Relation to Disclosure

Whatever happens in practice in Ireland, in this country there is no accepted legal definition of what constitutes appropriate explanation in relation to medical procedures. Generally the professional standard prevails. However, the Supreme Court argued in the case of *Walsh* v. *Family Planning Services Ltd.* (1992), which concerned the disclosure of risks in relation to surgery for a vasectomy, that the more elective the treatment, the greater the duty to disclose *all* material risks (all risks of grave consequences no matter how remote). Also, Justice Kearns, in a recent High Court case, *Geoghegan* v. *Harris* (2000), which concerned the disclosure of risks in relation to dental implant surgery, concluded in favour of the reasonable person standard. In that case, Justice Kearns observed:

> This Court is of the view that the 'reasonable patient' test, which requires full disclosure of all material risks incident to proposed treatment, is the preferable test to adopt, so that the patient, thus informed, rather than the doctor, makes the real choice as to whether treatment is to be carried out. (*Geoghegan* v. *Harris* 2000: 162)

Activity

In the case of Grace Wahlstrom, Jolene Tuma has to draw upon some standard of disclosure in order to decide on what kind of information she should give the patient about her treatment options. Take each of the three standards of disclosure and apply it to the situation.

a) Is Jolene Tuma obliged to discuss alternative treatments with Grace Wahlstrom under the professional standard? Would any similarly qualified nurse do so?

b) What is the nurse's duty under the reasonable person standard? Do 'reasonable' people want information about herbal remedies and natural cures?

c) What might the subjective standard demand of the nurse in this case? Would Nurse Tuma be obliged to respond to the patient's questioning about alternatives to treatment?

d) Consider the terms we have used above in relation to information provision: *exchange and dialogue* and *disclosure and monologue*. Write a list of characteristics that you associate with each of these sets of terms. Which set of terms do you think characterises the approaches of the doctor and the nurse in relation to Grace Wahlstrom?

e) It might be suggested that the problem in this case is not so much *what* information Jolene Tuma gave Grace Wahlstrom and her family but the fact that she did not involve the doctor in the process. Do you think that the conflict that arose in this case might have been avoided if the respective roles of the nurse and doctor in relation to patient care were made clearer at the outset? What approach would you take if you were Jolene Tuma?

Authorisation

One final condition of a valid consent in our view is that of authorisation. Following on the work of Beauchamp and Childress (2001) and Faden and Beauchamp (1986), we would argue that, ideally, the competent and informed patient *authorises* the professional to provide treatment or care. This view starts from the premise that the patient is the most authoritative decision maker in the situation and participates in decisions and/or directs their treatment (Madden 2002: 412–3). Beauchamp and Childress posit the notion of *autonomous authorisation* as one way of understanding consent:

> In the first sense, a person must do more than express agreement or comply with a proposal. He or she must authorize something through an act of informed and voluntary consent. (Beauchamp and Childress 2001: 78)

The authors distinguish this sense of consent from what they describe as *effective consent*:

> In the second sense, informed consent is analysable in terms of the social rules of consent in institutions that must obtain legally or

institutionally valid consent from patients or subjects before proceeding with diagnostic, therapeutic, or research procedures. Informed consents are not necessarily autonomous acts under these rules and sometimes are not even meaningful authorizations. (Beauchamp and Childress 2001: 78)

On this second understanding of giving consent, which is probably closer to what actually happens in practice, all that is required is that a person expresses consent within the terms of an institution's rules or guidelines.

Activity

a) Think of an example of consent that is autonomous but not effective.

b) Think of an example of consent that is effective but not autonomous.

Consent of Minors

The example that Beauchamp and Childress give to illustrate the differences between the two senses of consent is that of the mature minor who is not legally authorised to give consent under existing rules, but who may, nevertheless, be able to authorise a treatment or procedure autonomously. In such a situation, the minor can give *autonomous*, but not *effective*, authorisation to the treatment.

Generally, children are not considered legally competent to make decisions about their health care. Irish law vests decision-making power in the case of minors (under eighteen) in parents or guardians. Such power must be exercised in the context of the children's constitutional rights. However, in relation to health-care decisions, the Non-Fatal Offences against the Person Act 1997 states that a person over sixteen years can effectively consent to surgical, dental or medical treatment.

The Act is, unfortunately, unclear on whether or not what has become known as **Gillick competence** applies to some decisions that under sixteen-year-olds might be seen to be capable of making. This term refers to the UK case of *Gillick* v. *West Norfolk and Wisbech AHA* (1985/6) where chronological age was found not to be a sufficient indicator of 'maturity' to judge competence for consent to medical treatment. In making his decision in the Gillick case, Lord Scarman of the House of Lords argued that 'the parental rights yield to the child's right to make his own decision when he reaches sufficient understanding and intelligence to be capable of making up his own mind on the matter requiring decision.' (1986 AC 112 at 186. See also Chapter 9 for further discussion of the Gillick case).

Activity

a) What is your response to the claim that the maturity of children is more significant for consent to medical treatment than their chronological age?

b) Would you agree with Lord Scarman that parental rights should yield to children's rights in some instances?

c) Can you name any kinds of medical treatment that under sixteen-year-olds avail of today without the knowledge or consent of their parents?

Summary Learning Guide 7.2

The mode of securing informed consent can be:

- Explicit – consent is expressed verbally or in written form;
- Implicit – consent is informed, voluntary and intended but it is indicated by behaviour or gesture;
- Tacit – consent is informed, voluntary and intended but it is not indicated by either word or gesture.

The three elements of informed consent are:

Competence to consent
- Is generally viewed as the capacity to make a decision. A person is considered competent if they are able to understand a therapeutic procedure, can deliberate on its benefits and risks and freely decide in the light of this deliberation;
- Can be considered, from a legal point of view, in the light of the Mental Health Act 2001 and the UK *Re C* test.

Information
- Is disclosed according to three standards:

  professional standard – focuses on the health professional;
  reasonable person standard – focuses on the generalised 'reasonable' patient;
  subjective standard – focuses on the individual patient.

Authorisation
- Underlines the fact that it is the patient (not the nurse or doctor) who authorises procedures or care.

EXCEPTIONS TO CONSENT

Exceptions to the requirement of informed consent may be defended on grounds of emergency, incompetence, patient waiver and therapeutic privilege.

Emergency

In emergency life-threatening situations, when a patient is unable to consent or to appreciate what is needed and when it cannot be established whether an **advance directive** exists should such a situation arise, a health professional may provide treatment without consent (see below for more on advance directives). For example, the treatment, without their consent, of an unconscious patient following an accident is generally considered warranted.

Incompetence

In cases of doubt, health professionals and courts of law decide who is above or below the threshold of competence. When a person is deemed to be incompetent because they are very ill, confused or demented, young or mentally impaired, others make decisions on their behalf. A health professional may, themselves, override the person's decisions, they may ask informal surrogates to decide, or they may seek involuntary institutionalisation of the incompetent person.

In Ireland, an individual may also be designated a ward of court. In such a case, the President of the High Court or Circuit Court is considered the person's legal guardian. That court appoints a wardship committee to secure the welfare of the ward, though for serious treatment such as sterilisation or the withdrawal of hydration and nutrition, it is likely that the committee would refer back to the court for decision making (Madden 2002: 401–9). Courts usually give consent to or refuse medical treatment on behalf of an incompetent individual, using criteria such as **substituted judgement,** advance directives and the **best interests test**. Briefly, a substituted judgement is usually informed by a person or persons who know(s) the patient and understand(s) their beliefs and values. On the basis of that understanding, a decision is made to accept or refuse treatment in a way that is consistent with what the patient would decide if they were competent.

An advance directive (e.g. a living will) is a document that enables a competent person to make decisions about his or her medical treatment in the event that they become incompetent and, therefore, lose the capacity to make decisions.

Finally, appealing to a patient's best interests involves making a decision to accept or refuse treatment on the basis of whether or not the predicted outcomes will most likely promote the patient's wellbeing. (See also Chapter 13 of this text for a further discussion of the process of decision making for incompetent patients in relation to the *Ward of Court* case 1995.)

Waiver

In some circumstances, an individual might waive their right to information about their condition, diagnosis or prognosis. In such a situation, health professionals are obliged to respect the wishes of the patient and withhold the relevant information. This is often called 'paternalism with permission', where the patient effectively permits a health professional to act paternalistically on their behalf.

Therapeutic Privilege

A more controversial exception to the requirement of informed consent than the three we have just outlined – necessity, incompetence and waiver – is that of therapeutic privilege. A health professional might appeal to *therapeutic privilege* and withhold information from a patient on the grounds that it might psychologically harm them – in other words, concern for patient welfare seems to demand not giving them information about their diagnosis, prognosis or treatment options. The 'harm' envisaged here involves serious psychological harm – it does not refer to the fact that a patient might be temporarily upset on hearing the information or might refuse treatment as a result.

Summary Learning Guide 7.3

Justified exceptions to the requirement of informed consent include:

Emergency: In emergency life-threatening situations, when a patient is unable to consent or to appreciate what is needed and when it cannot be established what they would want if they were able to consent.

Incompetence: When a person is deemed to be incompetent because they are very ill, confused or demented, young or mentally impaired, others such as health professionals, surrogates or courts make decisions on their behalf. They usually decide by appealing to criteria such as substituted judgement, advance directives and the best interests test.

Waiver: In some circumstances, an individual might waive their right to information about their condition, diagnosis or prognosis.

Therapeutic Privilege: A health professional might appeal to therapeutic privilege and withhold information from a patient on the grounds that it might psychologically harm them.

Conclusion

The case of Jolene Tuma, examined in this chapter, draws attention to the challenges facing nurses in relation to protecting and promoting the autonomy of individuals who are patients under nursing and medical care.

The case highlights the meaning and significance of informed consent and indicates those exceptional circumstances where it might not be required. A central issue in that case also is Jolene Tuma's concern at the level of information with which the patient, Grace Wahlstrom, has been provided by her doctor. The fact that Nurse Tuma's attempts to address Mrs Wahlstrom's unique concerns almost cost her her job indicates the professional tensions that can exist in such situations and the price that some nurses have had to pay in the course of fulfilling what they see as their professional obligations.

What the case illustrates is that informed consent is a process of understanding which is not measured simply or solely in terms of indicators such as a 'yes', a nod of the head, a proffered arm or a patient's signature. Instead, the challenge of ensuring that a patient authorises a procedure is one that demands ethical understanding as well as communication skills and imagination.

With this understanding of the principle of informed consent and the challenges it presents to nurses caring for patients, we turn, in Chapter 8, to the additional challenges that the requirement of informed consent poses to nurses who undertake research that involves human participants.

The following terms are explained in the glossary:

advance directive

best interest standard

competence

Gillick competence

informed consent

professional standard

reasonable person standard

subjective standard

substituted judgement

therapeutic privilege

waiver

– 8 –

Informed Consent in Research

Objectives

At the end of this chapter, you should be able to:

- Discuss a research study drawn from recent history which failed to meet international ethical standards for the protection of research participants;
- Distinguish between therapeutic and non-therapeutic research;
- Discuss some of the challenges that research with children presents to nurses.

INTRODUCTION

Scientific research in health care is a form of inquiry that uses a variety of systematic approaches to pose and answer questions and provide and test solutions to problems that arise in relation to human health and illness. Where this research involves human participation, experimental and non-experimental tools of investigation are deployed, such as randomised control trials, observational instruments, surveys, and face-to-face interviews, and the research is carried out in diverse settings such as laboratories, hospitals and communities.

While it is generally acknowledged that research involving human beings is profoundly important to enhance understanding of human living and dying, it is also accepted that there is a limit to what researchers can be allowed to do; while history gives testimony to tens of thousands of research success stories that have impacted in small and large ways on human wellbeing, it also bears witness to darker tales where confusion, greed, carelessness, ignorance and malice on the part of researchers and research institutions have led to exploitation, injury and death.

Concern to prevent harm and to protect the human rights of research participants has led to the almost universal adoption in law and professional regulation of fundamental ethical principles such as beneficence, respect for human dignity and justice. Documents such as the *Nuremberg Code* (1949), the *Helsinki Declaration* (1964/2000) and the *Belmont Report* (1979) stipulate rules, based on these principles, that researchers are expected to follow. These rules relate, for example, to: participant voluntariness, self-determination, informed consent, confidentiality, anonymity, privacy and the right to fair treatment. While each of these rules is profoundly important and the subject of intense debate among researchers and ethicists, chief among them is the requirement of the informed consent of individuals to participate in research. This requirement is the focus of discussion in this chapter.

IN THE NAME OF RESEARCH

The international codes that emerged in the second half of the twentieth century, such as the *Nuremberg Code* and the *Helsinki Declaration* were, in part, a response to universal revulsion at the research experiments carried out by Nazi doctors and nurses in the concentration camps of the Second World War, but they also reflect a general concern with scientific research practices on human beings worldwide (Pellegrino 1997). Unfortunately, the Nazis were not alone in disregarding and ignoring the rights and welfare of participants in health-related research. In the twentieth century, there were many cases in different countries where research participants were exploited or mistreated, or where their consent to participate in the research was neither sought nor adequately gained.

One such example is that of a Cervical Cancer Study (1966–7) in New Zealand, which left women, diagnosed with cervical cancer in the National Women's Hospital, Auckland, untreated. This research was carried out without informing the participants, some of whom lost their lives, in order that the natural progress of their disease might be observed (Coney 1988).

In Ireland also, questions have recently been raised in relation to vaccine trials that were carried out in the 1960s and 1970s. These trials involved a number of children in residential care, and a recent Department of Health report (2000) was undecided as to whether or not consent to the trials was given in relation to these children (Donnelly 2002: 8).

Another example of research gone awry is the Tuskegee Syphilis Study (1933–72), carried out by US Public Health Service physicians in Macon County, Alabama. The randomised control trial involved 399 rural African American men who had syphilis and 201 who did not. In the 40-year period of the study, the purpose of which was to observe the progress of the disease, the men with syphilis – largely poor and illiterate sharecroppers – were not informed of the nature of their condition; in fact, they were deceived into thinking that they were being treated for 'bad blood'. Even when penicillin was identified in 1943 as an effective drug for syphilis, the public service did not administer the drug to the men unless they asked for it. By the time the study was discontinued in 1972, 128 men had died of syphilis or related complications, at least 40 women who were married to these men had been infected, and 19 children had contracted the disease at birth (Heller 1972; Jones 1993; Tuskegee Syphilis Study Legacy Committee 1996; Brandt 1978).

An interesting aspect of the project, from a nursing point of view, is the controversial role played by the African American, Eunice Rivers, who, as public health nurse, acted as a liaison between the black men who were being studied and the white doctors in the public health service who were leading the study. In her role, Rivers ferried the men to and from the clinic in which they were 'treated', gave them aspirin and hot meals, and encouraged those who were considering withdrawing from the study to keep attending. In a 1953 Public Health Report by Rivers and other investigators, Rivers' role was explained in the following way:

> Between surveys, contact with the patients was maintained through the local county health department and an especially assigned public health nurse, whose chief duties were those of followup worker on this project. The nurse also participated in a generalized public health nursing program, which gave her broad contact with the families of the patients and demonstrated that she was interested in other aspects of their welfare as well as in the project. The nurse was a native of the county, who had lived near her patients all her life, and was thoroughly familiar with their local ideas and customs. [. . .]
>
> It is very important for the followup worker to understand both patient and doctor, because she must bridge the gap between the two. The doctors were concerned primarily with obtaining the most efficient and thorough medical examination possible for the group of 600 men. While they tried to give each patient the personal interest he deserved, this was not always possible due to the pressure of time. Occasionally the patient was annoyed because the doctor did not pay attention to his particular complaint. He may have believed that his favorite home remedy was more potent than the doctor's prescription, and decided to let the whole thing go. It then became the task of the nurse to convince him that the examinations were beneficial. If she failed, she might find that in the future he not only neglected to answer her letters but managed to be away from home whenever she called.
>
> Sometimes the doctor grumbled because of the seemingly poor cooperation and slowness of some of the patients; often the nurse helped in these situations simply by bridging the language barrier and by explaining to the men what the doctor wanted. Sometimes the nurse assisted the physician by warning him beforehand about the eccentricities of the patients he was scheduled to see during the day. For example, there was the lethargic patient with early cancer of the lip who needed strong language and grim predictions to persuade him to seek medical attention. (Rivers, Schuman, Simpson and Olansky 1953: 391–5)

In the same report, it was observed about Rivers that '[a]mong her deepest convictions [was] the belief that rural areas desperately need[ed] good and sympathetic nurses to participate in and carry out effectively public health programs as well as private medical care' (Rivers, Schuman, Simpson and Olansky 1953: 393).

While Rivers' actions in relation to the study were well intended, commentators, since, have pondered how a nurse who was so clearly committed to the people in her community could have continued to participate in the study, and Rivers has been cast as a subservient figure who was simply obeying authority because of her status as a woman, African-American and nurse (Jones 1993). Other writers, such as Smith (1996) have challenged the stereotyping of Rivers as either victim or villain and have attempted, instead, to take a more context-sensitive view of her involvement in the research.

Activity

a) Reflect on the extract from Eunice Rivers' Report describing her conduct in the Tuskegee Study. Can you identify any actions on her part that might raise ethical concerns?

b) Consider the multiple roles of Eunice Rivers: public health nurse, researcher, 'bridge' between doctor and patient/subject. Can you think of a situation in your professional life where you had to reconcile the demands of multiple roles?

c) The story of Eunice Rivers inspired the film *Miss Ever's Boys* (1997) directed by Joseph Sargent and starring Alfred Woodard and Lawrence Fishburne. Watch the film and critically evaluate its treatment of the central character.

REGULATIONS GOVERNING CONSENT TO RESEARCH

As we indicated at the outset, the informed consent of human participants in health-related research studies is stipulated by such international codes as the *Nuremberg Code* (1949), the *Belmont Report* (1979), the *Council of Europe Convention on Human Rights and Biomedicine* (1996) and the World Medical Association *Declaration of Helsinki* (1964/2000). All of these codes prioritise the interests of the research participant over the interests of research and they stipulate the requirement of informed consent as a mechanism for ensuring that the rights of the research participant are protected. For example, Principle 22 of the Declaration of Helsinki insists that:

> In any research on human beings, each potential subject must be adequately informed of the aims, methods, sources of funding, any possible conflicts of interest, institutional affiliations of the researcher, the anticipated benefits and potential risks of the study and the discomfort it may entail. The subject should be informed of the right to abstain from participation in the study or to withdraw consent to participate at any time without reprisal. After ensuring that the subject has understood the information, the physician should then obtain the subject's freely-given informed consent, preferably in writing. If the consent cannot be obtained in writing, the non-written consent must be formally documented and witnessed.

In Ireland, the law does not address research studies generally. However, the Control of Clinical Trials Act 1987/1990 stipulates that every clinical trial must be approved by the Minister for Health and an ethics committee and it prescribes the composition of ethics committees, nationally and regionally. The Act also obliges the clinical researcher to adhere to the *reasonable person standard* of disclosure, declaring that it 'unequivocally adopts the standard of disclosure of all material circumstances' (1987 Section 9 General Note (a); See also, Chapter 7 in this text, for an explanation of the reasonable person standard).

In addition, the recent passing of the Clinical Trials Directive 2001/20/EC, promulgated by the European Parliament in May 2001, stipulates that the laws, regulations and administrative provisions of the EU Member States, relating to the implementation of good clinical practice in the conduct of clinical trials, are standardised across Europe. Ireland, like other European states, will have to bring its national laws in line with the provisions of the Directive and these are far more stringent and protective of the rights of research participants than existing laws.

In 2004, the Irish Council for Bioethics, located at the Royal Irish Academy in Dublin, published *Operational Procedures for Research Ethics Committees: Guidance 2004.* This set of guidelines takes cognisance of international best practice (ICB, 2004). Guidelines protecting research participants have also been adopted in the codes of a range of health-care organisations, including nursing and midwifery bodies such as the International Council of Nurses (*Ethical Guidelines for Nursing Research* 2003), Canadian Nurses Association (*Ethical Research Guidelines for Registered Nurses* 2002) and the Irish Nursing Board, An Bord Altranais. Specific guidelines for research with human participants are due for publication by An Bord Altranais in 2004 but the existing *Code of Professional Conduct for Nurses and Midwives* (2000) offers the following caution:

> In taking part in research, the principles of confidentiality and the provision of appropriate information to enable an informed judgement to be made by the patient, must be safeguarded. The nurse has an obligation to ascertain that the research is sanctioned by the appropriate body and to ensure that the rights of the patient are protected at all times. The nurse should be aware of ethical policies and procedures in his/her area of practice.

What is common to all of these regulations and codes is the recommendation that participants in a research study give their express consent (where possible) to their participation. (See Chapter 7 for an explanation of the different forms of consent.) Provision for such consent is often spelled out in a consent form. The presentation and detail of the form may vary but it generally includes clear and substantial information about the nature and scope of the proposed research and its risks and benefits to the participant. Also, the form usually guarantees just treatment, participant confidentiality and the option of withdrawing from the research without penalty. In signing a consent form, an individual indicates that they have read and understood the information provided in the form and that they freely agree to participate in the proposed research study.

THERAPEUTIC AND NON-THERAPEUTIC RESEARCH

An important consideration in the ethical evaluation of a proposed research study is the intention of the research itself. Research which is primarily

---

Summary Learning Guide 8.1

The informed consent in relation to research is regulated by:

International Codes such as
- Nuremberg Code (1949)
- Belmont Report (1979)
- Council of Europe Convention on Human Rights and Biomedicine (1996)
- Helsinki Declaration (1964/2000)

Irish Law
- Control of Clinical Trials Act (1987/1990)

Irish Guidelines
- Irish Council of Bioethics: Guidance 2004

European Law
- European Clinical Trials Directive (2001/20/EC)

Nursing and Midwifery Guidelines such as:
- *Ethical Guidelines for Nursing Research,* International Council of Nurses 2003
- *Ethical Research Guidelines for Registered Nurses,* Canadian Nurses Association 2002.

---

intended to help an individual patient or particular group is considered *therapeutic research* – for example, a study that tries an experimental drug on a patient for their benefit.

On the other hand, the primary aim of *non-therapeutic* research is to produce generalisable knowledge about a particular illness or intervention, not to benefit specific individuals – for example, the Tuskegee study aimed to add to knowledge about syphilis, not to benefit the men who participated in it.

Ethical concern in relation to therapeutic research focuses on questions of justice – on fair access to the research and to the benefits that might follow on participation. In cases of non-therapeutic research, the ethical focus is on the burdens and risk that the research might present to participants; the greater the risk, the greater the need to justify the research.

With few exceptions, the informed consent of participants is an ethical and legal requirement of both therapeutic and non-therapeutic research.

Activity

a) Can you think of any examples where an exception to the requirement of informed consent might be made in relation to therapeutic research?

b) One exception to informed consent in relation to therapeutic research might be where experimental treatment is carried out in emergency settings where the patient is unconscious or traumatised and there is no suitable surrogate to provide informed consent on their behalf. Would you agree that these kinds of circumstances are, justifiably, exceptional? List possible justifications for going ahead with the treatment and list objections to it.

c) Another exception to informed consent in relation to therapeutic research might be where experimental treatment is carried out on newborn babies with disabilities whose parents are so distraught that they are unable to comprehend the proposed procedures. Would you agree that these kinds of circumstances are, justifiably, exceptional? List possible justifications for going ahead with the treatment and list objections to it.

Summary Learning Guide 8.2

Therapeutic Research

is primarily intended to help an individual patient or particular group. Ethical concern in relation to therapeutic research focuses on questions of justice – that is, on fair access to the research and to the benefits that might follow on participation.

Non-therapeutic Research

is primarily intended to produce generalisable knowledge about a particular illness or intervention, not to benefit specific individuals. The ethical focus in relation to non-therapeutic research is on the burdens and risk that the research might present to participants; the greater the risk, the greater the need to justify the research.

With few exceptions, the informed consent of participants is an ethical and legal requirement of both therapeutic and non-therapeutic research.

NURSING RESEARCH

As we have seen from even a cursory glance at the history of health-related research, nurses who undertake research which involves human beings are faced with important challenges and, often, conflicting obligations. These challenges will increasingly arise as nurses not only participate in multidisciplinary health research initiatives, but also as nurses undertake, specifically, nursing research – that is, research that is related to nursing procedures and care.

Nursing research is a relatively new form of inquiry, driven, in part, by the shift in nursing education from training schools in hospitals to third-level institutions, and, in part, by the general recognition that best nursing practice is based on sound evidence as well as experience. With the advent of graduate, postgraduate and postdoctoral paths of scholarship in nursing knowledge and practice, there has been an accompanying drive to support that scholarship and practice with evidence drawn from empirical studies. The result is the development of a new discipline in nursing – nursing research, which uses the range of scientific research approaches and methodologies in order to expand nursing knowledge and enhance the effectiveness of nursing and midwifery interventions.

Nursing research may involve different kinds of participants – for example, individuals from the general population who are surveyed on their attitudes to health-promotion initiatives; nurses who are interviewed about their understanding of ethical issues; patients who are tested pre and post a particular exercise programme. While all research participants deserve protection and respect, however, there can sometimes be an ethical tension for the nurse who is, simultaneously, both nurse and researcher (this was the case for the public health nurse in the Tuskegee Study). On the one hand, the aim of nursing practice is to promote the health and wellbeing of individual patients. On the other hand, the aim of nursing and health research is to advance knowledge in order to improve treatment and care outcomes for everyone. This tension can be expressed in the following way:

> As [carer], the [nurse's] primary obligation is . . . her patient's welfare. Based on the best available knowledge and . . . her personal skills, the [nurse] has got to choose the most effective [care] that best promotes the patient's well-being and minimises the risk of harm for the patient. As researcher, the [nurse] is obligated to perform methodologically sound investigations to advance the body of generalisable and validated knowledge in the different domains of . . . health care. Knowledge about the efficacy and safety of new health care regimes, however, can only be advanced by conducting studies with human subjects. . . . Unlike [nursing] practice, which aims at helping individual patients, scientific research can disregard the individuality of each patient in order to gain generalisable knowledge about different classes of patients. (Boomgaarden, Louhiala and Wiesing 2003: 12–13)

Activity

If you were a nurse caring for a patient and you were also a member of a research team who was seeking the informed consent of that patient to participate in a research study, how might you determine that the patient/participant was genuinely free to give or refuse consent?

Research with Children

Research with vulnerable populations such as those who are socially or economically marginalised, disabled or gravely ill, institutionalised or imprisoned, very young or very old, must be undertaken with particular sensitivity and caution, because these groups are more open to being patronised, misunderstood, manipulated and exploited than others.

While nurse researchers might be on their guard in relation to the rights of vulnerable participants in experimental research involving some kind of clinical intervention, they also need to exercise care in relation to non-experimental research activities involving, for example, face-to-face interviews. While the wellbeing and dignity of the research participant is not as obviously at risk in non-experimental research as it is in experimental research, serious ethical concerns can, nevertheless, arise, especially in relation to informed consent.

The following case illustrates the ethical challenges that a nurse researcher must address in relation to research that involves interviews with children. It is drawn from the field notes of a doctoral study exploring children's and parents' perspectives on food and eating in the management of cystic fibrosis.

Case 8.1: The Reluctant Interviewee

When the nurse researcher, Eileen Savage, arrived at the home of seven-year-old Tadhg Murphy at the agreed time of two o'clock one afternoon, the boy's mother immediately invited her into the living room and called for Tadhg to come downstairs. As he came into the room, Tadhg appeared fretful and said that he had changed his mind about being in the project; he was 'too busy'.

The researcher attempted to reassure the child that he did not have to take part if he did not want to and she asked him about his planned activities, which included football, racing with his friends and watching TV, especially his favourite programme, *Buzz Lightyear*. (Inwardly Eileen worried as to what would happen if every child from thereon decided not to participate.)

Eileen confided that she had not seen *Buzz Lightyear* in a while because she herself had been occupied with her project. Tadhg grew very interested when she told him that her interviews with children would be taped to ensure that she remembered everything they said. This prompted her to take the tape recorder from her bag and show it to Tadhg who was keen to know how it worked. 'Wow, this is cool,' he exclaimed and told Eileen that he had changed his mind again and that now he wanted to talk to her about having cystic fibrosis. He stipulated, however, that they would have to stop the interview at four o'clock so that he could watch his programme. (Savage 2003a)

At the beginning of her visit, the researcher is caught in a dilemma between respecting Tadhg's expressed desire not to participate in the interview and her research goal which she believes would ultimately benefit children just like Tadhg. On the one hand, Tadhg and his parents have agreed to participate in the research. On the other hand, Tadhg has now explicitly refused to participate. The researcher in this case must consider:

- The ethical and legal regulations in relation to research with children;
- The ethical obligations on the part of researchers to respect and promote the autonomy of children in relation to their participation in research.

Regulations Governing Research with Children

As explained in Chapter 7, children in most western countries who are under eighteen (sometimes sixteen) years of age are considered minors and cannot generally give effective (legal) consent in relation to serious health-care decisions. However, even if they cannot legally consent, children's agreement to health-care procedures is generally sought as it is viewed as an ethical (if not a strictly legal) requirement. To this end, the United Nations Convention of the Rights of the Child, requires that:

> the child who is capable of forming his or her own views [be accorded] the right to express those views freely in all matters affecting the child, the views of the child being given due weight in accordance with the age and maturity of the child. (cited in Madden 2002: 473)

Similarly, children under eighteen years of age cannot generally give effective (legal) consent to participate in research studies, but, nevertheless, their consent is considered an ethical requirement. In relation to the involvement of children in research, the UK Royal College of Paediatrics, for example, argues that even when it is not legally required, the agreement of school-age children to participate in research should be obtained, and that researchers should always ensure that the child participant does not object to his or her participation (Royal College of Paediatrics 2000: 177–82).

Activity

a) From what you have read so far of Savage's field notes, would you describe it as therapeutic or non-therapeutic?

b) At the outset of Case 8.1, the research participant, Tadhg, clearly indicated his refusal to take part in the project. How would you ethically evaluate Savage's response to Tadhg's refusal?

Promoting the Autonomous Capacity of Children

Prior to the interview described in Case 8.1, Savage instigated a number of different measures in her efforts to respect and promote the autonomous choice of the children who participated in her research study. For example, in preparing both parents and children to participate in the research process, she designed information leaflets on her research that were specifically directed toward each group and sent to them in advance of seeking their consent. On meeting with children, Savage read the leaflets with them in a question and answer format in order to determine what children had gleaned from the leaflets in terms of their involvement. Further, parents were invited to sign consent forms, but consent forms were also provided for the children to sign. Savage comments on this process:

> Although children agreed to take part in the interview, I was cautious about making assumptions that they would be willing to talk openly about any topic that arose or that they would take the initiative to advise me of their preference not to talk about a sensitive topic. Therefore, I was mindful of cues that indicated their ease or discomfort in talking about issues that arose. (Savage 2003b: 76)

During the interviews, children were occasionally asked how they were finding them. In concluding her account of interviews, Savage commented that 'Consent was seen as an ongoing process and so I remained ethically sensitive to children . . . during the interviews to assess their willingness to stay involved in the study' (Savage 2003b: 98). Raising the issue of voluntarism – whether children felt free to participate or not – Savage suggested that she was concerned that children might agree to participate because their parents insisted that they do so. In reflecting on her experience, however, she concluded:

> [T]here were no indications from children that their parents made them take part in the study . . . They advised me that the decision to take part in the study was theirs and not their parents'. Some parents commented that their children responded favourably to the study information leaflets designed for them because they saw it as an acknowledgement of their views being as important as their parents'. The refusal of some children to take part in the study contrary to their parents' wishes was an indication of how children felt free to choose for themselves. (Savage 2003b: 98)

Activity

Make a list of the key consent elements in Savage's approach to research involving children.

You might have suggested some of the following:

1. The intent to promote the autonomy of children in relation to research agendas that affect them;
2. The belief that children are capable of giving their own consent to participate in research;
3. The design of information leaflets aimed directly at children;
4. The question and answer session which helped children to understand what the research was about;
5. The implicit acknowledgement in sharing information with children that *their* understanding of and views in relation to the research process was important to the researcher;
6. The consent form designed specifically for, and signed by, the children themselves;
7. The determination to ensure that informed consent was ongoing by asking direct questions about participation during the interview;
8. The recognition that children had the right to refuse to participate in the study even if their parents consented on their behalf.

Activity

Savage seems to have identified some very significant features of a research process that takes into account the importance of respecting and enhancing children's autonomy. Can you think of any other elements that would characterise best practice in relation to this issue?

CONCLUSION

This chapter has explained the different ways in which the requirement of informed consent protects and promotes the rights of research participants. We highlighted the controversial role of a public health nurse in one non-therapeutic research study and we explored some of the challenges that nurses are faced with in undertaking research involving children. In exploring Case 8.1, regulations governing the participation of adults and children in research are referred to but we also focused on the deeper ethical meaning of informed consent that emerged in the course of the researcher's subtle negotiations with the research participant, Tadhg. As the researcher in this case indicated, children's capacity to participate *autonomously* in research can be enhanced by taking a number of steps such as involving them directly in the process and genuinely respecting their right to refuse.

The evolution in understanding what is required in order that individuals participate fully and freely in health-care decision making or research has been won at the cost of the health and lives of, perhaps, many tens of thousands of people. It is ironic that health professionals who are, for the most part, wholly committed to the wellbeing of their patients, have so often ignored, abused or plain misunderstood the interests of the people in their care. As a response to mistakes or misconduct, there is little doubt that the principle of informed consent will challenge nurses involved in multi-disciplinary and nursing research to reflect critically on their activities and make greater efforts to protect and empower those who have placed their trust in them.

Section Two:
Living and Dying

Section Two focuses on the spectrum of ethical questions about living, suffering and dying. Chapters 9 through 12 concentrate on moral challenges in reproductive ethics. In Chapters 9 and 10, the lens is on the ethical questions of abortion.

Abortion has a long and complex history in Ireland, beginning with the prohibition of elective abortions under the Offences against the Person Act of 1861, continuing to the present time. Many nurses coming into third-level studies in Ireland are too young to have experienced the public debates over the past twenty-five years. Moral questions are delineated: nurse conflicts in assisting abortion; how to adjudicate the rights of women, the rights of the unborn; and the responsibilities of government in the sensitive issue of abortion.

While Irish law prohibits elective abortion, thousands of Irish women annually choose to leave the country to have abortions. The diverse narratives of women about their abortion experiences are presented, and the positions on the moral status of the embryo are explained and evaluated. In Chapter 10, the question of liberty of conscience in reproduction is introduced. The socio-political question is raised about whether the Irish State has an obligation to provide policies or laws to give citizens freedom of choice in reproduction.

Chapters 11 and 12 extend the discussion of procreative autonomy by examining the ethical implications in developments of Assisted Human Reproduction. The desire to have children of a specific sex is the focus of Chapter 11. New technology defines new moral issues both in reproduction and in end stages of living. The technology of sex-selection methods is explained. Sperm sorting, in particular, is discussed as one relatively effective method of achieving an offspring of a particular sex. Moral positions on sex selection are detailed, sharpening the question of whether the extension of parental autonomy to sex selection can be ethically justified. Justification brings to light a full discussion of sources of harm to human life that might follow on parental autonomy.

Chapter 12 continues the theme of procreative autonomy in the discussion of surrogacy, a practice that, in fact, has an ancient history, traceable to an Old Testament story of Abram. Surrogacy raises moral, legal and social challenges, with the splintering of 'mothering': genetic mother, gestation mother and nurturing mother. Chapter 12 sharpens the questions of whether moral limits on reproductive choice are warranted.

Chapters 13 and 14 move from the beginnings of human life to the ends of human living: chronic illness and dying. Medical technology offers increasing opportunities to prolong life. But this reality brings in sharp relief the ethical questions about one's moral obligations to prolong human life. Moral arguments for withholding and withdrawing life-support systems are explored in two cases: of a competent patient who chooses not to continue living and a patient who suffers from a permanent vegetative state (PVS). Special focus is given to several mechanisms for decision making when a patient cannot voice their preferences about living or dying.

Abortion and Moral Space

Objectives

At the end of this chapter, you should be able to:

- Explore the meaning of conscience as an internal sanction;
- Evaluate the various options of participation that a nurse might have in assisting with abortion;
- Explain the view claiming that the moral status of the unborn is 'indeterminate';
- Discuss and assess the idea of 'moral space' within health-care facilities.

INTRODUCTION: LABELS AS DIVERSIONS FROM MORAL REFLECTION

No issue in reproductive ethics is riddled with more fundamental moral disagreement than abortion. Giving emotionally loaded labels for diverse views on abortion is one of the methods commonly used to synopsise and dismiss opposing positions. It is shorthand for the message: 'I don't intend to listen because I know your views already.' Using this counterproductive method, we casually label persons who hold different views on abortion in mutually exclusive categories as 'pro-abortion' and 'pro-life' as if these labels can begin to approach the complexity of understanding, motivations and experiences that inform the diverse views on abortion. The labels effect the opposite: they project negative moral judgements and camouflage the genuine difficulties of the moral and political questions of abortion.

'Pro-life' and 'pro-choice or pro-abortion' labels are a mechanism for avoiding the intellectual work required in ethics to re-examine one's own views when faced with disagreement from others. The labels also fail to contribute toward clarification of what might be done to accommodate genuine moral diversity of cultures, races and religions. This diversity is increasingly a reality in the Republic of Ireland.

In the following case, a nurse is asked by her supervisor to help prepare for an abortion. The nurse is morally opposed to abortion and tries to be excused from the task.

Case 9.1: The Nurse Asked to Assist in an Abortion

Eileen Kinsella, a nurse of fifteen years, worked part-time in a small suburban hospital in Leeds. As she was familiar with the hospital's routines and the staff, she was often asked by the nursing supervisor to work in those patient-care areas short on nursing staff for that particular shift. Today, she was asked to work in the recovery room. Within an hour, however, the nurse supervisor called and asked her to report to A-4, the suite of rooms where elective abortions were usually performed. Hesitatingly Eileen told the supervisor that she did not believe in abortion. A devout Catholic, she considered abortion the killing of human life and a mortal sin. Would it be possible for the supervisor to find someone else to help out at A-4? The supervisor said she understood and would try to find another nurse.

In the meantime, however, Dr Michael Moran needed someone to prepare his patient and set up the room for the abortion. Since Eileen was not busy at the moment, the supervisor asked her if she could go to A-4 to assist at the set-up stage. Reluctantly Eileen agreed to this arrangement as long as the supervisor would send another nurse to replace her. The supervisor assured her that she would do this.

In A-4, after organising the equipment and room, Eileen prepared the patient, Sally, a fourteen-year-old teenager approximately 8 weeks pregnant. A business associate of her father's had raped Sally when he offered her a lift one day. Eileen told Michael that his patient was ready but that she would not participate in the proceedings. Another nurse would arrive shortly who would assist him. Michael objected to the delay, saying to Eileen, 'I don't think I should have to wait while the nursing staff sorts their conscience questions. Everyone – the patient, the community and the family – will be better off not having to deal with one more illegitimate child requiring public support.'

When Eileen stated that her religious and moral beliefs did not allow her to participate in an abortion, Michael argued that conscience should not be too sensitive here. The early embryo is 'a complex organ but not yet really human life'. The young woman had been raped and, he said, someone had to see that she was 'a victim in this situation'. Michael again asked that Eileen reconsider and assist him. When Eileen declined, he went down the hallway in search of the supervisor. He felt it was a sad day for patients when nurses decided they would not provide needed care.

(Adaptation of case from Fry and Veatch 2000: 35–6)

CONSCIENCE RIGHTS

A person's conscience may lead to resistance to the demands of others in the form of conscientious refusal or objection. In this situation of potential interpersonal conflict, Eileen had to determine not only how she would act in the light of her conscience but also how she would respond to the claims of conscience made by others, including Michael Moran, her supervisor and Sally. When people claim that their choices are coming from 'conscience', they sometimes mean they are compelled by conscience to resist demands made by others. That seems the case here. But let's take a moment to look at this idea of 'conscience'.

Many people believe in the slogan, 'Let your conscience be your guide'. This suggests that the voice of one's conscience is the final authority in moral justification. But rather than consider conscience as some special inner voice or self-justifying moral faculty, we might consider a different meaning where conscience is not a fixed 'collection' of one's moral beliefs.

Rather, 'conscience' refers to a form of self-reflection and judgement about one's acts: are they obligatory, wrong, good, prohibited? It also involves a certain willingness to reconsider views in the light of new insights or understandings. In this way, one's conscience is informed and subject to change.

> It is an internal sanction that comes into play through critical reflection. This sanction often appears as a bad conscience – in the form of painful feelings of remorse, guilt, shame, disunity or disharmony – as the individual recognises his or her acts as wrong. A conscience that sanctions in this way does not signify bad moral character. Indeed, this form of conscience is likely to occur in persons of strong moral character (Beauchamp and Childress 2001: 38).

This understanding of 'conscience' links it closely with the active and ongoing reflection that characterises a moral agent. Likewise, there is a strong link between respecting autonomy and respecting conscience claims:

> The right to have one's autonomy respected – the right of self-determination entails the right of conscientious action . . . It is therefore possible to justify overriding a person's conscientious action if that action imposes serious risks on others, invades the autonomy of others, or treats others unjustly. But individuals and the society bear a heavy burden of proof in arguing that coercion of conscience is necessary to protect others from harm, to respect others' autonomy, or to preserve fairness. (Beauchamp and Childress 1989: 390)

Activity

a) If nurses have moral objections to abortion, do you think this poses any obstacles to good nursing care for women choosing abortion?

b) If a woman who was coming in for an abortion raised a conversation about whether she was making the 'right decision', how would you respond?

c) As a nurse attending a young woman and providing follow-up care, would you consider raising with her the conversation of contraceptive practice?

d) Try to explain your reasons and any difficulties you might anticipate in engaging in this conversation.

THE CLINICIAN'S CONSCIENCE: ACTING-OUT OF BENEFICENCE

One reading of Michael Moran's response to Sally is to see that he is acting out of beneficence. He asks: what will contribute to the wellbeing of this patient? Beneficence, as you saw in previous chapters, requires that we choose actions that maximally promote patient welfare. Part of the doctor's view is that Sally was badly violated in being made involuntarily pregnant through rape. This indignation about the abuse on Sally reflects a certain respect for the patient and her vulnerability. In many jurisdictions where moral and legal guidelines exist for abortion, rape and incest are offered as defences for abortion as explained in the following text.

> It is commonly argued that abortion is justified when the pregnancy occurs as a result of rape or incest. It is argued that abortion under these circumstances is justified for two reasons: (1) abortion will safeguard the mental health of the woman which is undoubtedly at risk and of great value; (2) the pregnancy resulting from rape or incest is a grave injustice and the victim is therefore under no obligation to carry the embryo to viability. (Rumbold 1999: 113)

Activity

Rumbold argues here that *how* a woman conceives and becomes pregnant is morally significant and strongly influences one's moral view on a particular abortion decision. Some writers argue that if a woman conceives without consent and as a result of rape, this gives moral grounds for her to choose abortion if she so wishes.

a) Do you agree that how a woman conceives is morally significant and relevant to a decision about abortion?

b) Some would claim that Sally ought to continue with the pregnancy even if involuntarily pregnant through rape. How would you evaluate that view?

c) If a family member had to give consent for Sally's abortion, would you have a conversation with them or simply get their signature to the procedure? If you decide on a conversation with the parents, what would you discuss?

UTILITARIAN CALCULATIONS OF OVERALL GOOD RESULT

The doctor's reasoning about Sally's overall best interests, and about society's overall common good shows a consequential calculation characteristic of the moral theory of **utilitarianism**. The calculation calls on him to reflect on what might be the best overall outcome in this patient's situation. Such a calculation is not always easy. Such consequential calculations highlight the difficulties in carefully applying a utilitarian moral decision theory (See Section Four). Consequential calculation requires understanding of all of the individuals involved in a situation; it calls for intelligent projection of likely events to follow. These judgements require experience and reflection on similar situations in one's professional life.

RESPECTING A MINOR'S AUTONOMY

Michael Moran's conscience is not seriously troubled by Sally's need for an abortion. However, given that she is a minor, he knows that he would need to secure the parental consent mentioned above. If we can assume that Sally is competent, then Michael's decision to proceed with the abortion could be viewed as respecting the teenager's autonomy and self-determination. Michael is likely to be familiar with the now-celebrated Gillick case which was decided in the UK in the mid-1980s. In that case, the idea of chronological age was challenged (Mason and McCall Smith 1999). Chronological age was found not to be a sufficient indicator of 'maturity' to judge competence for consent to medical treatment including contraceptives and, by extension of interpretation, perhaps, abortion. The UK Department of Health at the time sent doctors a document giving criteria for their use in determining competence of minors. The criteria are referred to as a definition of **Gillick competence**. If the minor fulfils the criteria, the consent of parents is not needed (On Gillick Competence, See Appendix 1).

VALUATIONS OF HUMAN FOETAL LIFE

We have been discussing Sally, Michael and Eileen in this case narrative. But from Eileen's point of view, there is another human being to consider: the unborn embryo. The case study reveals a fundamental moral disagreement between Eileen and Michael; their disagreement rests on their different evaluations of two important elements:

1. The status of the human embryo.
2. The primary right of a woman to decide whether she can or will continue her pregnancy.

We will postpone the discussion of a woman's right to decide here as it is analysed further in Chapter 10. Instead we will focus, first, on the status of the embryo. Eileen views the unborn embryo very differently from how Michael views it and perhaps Sally's view is different again. We don't have insight into Sally's thoughts on this matter, but from her decision, is it obvious which position she would hold?

There are three commonly stated views about the moral status of the embryo during the period between conception and birth. As you read, consider which position might be attributed to Michael, Eileen and the young girl, Sally, and, indeed your own view.

1. Fertilisation View

This view rejects the validity of any attempt to make morally significant distinctions after fertilisation. It claims that it is fertilisation that is the non-arbitrary point marking the inception of a human life. In scientific terms, the fertilisation view holds that an individual's DNA – genetic profile – is determined at fertilisation when ovum and sperm join together and form a single entity that normally endures as a single entity. The fertilisation view also argues that the embryo is, throughout pregnancy, entitled to serious moral consideration and, therefore, protection because it is a human being with special reference to its first nine months of history.

2. Gradualist View

The gradualist sees the human embryo as a *potential* human life. The seriousness and moral gravity of abortion increases as the embryo develops from fertilisation to birth. An early embryo would have less strong rights to protection than a 28-week embryo that, with neonatal help, is capable of independent existence. In different variants of this gradualist view, various 'moments' in foetal development are referred to as a transition to a stage in which the embryo would be more worthy of protection – the appearance of the primitive streak, for example, or the commencement of brain activity.

3. Embryo as Organ

The embryo throughout pregnancy is best understood as an 'organ' of the mother. According to this view, there are few, if any, moral conflicts in removing the embryo if the mother so chooses. Being dependent on the woman for its nourishment, it bears no rights on its own.

Summary Learning Guide 9.1

Three main positions on the status of the embryo are:
- The *fertilisation* view: conception is the point at which a human being is formed and merits rights of protection;
- The *gradualist* view: the embryo is a potential human being and obligations to protect it increase as development progresses through to birth;
- The *organ* view: the embryo is most analogous to an organ of the pregnant woman and bears no rights on its own.

THE INDETERMINATE MORAL STATUS OF THE UNBORN

To many, these moral positions about the status of the embryo and the morality of abortion may *seem* to be a straightforward assessment of empirical, factual information about the gestation of the unborn during nine months. It would be relatively easy if that were the case – somehow the facts of gestation would speak their significance. But Sissela Bok challenges this assumption. She argues that deciding the moral status of the unborn is not a scientific, factual matter:

> The different views as to when humanity begins are not dependent upon factual information. Rather, these views are representative of different world-views, often of a religious nature, involving deeply held commitments with moral consequences.
>
> There is no disagreement as to what we now know about life and its development before and after conception; differences arise only about the names and moral consequences we attach to the changes in this development and the distinctions we consider important.
>
> Just as there is no point at which Achilles can be pinpointed as catching up with the tortoise, though everyone knows he does, so too everyone is aware of the distance travelled, in terms of humanity, from before conception to birth, **though there is no one point at which humanity can be agreed upon as setting in**.
>
> Our efforts to pinpoint and to define reflect the urgency with which we reach for abstract labels and absolute certainty in facts and in nature. (Bok 1974: 38–9).

Consider Sissela Bok's analysis. How does it apply to Eileen Kinsella and Michael Moran? They have very different views and moral positions on abortion yet both say that they value human life. Bok tries to explain how these differences arise. It is not that Eileen values human life and Michael doesn't. They have very different appraisals of the unborn reality that Sally carries. They attach profoundly different values to this reality. Bok further explains that deciding on the moral status of the embryo is not a straightforward task of looking at facts in the embryology of reproduction.

To think that the facts deliver the moral judgement is to equate moral judgements with empirical data. This is widely viewed as an error in reasoning, famously known as the 'naturalistic fallacy'. This error of reasoning occurs when we make an inference from known facts to moral assertions without showing the value assumptions that are usually hidden premises but are needed to support our inference.

Activity

a) Consider the fertilisation view again. Are there any difficulties in the claim that 'fertilisation is a non-arbitrary point'?
   One objection to this position, for example, is that fertilisation is a process rather than a point and that, on occasion, 'twinning' can occur where the fertilised egg can divide and become two individuals.

b) Consider the gradualist view. Do you see any difficulties with this position?
   One objection might be that it seems arbitrary (and therefore morally unacceptable) to distinguish between an embryo at 28 weeks and an embryo at 26 weeks.

c) Critically consider the organ view.
   This position is often critiqued because of the false comparison drawn between the embryo and other vital organs of a person in terms of their potential for development into a fully-fledged human being.

d) Some argue that even if one were to accept the fertilisation view of the status of the embryo, there remain certain circumstances where abortion is morally acceptable. Can you think of any such circumstances?

MORAL OBJECTIONS TO ASSISTING WITH ABORTION

Eileen does not respond to the situation she finds herself in solely out of a benefit-producing principle or calculations aimed at the best overall consequences. She responds out of a set of personal moral values developed from her own background, education, cultural experiences and religious beliefs. These beliefs reflect the *fertilisation view* explained above, claiming that human life begins at conception. For Eileen, the embryo is a human life, destruction of human life is murder and, as such, if she were to participate in the abortion, she would be an accomplice in a grave sin.

Even while believing that human life begins at fertilisation, Eileen might still be able to agree with some of Michael Moran's assessment of 'net benefit' to be produced by the abortion. Sally might not be able to rear a child, her life would be drastically altered or her family might feel obliged to take the baby for rearing.

However, the crucial difference in Eileen's position – a position that comes from a **deontological** perspective – is that the mere enumerations of 'net benefit' do not make abortion right. **Deontology** refers to duty-based systems of ethics that maintain that the morality of actions is to be judged in terms of their conformity with moral rules, obligations, rights and so on. Deontology rejects the claim that evaluation of good consequences is ever sufficient to determine the moral value of an action. There are categorical values that cannot be compromised. Eileen's position is an example of such a deontological moral perspective on abortion. For Eileen, the good effects and consequences for either Sally or society do not make abortion right.

Summary Learning Guide 9.2

To say that the moral status of the embryo is 'indeterminate' means that:

- There are no empirical, scientific facts that will, on their own, establish a conclusion about the morality of abortion;
- The diverse views about the moral nature of the human embryo are based on diverse world-views often of a religious nature;
- If we assume that the facts of nature are sufficient to make a moral judgement about anything, we erroneously infer moral judgements from empirical data;
- In making such an inference, we fall into the reasoning error called the 'naturalistic fallacy'.

PERSONAL VALUES AND NURSE PARTICIPATION IN ABORTION

Eileen's refusal to participate in abortion comes from strong moral rules, generated and supported by religious beliefs that were inculcated from an early age. Those religious beliefs would have reinforced the fertilisation position on abortion. However, Eileen and Michael both have to negotiate their opposing views respectfully in order to decide how to proceed. Where does tolerance for opposing perspectives come into their overall moral positions? Providing some kind of support mechanism in the hospital unit might facilitate further discussion of conscience conflicts of this nature, since they are likely to occur again.

If a nurse is not morally opposed to abortion as a choice for women, then she is, in general, without conscience conflict in assisting with elective abortions. Yet, some inner conflict may be felt in assisting. For example, a nurse may be saddened by the need for abortion as a solution and, in fact, may not personally endorse abortion choice as her own moral position. She might, nevertheless, argue that other women who have different ethical perspectives on abortion should be entitled to make their own choice. In this instance, liberty of choice or respect for the moral autonomy of women would be the dominant principle.

A different situation occurs if a nurse has strong moral opposition to abortion and feels that she would be an accomplice in serious wrong if she assisted in the abortion surgery. Where this is so, the nurse may be in conflict with institutional assumptions about her professional obligations. This depends to a great extent on what provisions the health-care institution makes for conscientious objections in various areas.

On what basis and to what extent should personal moral values and beliefs influence performance of professional duties in routine nursing care?

There are at least four responsibilities that Eileen might be expected to carry out:

1   Set up the room for the abortion;
2.   Prepare the woman having the termination;
3.   Take part in the actual abortion;
4.   Aftercare of the woman.

Activity

Reflect on the four responsibilities mentioned. Are there others that you think are overlooked here?

a) Since Eileen is morally opposed to abortion, would she be morally complicit if she took part in all of these different nursing tasks? Some of them?

b) If Eileen said she could help with 1, 2, and 4, but not 3, how could you explain her moral position in making these decisions?

c) Consider: Would it be possible for a nurse to assist in the abortion throughout the procedure but simply reassure herself that 'in her conscience' she does not approve? In brief, is the nurse complicit (or guilty by cooperation) because she assists as a professional nurse?

CONSCIENCE CONFLICTS AND MORAL SPACE

Eileen was prompt in explaining to her supervisor that she had conscientious objections to participating in the abortion procedure. She requests, if possible, that another nurse be found who does not object. The supervisor was responsive and said she would try to find a replacement.

Eileen further agreed that she would prepare Sally and the room for the abortion but that she could not take part in the actual abortion procedure. This is a classic example of a situation where the nurse professional wonders, on conscience grounds, about their degree of participation and complicity in a situation they take to be a moral wrong. Where total dissociation may be impossible, conscientious agents have to decide how far they can cooperate without violating their consciences (Dooley 1994: 622–3). One position on nurse participation when moral objections to abortion exist is given as follows:

> A woman who is having an abortion or a patient who has refused treatment with suicidal intent still needs ordinary nursing care, and

nurses can give such care – feeding, comforting, administering pain-killing drugs – without adopting any proposal that the unborn or the suicidal patient should die.

It is even possible to imagine situations in which nurses might prepare patients for operations. If they do not adopt the immoral purpose as their own, nurses might possibly and blamelessly help physicians carry out abortions. (Grisez and Boyle 1979: 435–6)

In trying to negotiate the conflict for Eileen Kinsella, the supervisor responds with respect. She actively tries to provide what, in Chapter 4, we call 'moral space' for conscience. To recap, 'moral space' is not an identifiable physical place (like a room) but is rather a term we use to refer to:

- an institutional health-care context
- where a philosophy of respect for moral autonomy is fundamental,
- where communication of conscientious objections can be facilitated by designated nurse personnel,
- where discussion and non-intimidating recognition of conscience differences regarding work practice are made possible,
- where discussion of moral differences are facilitated through an informal forum;
- such a forum is a readily available mechanism for review of cases that bring ethical challenges to the fore.

The supervisor also offers moral space by negotiating with Eileen on those elements in patient care that she can perform without serious moral unease. For Eileen, preparing Sally, the room and giving attentive post-abortion care are activities that she believes do not cross the line into complicity with the actual abortion surgery. In Eileen's conscience, those activities would be morally right for her.

CONCLUSION

The availability of abortion in many countries around the world elicits moral dissent from some professionals who are asked to assist in the abortion process. The dissent calls for an understanding of conscience as an internal sanction but one that comes into play and is reassessed with critical reflection. Moral differences about abortion require institutional provision of moral space. This latter concept was introduced in this chapter to show the multiple elements needed to be put in place if respect for conscience is to become a reality within health-care contexts.

We explained three diverse evaluations of the status of the embryo indicating that they are each based on radically different world-views and value priorities. The text of Sissela Bok showed the indeterminacy in the question of the moral status of the embryo. The 'naturalistic fallacy' was explained, indicating the hazard of drawing inferences from facts of nature. To escape this basic error of reasoning, one must be prepared to lay out the value assumptions that move us in argument from facts to judgements of moral value.

The following terms are explained in the glossary:

deontological theory

Gillick competence

gradualist position on moral status of
    the human embryo

moral space

utilitarianism

– 10 –

Personal Conscience and Public Policy

Objectives

At the end of this chapter, you should be able to:

- Explain the religious history and constitutional position on abortion in the Republic of Ireland;
- Evaluate the divergent positions on the primacy of women's conscience in abortion decisions;
- Clarify the relationship between individual conscience and support for a public policy on abortion;
- Assess the challenge of creating moral space.

INTRODUCTION

The question of abortion has had a stormy history in the Republic of Ireland though many nurses coming into nursing studies at third level in Ireland would not have been born when public debate on abortion came to prominence in the early 1980s. Working as professionals in acute-care hospitals, nurses here have not had to confront directly the moral challenges raised by abortion. They may have faced the difficulty of a personal decision about a pregnancy but, to date, hospitals do not perform elective abortions. Measures are taken to save the lives of women only if this is absolutely necessary, but such situations are infrequent.

In Chapter 9, we looked at a case where a nurse who was asked to assist in abortion faced moral dilemmas in relation to what her obligations were – professionally and personally. In this chapter, we begin with a Supreme Court case central to Irish public debate in the early 1990s. It is also a case of a young woman raped. When she was not allowed to go to the United Kingdom for an abortion, the public discussions led to a careful scrutiny of women's conscience rights in the area of reproductive choice. The relative silence of women who have experienced abortion will be the first focus of this chapter. Secondly, we examine the question of a state's obligations to respond through policy or legislation to the moral diversity of views about abortion. The facts about the history of abortion in Ireland from 1861 to the present are provided in Appendix 2.

THE REALITY OF ABORTION IN IRELAND

In order to tease out some of the ethical issues that arise in relation to the history of abortion in Ireland, consider the following Irish legal case which arose following the rape of a young girl; it is not unlike the case discussed in Chapter 9.

Case 10.1: *Attorney General* v. *X and Others* **(March 1992)**

A fourteen-year-old girl became pregnant as the result of an alleged rape. Her parents wished to take her to England for an abortion. They asked whether genetic fingerprinting would help a prosecution of the alleged rapist. The gardaí referred the issue to the Director of Public Prosecutions who informed the Attorney General (AG). In turn, the AG obtained interim injunctions in the High Court to prevent the girl and her parents from procuring an abortion within or without the jurisdiction – and indeed from leaving the jurisdiction for nine months.

At a full hearing, a psychologist testified that there was a risk that the girl might commit suicide as she had repeatedly threatened. The Supreme Court allowed an appeal and thus lifted the injunction. The Justices argued that the risks to the life of the mother included a real and substantial risk that she might commit suicide. In their Supreme Court Judgement, they urged the Government to draft legislation that would stipulate terms for permissible abortions. As of now, this legislation has not been drafted.

As Case 10.1 indicates, the Supreme Court gave a judgement of 4–1 in March 1992 that abortion is not always unlawful in Ireland. The Court argued that abortion is legal in limited cases. In what has become known as 'the X case', the Supreme Court decided:

> If it is established as a matter of probability that there is a real and substantial risk to the life as distinct from the health of the mother, which can only be avoided by the termination of her pregnancy, that such termination is permissible, having regard to the true interpretation of Article 40.3.3. [of the Irish Constitution]. (*Attorney General* v. *X and Others*)

The decision was embraced by some in Ireland as a breakthrough of civil liberties and the reproductive rights of women. Others lamented the judgement as a lapse of judicial discretion and predicted that abortion on demand would become a reality in Ireland. This has not happened to date.

While legislation does not permit abortion in Ireland, Irish women nevertheless choose abortion. In their extensive survey of Irish abortion, Evelyn Mahon, Catherine Conlon and Lucy Dillon estimated that 8.5 per cent of all Irish pregnancies result in abortion.

> British statistics show that the recorded numbers of Irish women having abortions has been steadily rising and that in 2000, 6,381 women having abortions in Britain indicated that they were resident in this State. It is widely accepted that many Irish-resident women do not give

their real addresses when obtaining abortions in Britain and therefore it is impossible to estimate with accuracy the real number of Irish women availing of abortion services, except to say that the true figures are higher than the 'official' statistics indicate. (Irish Council of Civil Liberties 2002: 12)

Irish women who do not give their address as living in Ireland often use addresses of relatives living in Britain or elsewhere. The reason for this is the social stigma attached to an unwanted pregnancy and the fear of being discovered as having had an abortion.

The Mahon report is the best available qualitative study of the reasons why Irish women decide to terminate their pregnancies. The reasons given by the women include: career and job-related concerns, concerns about education and continuance in training courses, fear of the stigma of lone parenthood on the women themselves and on their families, concern for existing children, financial difficulties, feelings of being unable to cope with a child, concerns that they were too young or too old to have a child, and the desire to exercise the right to control their fertility. There is no evidence that the lack of legalised abortion in Ireland has had any effect on the Irish abortion rate, except that the expenses involved in travelling to Britain, accommodation and the abortion procedure are likely to cause significant difficulties for less well-off women (Mahon cited in ICCL 2000: 13).

The failure of successive governments to develop a legislative and social framework to cope with Ireland's abortion reality is understandable in terms of political pragmatism: it is perceived to be at odds with the views of the current population in the country. Even so, the Irish abortion reality is a striking example of the divergence between, on the one hand, our national attitude, and, on the other hand, our actual practice. The abortion rate of Irish women is a curious phenomenon given the avowed differences in the religious and moral thinking on abortion in Ireland and the United Kingdom.

Summary Learning Guide 10.1

In the case of *Attorney General* v. *X and Others* (Ireland 1995)

- A young teenager was raped and, feeling suicidal, wished to go to the UK for an abortion;
- The Attorney General issued an injunction restraining her from leaving the country;
- The Supreme Court judgement ruled 4–1 that an abortion is not always unlawful in Ireland;
- The Court reasoned: a substantial risk of suicide was a real and substantial threat to the mother's life.
- Thus, abortion was stated to be legal in limited cases.
- Supreme Court Justices urged the Irish Government to draft legislation. As of 2005, this has not occurred.

RECORDING THE SILENT VOICES OF WOMEN

Irish women have been going to England for abortions for many years because this choice was a criminal offence in Ireland. The women remained secretive and quiet about their decision. Often, neither family nor friends knew that they had 'taken the boat' to England. A combination of secrecy and shame combined to keep them silent about what often proved a very difficult decision to make. Stories of women who had abortions have been recorded in *The Irish Journey*. The book is dedicated 'to the women who bravely contributed their stories of abortion and to all women who experience crisis pregnancy' (Irish Family Planning Association, 2000). The publication corroborates research by Mahon et al. on **crisis pregnancies** in Ireland. According to their research, the decisions of many women to have an abortion are seldom simple and are based on a complex set of emotional, psychological, religious, cultural and financial considerations (Mahon et al. 1998; Petchesky 1986; Edmondson 1992; Fletcher 1993).

There is a wide diversity of situations where women experience crisis pregnancies. If we try to generalise and make universal statements about how *all* women feel and what *all* women think when considering the abortion path, we may easily misunderstand the differences that exist – differences of moral conflict or reasons for the decision. Recognising the diversity of moral consciousness among women requires an understanding of women's perceptions of abortion.

> We cannot assume a reproductive consciousness that is universal among women. No universal consciousness grows out of the conditions of reproduction, for abortion, pregnancy, and childbearing are different in different social circumstances and consciousness will reflect those differences . . . Class and ethnically divided policies of the state in regard to reproduction may contribute to this varied consciousness. Even within the same circumstances and the same woman, consciousness about abortion is likely to be multilayered or contradictory. The same woman who avers that abortion is 'terrible' or 'wrong' may also insist on her need or right to have one. (Petchesky 1986: 364–5)

This text suggests that, for many women, different levels of consciousness are operating at once and people's understanding of the dictates of morality and their understanding of their own situation and needs are in conflict.

Activity

a) List some of the factors that might come into play when a woman considers terminating her pregnancy. In your opinion, are some of these 'common factors' – that is, do they occur more regularly than others?

b) Can you propose an argument explaining how a woman who strongly believes that abortion is generally wrong could, in good faith, justify her own decision to proceed to termination?

c) Is (b) an example where a general moral principle is held but there arise exceptions to this general norm? If this is so, what reasons would you propose to justify the exception?

Alternatively: consider whether you want to reason in a Kantian deontological mode that no reasons could justify abortion (revise Chapter 3 on truth telling).

THE IRISH JOURNEY

Consider Petchesky's account of reproductive consciousness in the light of the following passage from *The Irish Journey*. The two dominant emotions recorded by many Irish women who choose abortion are a feeling of 'isolation' or 'shameful secrecy' and ambivalence about the unborn. Sherie de Burgh writes:

> Carrying a sense of shame for your country is a terrible burden. Ireland's refusal to accept the reality of abortion, and acknowledge the humanity and rights of the individual woman behind the statistics, bestows a sense of shame on women and creates secrecy and isolation to reinforce that feeling. The individual decision that a pregnancy that is a crisis will end in abortion is no less painful and sad for an English woman than for her Irish counterpart. But she [the English woman] does not carry the weight of her country's judgement – she is acknowledged by the provision of services which she may decide she needs. Her crisis and decision is private, but not necessarily secret. (Sherie de Burgh in IFPA 2000: 4)

Because abortion has been criminalised in Ireland, the isolation and secrecy prevail. Because secrecy prevails, people cannot hear women tell of their decisions, nor realise the complexity of many such decisions. Secrecy does not help us to revise our understanding of women who are in crisis pregnancies. We may fall into a habit of **dichotomous thinking**, thinking that it is the pregnant woman against the unborn life. Thinking in terms of either/or options is something of a rhetorical move. It is used more often with the aim of simplifying an emotionally weighted discussion than of clarifying it. The deficit in dichotomous thinking is that we sacrifice creative thinking to simple terms. Creative reflection would have us consider other alternatives in trying to understand a difficult question.

The lifting of secrecy could help reduce dichotomous thinking about the abortion choices of women. For example, on the basis of listening to the many stories of women in Ireland who have had abortions, de Burgh further explains:

> I have never met the woman for whom this [abortion] was an easy or lightly taken decision. It is my experience that women have abortions because they feel that they cannot give a quality of life to that child, whatever their own personal reasons may be. They are not at war with their embryo. They are distressed and saddened by their knowledge that it is the born child they cannot have. It is the commitment to

parenting this child that they cannot make at this time. (Sherie de Burgh in IFPA 2000)

WOMEN AS PRIMARY MORAL AGENTS

Those who believe that a legal and political resolution of abortion should put decisions about abortion into the hands of pregnant women may, at the same time, accept that unborn life is humanly valuable and not to be thought of simply as tissue globules. For many centuries, the abortion debate has been discussed as an adversarial contest between women and the unborn. In some countries – including Ireland – a strong **pro-natalist** position prevailed in much of the public debate. A pro-natalist position refers to a viewpoint that says that women must relinquish their freedom to control their reproductive powers and cede, to the child conceived, the right to be born. From the pro-natalist perspective, women are represented as having a proper maternal function and, where a pregnancy occurs, the responsible moral choice would be to proceed and give birth. The focus of this position is mainly on the moral protection required for the innocent unborn.

The progress of civil and political rights for women over the last two centuries has changed the perception and reality of women's options. From the pro-natalist position that implies a limitation on women's liberties of choice in reproduction, developments in civil and political rights have allowed women to assume birth decisions as their own. With these developments there is an increasing reluctance to allow 'legal experts' or 'medical professionals' to make the abortion decisions instead of women (Smyth 1992). The public debates about abortion in most Western countries have echoed similar concerns about co-opting women's moral choices and liberty of conscience.

Affirming the primacy of women's moral agency is not intended to encourage women's evasion of responsibility. It is rather to encourage women to take 'responsibility' for their own decisions. Any decision by a woman for abortion takes account of all human factors: economic, social, psychological, emotional and moral. All of these factors contribute to any woman's abortion decision. Once this is clarified, moral differences are explained by reference to all of these factors.

MORAL DISAGREEMENT

It is routine in our experience to meet rational, well-meaning and sincere individuals who nevertheless disagree on moral issues. Some people believe that capital punishment is immoral while others think it is morally acceptable. Some argue that tax evasion is unjust while others consider it perfectly acceptable to evade taxes properly due.

Many people believe that abortion is immoral. Others disagree. Some think it is immoral in general and yet judge that women may need to choose abortion for many complex reasons. Many available examples show clearly that the fact of moral disagreement is a fundamentally obvious one in our world. The disagreement about abortion is complicated by different judgements about the extent to which legislation should be used to enforce moral values.

A person might agree that something or other is immoral and still believe that legislation should not make it illegal (Clarke 1982: 10). How a state responds politically to the fact of moral disagreement is revealing of the extent to which democracy in that state can justly accommodate and respect minority views on controversial issues. If moral disagreement about reproductive issues is inevitable, as it seems to be worldwide, we need to look to a more general value that offers us a principle for proceeding toward political accommodation of moral diversity. In the concluding section of this chapter, the principle of tolerance is offered for discussion as one way of recognising cultural diversity and proceeding with amicable political negotiations.

If we agree that moral disagreement is a reality among equally sincere, thoughtful and well-intentioned individuals, an important task for nursing ethics is to develop a theory that does at least two things:

1.   That recognises and leaves room for moral disagreement;
2.   That acknowledges that mutually incompatible moral views may be equally valid.

Religious Beliefs and Public Policy

In Chapter 9, we discussed the moral status of the embryo. We explained that it is impossible to get a definitive answer about the morality of abortion by following rational arguments alone to arrive at infallible answers about the status of the unborn. If this is so, perhaps we can rely for guidance on the religious beliefs of the people in a country.

For some individuals, their religious beliefs will fill in the value gaps in appraising the moral status of the unborn. But religious beliefs take many forms and the reality of multiculturalism is undisputed in Ireland today. Along with ethnic diversity is religious diversity and choosing to install one (numerically dominant) religious position into law may strike people as simply discriminatory against minority religions.

Desmond Clarke writes about the complexity of relations between Church and State. In his view, there are fundamental difficulties if a state allows one religious viewpoint to determine public law. Consider Clarke's explanation of the problems:

1. If the majority in a country believed, for religious reasons, that blood transfusions are immoral, we would not think they are justified in forbidding blood transfusions by law. Or if the majority believed for religious reasons, that Roman Catholic services are idolatry, we certainly would not agree that they could justifiably make them illegal.

2. If we once agree that a majority of religious believers may decide civil legislation simply because they are in the majority, we thereby surrender the right to religious and political freedom.

3. So, the mere fact that a numerical majority of the population believes something or other hardly makes it just or moral: and the claim that they believe it for religious reasons does not strengthen the case especially if religion is used to excuse the need for some kind of moral argument. Religious faith alone cannot provide a rational basis for deciding questions of justice. (Clarke 1982: 12–13)

In brief, we cannot define what is moral or immoral simply by reference to the local community, whatever the nature of their religious beliefs or lack of such beliefs may be. Nor can we derive moral guidance from counting the numbers who support various beliefs. The mere fact that a majority of an electorate shares a belief tells us nothing about its validity or reasonableness. We need to argue for norms that could be agreed by those without any religious faith, or by those who differ profoundly in religious traditions. This task asks us to think about the relationship between one's private moral views and provisions in civil law or public policy.

Summary Learning Guide 10.2

Appealing to the majority religious views to decide abortion policy has the following problems:

- The idea of a clear 'majority view' camouflages many differences of individual viewpoints;
- Adoption of a majority view sacrifices the rights of minorities to religious and political freedom;
- The number of persons holding a position does not amount to moral justification of that view.
- Therefore: we cannot coherently define what is moral or immoral simply by referring to the views of a local community. Attempting to do this confuses numerical fact with moral arguments.

TOLERANCE: PERSONAL CONSCIENCE AND PUBLIC POLICY

It is one thing for individuals to hold their own religious views on abortion. It is another political and moral question as to how a state should legislate regarding abortion. Ronald Dworkin offers one analysis of the value of tolerance. He considers tolerance to be a basis for a democratic society that cherishes human dignity.

> 1. The most important feature of Western political culture is a belief in individual human dignity: that people have the moral right – and moral responsibility to confront the most fundamental questions about the meaning and value of their own lives for themselves, answering to their own consciences and convictions. That assumption was the engine of emancipation and of racial equality, for example . . . The principle of procreative autonomy, in a broad sense, is embedded in any genuinely democratic culture.
>
> 2. **Tolerance** is a cost we must pay for our adventure in liberty. We are committed, by our love of liberty and dignity, to live in communities in which no group is thought clever or spiritual or numerous enough to decide essentially religious matters for everyone else. If we have genuine concern for the lives others lead, we will also accept that no life is a good one lived against the grain of conviction, that it does not help someone else's life but spoils it to force values upon him he cannot accept but can only bow before out of fear or prudence. (Dworkin 1993: 167–8)

These discussions assist in trying to consider whether majority views (cultural or religious) are sufficient to decide what legislative provision a state should make in relation to abortion. Assume that we wish all citizens of a state to be given freedom of their beliefs. Clarke and Dworkin suggest that, to achieve this, public policy or civil law needs to afford flexibility for a range of individual choices. Some of these choices might be thought immoral to many people in a country. But this is precisely what moral disagreement means in a civil society endorsing tolerance.

Activity

a) List three arguments you would offer to defend a government decision to prohibit abortion.

b) List three arguments you would offer to defend a government decision to allow for abortion *even if* the moral views of a majority in the state reject abortion.

RELIGION, TOLERANCE AND LIMITS

Writers down through the centuries have stressed the necessity for a free state to protect the value of religious tolerance.

One Christian theologian, Bernard Haring, argues that:

> We should not oppose legislation of the pluralistic state that leaves freedom in these cases to the physicians and the mothers to decide. . . . (Haring 1978: 34)

Different writers disagree with Haring, especially the philosopher, Germain Grisez, who thinks that there are certain limits that politicians must never transgress. Grisez argues that specific basic norms are inviolable and certain compromises (especially in areas such as abortion and nuclear deterrence) are not permitted. At the heart of Grisez's theory is his strong deontological belief that persons must not act directly against certain basic goods (Grisez and Boyle 1979). According to this view, because the taking of an innocent human life acts against a basic good, direct abortion is always prohibited. For example, Grisez thinks that public officials cannot, in good conscience, support legislation to fund abortion.

Haring, on the other hand, believes that politicians can support legislation allowing for abortion choice. This position is in recognition of genuine moral disagreements about abortion and respect for the moral conscience of sincere people. Grisez and Haring illustrate that the moral differences that exist about the relationship between individual conscience and public policy go to the heart of religious traditions. Both of the authors represent a theological and philosophical position within the Roman Catholic religious tradition.

1. The principle enunciated by Haring is: where profound and widespread moral disagreement exists on an issue, civil law should reflect this by allowing liberty of choice on that issue.

2. The principle enunciated by Germain Grisez holds that even if widespread disagreement exists, some liberties should not be tolerated. He believes the freedom to choose abortion is one of those liberties that should not be tolerated.

Grisez's position raises the question about the source of such moral certainty. If the source of the certainty is theological, there is a vicious circle here. How can one appeal to their religious beliefs as the basis for the civil legislation that would apply to a religiously diverse people?

CONCLUSION

In this chapter, we presented the case of the fourteen-year-old Irish girl who was raped and, subsequently, was refused leave of the country to procure an abortion. This ultimately led to a Supreme Court judgement that abortion is not always illegal in Ireland. The criterion the court gave was that a woman's life must be threatened substantially and such a threat could be a danger of suicide over the abortion.

The sequence of events over the past twenty-five years has brought to public prominence the 'criminal' mark assigned to women who went outside the state for abortions. Because of the criminalisation of abortion, many women have been silenced about their abortion choices. Silent though these women may be, statistics indicate that some 12,000 of them travel to the United Kingdom for abortions each year.

We also explored the political and ethical notion of freedom to live according to one's conscience, and freedom to exercise moral agency within civil society. Texts from writers such as Grisez, Clarke, Dworkin and Haring offered alternative views on the liberty of conscience that a civil state can justify. We suggested that agreement and certainty do not obtain in this debate but the very fact of profound moral disagreement may be seen as evidence that more serious thought must be given to this question: Can a reasonable person agree to support civil legislation to allow for choices by others where the choices are ones they cannot personally defend? This is the question at the heart of much social ethics and public policy.

Finally, many nurses coming into third-level studies in Ireland will be too young to have experienced the public debates in Ireland in the 1980s. In recognition of this, we provide an Appendix of the significant dates of this debate since 1861.

The following terms are explained in the glossary:

Attorney General v. *X*

crisis pregnancy

dichotomous thinking

Pro-natalism: within the context of abortion positions

tolerance

Selecting for Sex

Objectives

At the end of this chapter, you should be able to:

- Outline some of the key ethical issues that arise in relation to Assisted Human Reproduction (AHR);
- Define new terms such as procreative autonomy, sex selection, the harm principle, instrumentalisation;
- Distinguish between medical and nonmedical reasons for selecting the sex of future children;
- Consider arguments for and against the availability of sex selection for nonmedical reasons

INTRODUCTION

Assisted Human Reproduction (AHR) is an umbrella term for a range of different technologies and procedures that have been developed in response to human conditions such as infertility, childlessness and disease. They are intended to assist individuals or couples to conceive a child (e.g. **donor insemination**, *in vitro* **fertilisation** (IVF), and surrogate childbearing). They have also been combined with genetic knowledge and can intervene in the development of the gametes (sperm and ova) and the **embryo** (e.g. **preimplantation genetic diagnosis** (PGD), **prenatal diagnosis, embryo therapy** and **stem-cell research**). Such interventions are, primarily, intended to avoid the transmission of congenital diseases or conditions and to treat disease in the wider population. They can also, in principle, be used to select for particular features that parents might desire their offspring to have.

The rapid development of technologies for AHR and unprecedented advances in genetic knowledge have created a profound sense of moral dislocation and uncertainty about what it is to be human and how we humans are to relate and reproduce responsibly. On the one hand, human fertilisation can take place outside the womb and an embryo can be grown in a test tube (*in vitro*). On the other, the mapping of the human genome is providing increasingly specific understanding of which genes are implicated in conditions such as Huntington's disease, cystic fibrosis, Duchenne muscular dystrophy, breast cancer, diabetes and deafness. The combined potential of reproductive and genetic technologies entails a seismic shift from a situation where birth, death, disease and disability happen by chance, to a situation where choices allow us to avoid or modify the seeming 'inevitable' nature of our human world.

The pace of development calls for a rethinking of fundamental ethical concepts and a re-evaluation of traditional assumptions and positions. Some of the key ethical problems that arise in relation to AHR include the following:

1. The procedures involved in AHR radically interfere with the ordinary course of nature and there is debate as to whether or not such interference is morally acceptable.

2. Some procedures associated with AHR involve the destruction of prenatal life, and there is widespread disagreement about whether or not, and to what degree, the early stages of human life ought to be protected.

3. There is concern because the processes of AHR impact directly on the welfare of the offspring involved and have far-reaching effects into the future.

4. The separation of genetic, gestational and rearing dimensions of parenthood that AHR entails profoundly challenges existing notions of motherhood, fatherhood, responsible parenthood and family.

5. There are worries about the physical, psychological and emotional impact of these technologies on women. According to one theorist, most of them 'operate on a woman's body in some way, turning it into a battleground of competing interests' (Robertson 1994: 14).

6. There is debate as to who should be allowed access to the processes of AHR: Married couples? Single women? Stable heterosexual couples? Lesbian and gay couples? Single people? People with disabilities or serious illnesses? Older people?

7. There are economic considerations concerning who pays for, and who profits from, the provision of AHR. Should the costs associated with AHR be market driven? Should the individual or the state, or both, pay for AHR services?

Granted the serious ethical questions that arise in relation to AHR procedures, societies must now decide whether or not to permit the development of these techniques, and they must determine the circumstances in which they are used, and the conditions and restrictions for use.

Currently in Ireland, there is no specific legislation governing the provision of AHR services. The only regulation that exists has come from the Guidelines of the Irish Medical Council (2004), which are directed towards medical practitioners but have no authority over scientists, researchers, therapists and other professionals working in the area of AHR. However, public debate on the ethical issues at stake in AHR is growing in Ireland, and some progress has been made toward the development of public policy in the area. For example, in 2000, the Minister for Health and Children, Micheál Martin, established the Commission for Assisted Human Reproduction, chaired by Dervilla Donnelly, Professor of Chemistry in Trinity College Dublin, to prepare a report on possible approaches to the regulation of assisted human reproduction and to determine the social, ethical and legal factors that should be taken into account when determining public policy in the area. At a public conference in Dublin organised by the Commission, in February 2003, the Minister indicated his support for an appropriate framework to regulate AHR provision in Ireland:

> It is clear that the application of science to the human reproductive sphere has brought with it many benefits. For example, allowing couples who have difficulties in conceiving to have children. Techniques such as in-vitro fertilization, the freezing and storage of sperm and artificial insemination by donor are available in Ireland and have undoubtedly enhanced the quality of life for many people. It is vital that such techniques are conducted within an appropriate regulatory framework which safeguards the interests and dignity of all concerned, and ensures that quality standards are in line with best practice. It is also however clear that the ability of science to intervene in, control, or even alter the natural process of the creation of human life poses fundamental ethical problems for all of us. (Micheál Martin, CAHR, Conference Proceedings 2003: 6)

The fact that in the course of its work, the Commission received in excess of 1,600 written submissions from members of the public, professional and voluntary organisations in relation to AHR indicates the strong level of public interest in this area.

Because of the range of AHR procedures and the complexity of the ethical problems that they give rise to, this chapter will focus on one technique that has been recently developed in the United States – sperm sorting, a procedure that enables an individual or couple to choose the sex of their future child. What is particularly interesting about sperm sorting is that, while it is a relatively simple technique, the arguments for and against its general availability shine the spotlight on two fundamental ethical values that are at stake in many reproductive decisions: procreative autonomy and the welfare of future children.

Activity

a) Before we explore in more detail some of the ethical issues in relation to AHR, take a few moments to consider your own views on infertility and childlessness. Do you think that the state has an obligation to assist some individuals to have children?

b) Reread the list of ethical concerns listed above. Do you think that some of these are more ethically significant than others? Choose two out of the seven that you think are of most moral concern, and give reasons why you believe this is so.

SEX SELECTION

The Methods

The chance of having a boy or having a girl after natural conception is around 50 per cent. However, since the beginning of recorded history, folk remedies testify to the fact that some individuals and couples want to choose the sex of their future child for various reasons. Up until the 1970s, folk remedies aside, the means to select the sex of offspring successfully have not been available. Since then, advances in reproductive technology have made it possible.

The first method that became available involves the prenatal diagnosis of the sex of the embryo in the womb and, possibly, abortion. The second involves *in vitro* fertilisation (IVF), analysis of the resulting embryos through pre-implantation genetic diagnosis (PGD) and, possibly, embryo destruction. The third and most recent method, which is the focus of this chapter, involves a procedure that is carried out prior to conception: sperm sorting.

What is Sperm Sorting?

Sperm sorting is a procedure which sorts sperm according to whether they carry male or female chromosomes. The resulting sample of the chosen sex can be used to inseminate a woman (AI) or to create embryos *in vitro*. .

Sperm Sorting: Flow Cytometry

The most successful sperm-sorting procedure, flow cytometry, was first patented by the United States Department of Agriculture in the 1990s and licensed to the Genetics and IVF Institute in Fairfax, Virginia, for clinical trials. The process involves adding a fluorescent dye to the sperm, which enables sperm sorting, since X sperm carry more DNA than Y sperm. When the sperm is sent through a flow cytometer in which a laser beam causes the dyed DNA to glow, X sperm glow brighter than Y sperm. The sperm are then sorted using a cell sorter.

Sperm sorting is reported to be 98.2 per cent successful for selection of females in 27 patients and 72 per cent successful for selection of males (Fugger, Black, Keyvanfar and Schulman 1998). While this method is still at the clinical trial stage, there are worries that the fluorescent dye added to the sperm (which attaches itself to the sperm's DNA) might cause damage.

What distinguishes sperm sorting from other sex-selection procedures from an ethical point of view is that, unlike prenatal diagnosis and pre-implantation genetic diagnosis, sperm sorting is a procedure that happens prior to conception. Should sperm sorting be determined to be safe, ethical objections to sex selection on grounds that it might involve abortion or embryo destruction would not apply to it.

Nevertheless, important ethical concerns remain. The following case illustrates some of the ethical challenges that an individual or couple must address if they are considering selecting the sex of their future child through sperm sorting.

Case 11.1 Family and Farm

Mary and Martin Murphy, live on a 200-acre farm in north Tipperary. The ownership and development of farmland is taken very seriously by the rural community in which they live and the practice has traditionally been for farmers to leave their land to one of the sons of the family.

Mary and Martin already have four children, all girls. All of the pregnancies have been difficult and have taken their toll on Mary's health. Her last pregnancy was particularly arduous but she and Martin are still anxious to have a son. They have heard that it is possible to select the sex of babies through a sperm-sorting technique, and they have downloaded information about the procedure from the web. As the procedure is not available in Ireland, they are contemplating travelling to a clinic in the United States which provides a sperm-sorting service.

Both Mary and Martin believe that their parental relationship with a son will be different from that which they have with their daughters. They also have concerns about what will happen to the farm; it is land that has been in the Murphy family for five generations.

Mary and Martin are two sincere people, good parents and neighbours who are committed to their family and community. It is clear from Case 11.1 that they have given serious consideration to sex selection through sperm sorting and that they have, for them, sound reasons for wanting to choose the sex of the next baby: concerns about Mary's health, the desire to balance the family, the wish to parent a son, worries about the future of the farm. Their choice raises a number of ethical questions, including:

- Are the couple's reasons for sex selection sound reasons from an ethical and legal point of view?
- Does the couple have a right to choose the sex of a future child?
- If the couple has such a right, will exercising that right involve harm to anyone?

Activity

Consider how you might respond if Mary and Martin came to you for advice. Do you think that their preference for a boy ought to be respected and facilitated?

Why Select for Sex?

The reasons why people try to choose the sex of their future child generally fall into the following two categories:

Medical Reasons

It is intended to avoid the passing on of known genetic diseases that are linked to a particular sex. For example, a couple at risk of passing on Duchenne muscular dystrophy (which affects only boys) might try to have a girl.

Nonmedical Reasons

1. An individual or couple may prefer a child of a particular sex for social, religious, economic or personal reasons. Like Mary and Martin in Case 11.1, they might want to continue traditional farming practices.

2. An individual or couple might prefer a child of a particular sex in order to balance their families. Like Mary and Martin in Case 11.1, they might have all girls and want a boy.

The Legal Situation

Sex selection, for medical reasons, is permitted in many countries, such as the United Kingdom, the United States, Sweden, Spain, Italy, the Netherlands and Australia. However, selecting the sex of children for nonmedical reasons, such as those of Mary and Martin, is not. For example, India introduced an Act, in 1994, prohibiting nonmedical sex selection; the UK Human Fertilisation and Embryology Authority (HFEA 2003) decided, after wide consultation and public discussion, to ban the use of sex selection for nonmedical reasons; and the Council of Europe's Convention on Human Rights and Biomedicine (1997) provides, in Article 14, that:

> The use of techniques of medically assisted procreation shall not be allowed for the purpose of choosing a future child's sex, except where serious hereditary sex-related disease is to be avoided.

However, the debate about nonmedical sex selection is far from settled. It is possible that sperm sorting (if flow cytometry proves to be safe) or other similar procedures may become widely and easily available at relatively little expense from the many fertilisation clinics or individual doctors (at least in the United States) willing to invest in the equipment needed to carry out the procedure.

Those who are in favour of allowing individuals and couples to avail of nonmedical sex selection generally defend their view on the following grounds:

-   That sex selection is based on the right of individuals to make reproductive decisions without interference from the state
-   That there is no compelling evidence that sex selection (i.e. sperm sorting prior to conception) will harm anyone

We will consider the force of each of these claims in turn.

Sex Selection and Procreative Autonomy

The strongest argument in favour of sex selection is that, in enabling prospective parents to choose the sex of their child, it promotes procreative autonomy. Procreative autonomy is a broad term that contains the idea that prospective parents should be permitted to make autonomous decisions about whether, with whom, when, how, and how many children they bear. It is valued because the reproductive process is generally viewed as core to human meaning and identity.

In its general sense, procreative autonomy is widely accepted as a basic human right and it is protected by the Universal Declaration of Human Rights (United Nations 1948: Article 16) and the International Covenant of Civil and Political Rights (United Nations 1976: Article 23). Echoing the protection afforded procreation by the United Nations, the Council of Europe declares that, 'Men and women of marriageable age have the right to marry and to found a family' (Council of Europe 1950: Article 12).

The key problem for proponents of procreative autonomy is to determine its precise scope: how far does the right to choose extend? Does it, for example, protect only choices about whether or not to have children, or, does it also protect choices about the number of children to have? Or can it also include choices about the characteristics of children, such as their sex? To address the problem, proponents of procreative autonomy generally appeal to the **harm principle** as the measure of the scope of procreative autonomy.

Harm Principle

The harm principle stipulates that individual freedom can be limited only on the basis of harm to others.

It was articulated in his thesis on liberty by the philosopher, John Stuart Mill, in the following terms:

> [T]he only purpose for which power can be rightfully exercised over any member of a civilized community, against his will, is to prevent harm to others. (1981 [1859]: 68)

Applying the harm principle to procreative choice, John Robertson, who might be described as one of the architects of the liberty thesis in relation to reproduction, makes the following claim:

> Such a presumption [in favour of most personal reproductive choices] does not mean that reproductive choices are without consequence to others, nor that they should never be limited. Rather, it means that those who would limit procreative choice have the burden of showing that the reproductive actions at issue would create such substantial harm that they could justifiably be limited. (Robertson 1994: 24)

Such a standard, Robertson argues, can be used to decide on which prohibitions, limits and regulations are appropriate for different procreative activities.

Importantly, Robertson distinguishes between two kinds of harm: harm to individuals and harm to ideas about what is a good society ('personal conceptions of morality, right order, or offence' [Robertson 1994: 41]). For him, only the first kind of harm – substantial and measurable harm to individuals – can, justifiably, limit procreative freedom.

> To take procreative liberty seriously, then, is to allow it to have presumptive priority in an individual's life. This will give persons directly involved the final say about the use of a particular technology, unless tangible harm to the interests of others can be shown. (Robertson 1994: 41–2)

Using this understanding of the harm principle, Robertson argues that sex-selection techniques, such as sperm sorting, if safe, should be made available to couples, on the grounds that they are not likely to cause serious harm to any individuals.

Sex Selection and Harm
Robertson's defence of sex selection hangs on his claim that it is a means to fulfilling a reproductive choice that will not lead to tangible harm. In defending his claim, however, Robertson must address two possible sources of 'harm': that sex selection instrumentalises children and that it promotes sexist norms.

Sex Selection Instrumentalises Children
The first worry is that allowing parents to choose particular traits or characteristics for their offspring, such as their sex, profoundly disrespects the future child. It treats her as a product of parental design and values the child because she meets parental specifications, not because she is valuable in herself. In making any selection of this nature, parents are making assumptions based on preconceived notions about the characteristics and inherent worth of a particular sexed child. In effect, permitting sex selection, in this view, instrumentalises children. It runs counter to Immanual Kant's ethic of respect for human beings which argues that no person should ever be reduced to an object or solely a means for another person's use. Referring to children born with the help of assisted reproductive technology, a recent report of the US President's Council on Bioethics reflects this general concern:

> [W]e do not in normal procreation command their conception, control their makeup or rule over their development and birth. They are in an important sense 'given' to us. Though they are our children, they are not our property. [. . .] Though we may seek to have them for our own self-fulfilment, they exist also and especially for their own sakes. Though we seek to educate them, they are not like our other projects, determined strictly according to our plans and serving only our desires. (President's Council on Bioethics 2002: 5)

However, granted that the instrumentalisation of children is a concern, it could be argued that the worry that children will be used solely as a means to others' ends is exaggerated. If a child is conceived just to benefit another person, the child is wronged; she is treated as a means to another's end. However, a child might be considered as a means, but also, as a value, in herself.

What Kinds of Things are Good or Valuable?
In trying to understand what is meant when someone is concerned that a child is being 'instrumentalised', we might begin by asking, 'What kinds of things are good or valuable?' Two kinds of goods are often discussed in ethics:

1) Purely *intrinsic* goods, good or desirable in themselves, independently of what other goods they might lead to (of which joy or health are examples);

2) Purely *instrumental* goods, good because they promise to lead to other good things (of which sport and money are examples).

Notice that, depending on the context, health can be considered as both an intrinsic and an instrumental good. We seek to be healthy for its own sake, but also because being healthy enables us to do the things we like doing, such as surfing off the Kerry coast or hang-gliding in Connemara.

So, some goods have a *combined* value – they are both intrinsic and instrumental.

If we have children because we hope to have companionship or care in later years, or because they might be a source of income, or a bulwark against mortality, or because we want to replace a previous child who has died, are we instrumentalising them or wronging them, treating them simply as means to our ends? While wanting children for their own sake without conditions might be the ideal, it seems evident that women or couples have children for all kinds of reasons – and for no reason at all. What is important is that, whatever their motivation, parents act for the best interests of their children once they are born.

In sum, children are wronged if they are treated solely as a means to some other end. However, it is not, in principle, morally unacceptable to consider that children have both intrinsic *and* instrumental value.

Activity

Take the following list of 'goods': this book, the chair you are sitting on, your eyes, money, your nursing career, your love for a significant other.

Consider each of these and decide whether it is best described as an instrumental, an intrinsic or a combined good.

Sex Selection Promotes Sexist Norms

Leads to Sex Ratio Imbalances
A second worry in relation to sex selection is that it is inherently sexist and is likely further to entrench existing sexist social norms. It is anticipated that

in many societies its widespread availability will affect sex ratios because in any **patriarchal** (or male-dominated) society, son preference is almost inevitable. In many such societies, sons have greater earning power, remain in the family home, pass on the paternal name and inherit the family property. Daughters, on the other hand, earn less, often require dowries, leave their family of birth on marriage, and remain dependent on their husband and his family (Warren 1999). Because of cultural and social practices such as these, sex selection through prenatal diagnosis and pre-implantation genetic diagnosis have already been widely used to favour the birth of sons. In doing so, they have contributed to the devaluation of girl children and the continued inferior status of women in the countries where they have been used. In some rural provinces in China, for example, the birth rate is currently 144 males to 100 females (Robertson 2002: 42).

In response to worries about sex ratios, defenders of sex selection appeal to empirical research which suggests that, at least in some Western countries, there is no demonstrable pro-male bias in sex selection. The 1993 Royal Commission on New Reproductive Technologies in Canada reported, for example, that:

> contrary to what has been found in some other countries, a large majority of Canadians do not prefer children of one sex or the other. Many intervenors [. . .] assumed that Canadians have a pro-male bias with regard to family composition; we found that this assumption appears to be unfounded. (cited in Dickens 2002: 335)

Even if it were the case that sex ratios changed following on sex selection, one defender of sex selection, Bernard Dickens, takes a positive view of the implications for women:

> Son preference has produced, but might also mitigate, the sex-ratio imbalance. [. . .] While ominous for the present generation of children, these figures offer a promise of future redress. If sons wish, as adults, to have their own sons, they need wives. The dearth of prospective wives will, in perhaps a short time, enhance the social value of daughters, reversing their vulnerability and the force of male dominance. (Dickens 2002: 336)

In a similar vein, while Robertson acknowledges that sex ratio imbalances would be so serious a threat of harm as to justify limits on procreative liberty, he considers that concerns about possible imbalances can be addressed:

> If use patterns did produce drastic changes in sex ratios, self-correcting or regulatory mechanisms might come into play. For example, an over-abundance of males would mean fewer females to marry, which would make males less desirable, and provide incentives to increase the number of female births. Alternatively, laws or policies that required providers of PGS to select for males and females in equal numbers would prevent such imbalances. (Robertson 2001: 4)

However, the optimistic view of Dickens and Robertson that a smaller female population might prove advantageous to women in the longer run is not well-founded. At least some empirical studies of populations with sex ratio imbalances have shown that such societies are characterised by

> bride-price and bride-service, great importance attached to virginity, emphasis on the sanctity of the family [. . .] proscriptions against adultery [. . .] marriage at an early age, and [prejudice against] women [. . .] regarded as inferior to men [in] reasoned judgement, scholarship and political affairs. (Guttentag and Secord 1983: 79, cited in Madden 2002: 166)

More research needs to be done in this area but, as it stands, the indications are that the widespread availability of sex selection would have the effect of furthering the imbalance of power and ultimately benefiting men at the cost of women. Having said that, it is also fair to make clear that the cost – $2,500 at present – and the invasiveness of the procedure will deter most people in Western countries from availing of it.

Activity

Consider the report of the Canadian Commission on New Reproductive Technologies in 1993, which concluded that Canadian couples do not favour one particular sex over the other. From your experience of family life in Ireland, do you think that Irish individuals and couples are similarly neutral about the sex of their children?

Reinforces Sex and Gender Roles

Even if worries about unequal sex ratios turn out to be unfounded, or are successfully addressed, there remains the charge that sex selection reinforces existing sex and gender roles and that children whose sex is selected will be expected to behave in perceived sex-appropriate ways (Berkowitz 1999: 415–7). For example, a child might be encouraged to pursue only activities that are considered appropriate for their sex. Or a child who expresses interest in the activities usually associated with the opposite sex might not only disappoint his or her parent(s) but might be specifically prevented from engaging in such activities. In this way, sex selection may lead to a diminution of the autonomous choices of children.

Defenders of sex selection must determine whether or not these fears are baseless. Further, if they accept that sex selection could exacerbate existing sex and gender differences, they must determine whether or not this is harmful to anyone's interest. In short, will sex selection lead to trivial or tangible harm? Again, Robertson is optimistic. He appeals to nature and claims that the fact that there are biological differences between males and females means that it is morally acceptable to want to choose a child of a certain sex. Noting that there are different physiological characteristics, he also appeals to psychological research which indicates that boys and girls differ in a variety of domains such as aggression, activity, toy preference, psychopathology and spatial ability. He also relies on the authority of one feminist, Supreme Court Justice Ruth Bader Ginsburg, who claims that 'Physical differences between men and women [. . .] are enduring [. . .] "Inherent differences" between men and women, we have come to appreciate, remain cause for celebration' (cited in Robertson 2001: 6). In Robertson's view, it would not be sexist to select a female child because of a parental expectation that the experience of having and rearing a girl would be different from that of having a boy (Robertson 2001, 5).

Robertson's appeal to supposedly natural or inevitable physiological differences between males and females, combined with his description of *sex* selection as *gender* selection, indicates that he seems oblivious to the now widely accepted distinction between the meanings of sex and gender. This distinction is articulated by Simone de Beauvoir in the 1949 feminist classic, *The Second Sex*, in the words, 'One is not born, rather, one becomes a woman'. This claim draws attention to the fact that while there are physiological differences between males and females, the level of significance that is attributed to these differences is a socio-cultural matter (De Beauvoir 1997: 295). In this view, an individual may be born female, but she constitutes herself as a girl and as a woman in a specific cultural context, which both enables and limits the kind of woman it is possible for her to be.

Consider how Western women can now wear men's style of clothing with almost complete impunity, while a man cannot wear a dress on most occasions without suffering ridicule. This indicates the rigid boundaries of the male gender (as opposed to their sexual) role in the West. So, sex is not simply a natural feature of an individual human being. Humans may be (mostly) males and females as other animals are. However, the difference with humans makes all the difference. Humans are interpreters who 'move in a certain space of questions' and it is in this interpretative space that significance is attached to different natural features of the world such as sex (Taylor 1989: 34).

On the one hand, Robertson argues that we no longer simply have to accept the dictates of nature and that interfering with and trying to control nature is not always wrong. On the other hand, to defend sex selection, he relies heavily on an appeal to supposedly natural differences, the significance of which is the subject of much debate. What are natural sex differences between males and females and what are socially constituted differences between men and women cannot, in principle, be decided. Sex and gender are inextricably bound together.

CONCLUSION

This chapter has described some ethical concerns arising out of the development of processes to assist human reproduction. Specifically, we considered ethical arguments for and against the availability of the sex-selection method, sperm sorting, for nonmedical reasons. These arguments revolve around whether or not sperm sorting might result in harm.

As we have seen, some theorists argue that any restriction of parental autonomy needs to be justified on the basis of empirical evidence. Such

Activity

Take a few moments to consider the effects of gender expectations on the lives of human beings.

a) Make a list of the ways in which gender expectations enable or limit the lives of girls/women.

b) Make a list of the ways in which gender expectations enable or limit the lives of boys/men.

c) Given the concerns raised in relation to sex rations and sexist practices, do you think that sex selection should be made available for nonmedical reasons at the present time? After further research to assess its likely familial and social impact? Never?

Summary Learning Guide 11.1

Sperm sorting is a method that

- Provides a means to select the sex of future children;
- Is used prior to conception.

The reasons for choosing a child's sex include

- Medical reasons – to avoid transmitting sex-linked diseases;
- Nonmedical reasons – to meet social, religious, economic, personal or family-balancing needs.

Key arguments *in favour* of making sperm sorting available for nonmedical reasons:

- It enables parents to make autonomous procreative choices;
- It does not cause serious harm to any individuals.

Key arguments *against* making sperm sorting available:

- It instrumentalises children;
- It promotes sexist norms – i.e. leads to sex ratio imbalances and reinforces sex and gender roles

---

evidence must show that the exercise of procreative autonomy causes tangible harm to individuals. We considered two possible sources of harm – the instrumentalisation of children and the perpetuation of sexist norms. We concluded that the instrumentalisation of children need not lead to harm in all instances. However, we raised some concerns that sex selection might perpetuate sexist practices and thus restrict or harm the lives of both sexes, but, especially, the lives of girls and women.

The following terms are explained in the glossary:

donor insemination (DI)
embryo
embryo research
gender
in vitro fertilisation (IVF)

pre-implantation genetic diagnosis
    (PGD)
prenatal diagnosis
sex
stem-cell research

— 12 —

Surrogate Pregnancy

Objectives

At the end of this chapter, you should be able to:

- Define surrogacy and describe its legal status;
- Discuss surrogacy in relation to procreative autonomy and potential harm;
- Consider different motives for surrogacy: altruism and remuneration;
- Evaluate arguments for and against commercial surrogacy.

INTRODUCTION

Surrogacy is a form of assisted human reproduction that is best described as social rather than technological, because it addresses infertility through an arrangement between collaborating individuals: the activity of collaboration rather than technological intervention is central to its meaning. In surrogacy, also described as 'contract pregnancy', a woman undergoes pregnancy and childbirth in order to provide a child for another couple who might, otherwise, remain childless. The surrogate mother may or may not get money for this undertaking.

Surrogacy has become the focus of public debate in recent years, largely because of the way in which it challenges our conceptions of links between maternity and motherhood, reproduction, parenting and childrearing. While it is, currently, the subject of debate, however, one type of surrogate pregnancy has a long tradition stretching back to ancient times. The Bible gives a very old example:

> Abram's wife Sarai had borne him no child, but she had an Egyptian slave-girl called Hagar. So Sarai said to Abram, 'Listen now! Since Yahweh has kept me from having children, go to my slave girl. Perhaps I shall get children through her.' And Abram took Sarai's advice [. . .] And once [Hagar] knew she had conceived, her mistress counted for nothing in her eyes [. . .] Sarai accordingly treated her so badly that she ran away from her [. . .] Abram was eighty-six years old when Hagar bore him Ishmael. (*Jerusalem Bible* 1985)

As the Biblical case illustrates, surrogacy arrangements present a range of different ethical issues, such as concerns for the welfare of the surrogate mother and the future child. These issues have become even more complicated since advances in reproductive technology have added to the ways in which surrogate pregnancy is achieved. In the more recent traditional method, the surrogate mother is inseminated, usually artificially, with the sperm of the commissioning man. Today, however, surrogacy can take a number of different forms. For example, with the help of *in vitro* fertilisation (IVF), it is possible to implant an embryo in the surrogate mother that is created by the gametes of both members of the commissioning couple. In this case, the role of the surrogate mother is purely gestational, and the child is genetically related to both of the commissioning parents. In another situation, where the egg is donated, three women will mother the child in different ways: genetic, gestational and nurturing.

Just as our discussion on sex selection in Chapter 11 considered procreative autonomy and its limits, this chapter also touches on similar issues as they arise in relation to surrogacy. In addition, we consider the ethical tensions that can sometimes emerge in situations involving assisted human reproductive processes, between the personal beliefs of a nurse or midwife and her professional obligations.

Activity

Take a few minutes to jot down your present views on surrogacy. Do you think that it is an acceptable solution to the problem of infertility that some couples have to deal with? Do you think that surrogacy arrangements should be undertaken solely for altruistic reasons? Should commercial surrogacy be prohibited?

THE LEGAL SITUATION

Countries in Europe and states in America take varying legal approaches to surrogacy, or contract pregnancy, arrangements. They are completely prohibited in Germany, Austria, Sweden and Norway, while in France, Denmark and the Netherlands only payment in relation to surrogacy is prohibited. In the United Kingdom (UK), surrogacy is regulated and the payment of reasonable expenses is allowed. In most of the US states, surrogacy is regulated; for example, Arizona, Michigan, Utah and Washington consider it a criminal offence, while Florida and California permit it with conditions (MacCallum and Madden 2003: 66).

In any situation where a surrogate mother might decide to keep the child, or where a commissioning couple might decide to refuse the child once born, a court might have to determine who should be considered the legal mother of the child – the commissioning mother (the woman who contracts or commissions the child), the genetic mother (the woman who provides the egg), or the gestational mother (the woman who carries the child and gives birth). In most of the jurisdictions in Europe, the United States and Australia, courts and laws have held that the woman who gives birth to the child is the legal mother, irrespective of the presence, or lack, of any genetic relationship she might have with the child (MacCallum and Madden 2003: 67). For example, the UK law states:

> The woman who is carrying or has carried a child as a result of the placing in her of an embryo or of sperm and eggs, and no other woman, is to be treated as the mother of the child. (Human Fertilisation and Embryology Act 1990, Section 27, 1)

Surrogacy takes place in the absence of any legislative provisions or ethical guidelines in Belgium, Finland, Greece and Ireland.

If one believes that the gestational role of the carrying woman is fundamentally important, one might favour considering the gestational mother as the legal mother. One reason for taking this position is that she is the one who nurtures the foetus in her womb for nine months and then goes through the birthing process. In addition, if the child's welfare is considered, the gestational mother needs to look after the health and safety of the foetus she carries: she has the responsibility of knowing that her lifestyle and choices will have permanent effects on the developing child. The argument would be that if the genetic input of the commissioning parents is recognised because of its effects on the child, then the contribution of the gestational mother must also be recognised. What is at stake with regard to both genetic and gestational input is the degree to which each of these affects the development of the child. It might well be argued that, of the two, the gestational input is by far the most significant (Dooley, McCarthy, Garanis-Papadatos and Dalla-Vorgia 2003: 69).

Alternatively, one might favour the intent basis for determining maternity, rather than a presumption in favour of the gestational mother. This has been the conclusion of a court in California which declared, in one contested case, that without the intention of the commissioning couple, the child would never have come into existence. The court concluded that, 'She who intended to procreate the child – that is, she who intended to bring about the birth of a child that she intended to raise as her own – is the natural mother under Californian law'. (*Johnson* v. *Calvert* 1993, 782).

Activity

Assume that there are five contributing parents: genetic mother, genetic father, gestational mother, social/intentional mother, social/intentional father. Which do you think is the more 'valuable' or 'important' parent? Is one more of a 'parent' than others? Do deep-rooted assumptions about mothering and fathering as biological get pronounced here? Support your conclusion with reasons.

CHANGING RELATIONSHIPS

While surrogacy is not regulated in Ireland, the following case focuses attention on the ethical challenges a midwife faces when she must negotiate the changes in relationships that come about as a result of surrogacy.

One ethical challenge that arises in this situation is that the procreative autonomy of Teresa and Tom must be considered in the light of any potential harm to Julie and the future child. A second ethical concern that

---

Case 12.1: Conceiving Cousins

Anne Forde is a staff midwife working in St Helen's Maternity Hospital in Cork city. She met with Julie Murphy, a thirty-three-year-old mother of two, on her admission into hospital. Julie was 35 weeks pregnant and had been experiencing mild contractions for the previous twenty-four hours. On examination, all seemed well with Julie and her baby, and Julie's consultant was happy with her progress.

While Anne was taking Julie through the details of her birth plan, Julie's visitors, Teresa and Tom, arrived and seemed very anxious about her. When the couple left the room, Julie told Anne that Teresa was a cousin of hers. Anne had to compose herself quickly when Julie went on to say that she was pregnant with Teresa's husband's child. It seemed that Teresa was infertile and that Julie had agreed to become impregnated with Tom's sperm and to bear a child so that the couple could have a family. Julie asked that Anne be sensitive to this situation if she were present at the birth. In particular, she wanted to involve Teresa as much as she could in the event, and she intended to hand the baby over to Teresa as soon as possible after the child was born.

While Anne had read in the papers about surrogacy arrangements, she was shocked to be faced with Julie's situation. She completely disagreed with Julie's decision to act as a surrogate mother because she felt that it was flying in the face of nature and that what she had done was an insult to God's plan. Reassuring Julie that she had noted her concerns about the birth, she went immediately to the Director of Midwifery and asked to be assigned to another woman. She felt that she could not give appropriate midwifery care to Julie when her conscience told her that what Julie was doing was morally wrong.

---

arises is the conflict between the professional obligations and personal beliefs of the midwife, Anne. We will address each of these issues in turn.

Procreative Autonomy and Potential Harm

Given the shortage of children available for adoption and the difficulty of qualifying as adoptive parents, Teresa and Tom's arrangement seems to be the only hope for them to have and raise a family. At present, their freedom to have such a family is constrained by adoption laws and other state practices. For this couple, surrogacy seems to be the only means of realising a good which is considered profoundly important to many people – giving individuals the chance to be born and parents the chance to nurture children.

However, as we pointed out in Chapter 11, procreative autonomy is constrained by the harm principle which permits individual freedom only so long as it is not likely to result in specifiable and tangible harm to other persons. The question arises as to whether or not the exercise of parental autonomy in this case will lead to any harm to others.

One objection to surrogacy arrangements generally is based on a concern about the possible instrumentalisation of the surrogate mother and child. This concern appeals to the Kantian ethic of respect, which we explored in relation to sex selection. To recap, Kant argues that no person should ever be reduced to an object or thing for another person's use. The essence of this claim is that each person is as valuable as any other person and each of us has an absolute duty to respect all persons, including our own selves. To disrespect persons is to treat them as conditionally valuable things – that is, as instruments or tools with no value in and of themselves. When I treat someone as a mere means, I ignore or trivialise that person's fundamental interests in freedom and wellbeing, in order to secure my own interests. Similarly when I treat myself as a mere means, I show little or no regard for my own fundamental interests in freedom and wellbeing.

In Julie's case, a Kantian objection to the surrogacy arrangement might be that Teresa and Tom are treating both Julie and the child as instruments of their desire to parent. In this view, their interest in Julie's labour in pregnancy and birth is solely instrumental – its purpose is to satisfy their desires rather than for the end of giving life to a child. In addition, it could be objected that when Julie agrees to bear a child with the intention of giving over personal responsibility for it, she treats the child more like a thing than a person. This goes contrary to a deep value assumption that a gestating mother should desire the child for its own sake and not as a means to attaining some other end – for the sake of Teresa and Tom (Anderson 1993).

However, it could be argued that, in Julie's situation, the Kantian objection lacks force. Here, the surrogate mother is a very willing and informed participant in the arrangements; she already has two children of her own and can anticipate her level of emotional attachment during pregnancy and childbirth. She also has a birth plan and has indicated to the midwife what she wants to happen as soon as her child is born, so she seems prepared psychologically and emotionally to hand over the child to Teresa and Tom after the birth. Teresa and Tom also seem to be genuinely concerned for Julie and appear prepared for what is about to happen. Given that Teresa and Julie are cousins, it is likely that they have known each other for a long time and that their relationship will continue after the birth. The fact that they are related may strengthen the bonds between them and their future child. Julie's decision to become a surrogate mother is grounded in purely altruistic motives. It could be understood as a labour of love to enable Teresa and Tom to have a family.

Activity

a) Do you think that the Kantian inspired objections to surrogacy apply to the case of Julie, Teresa and Tom?

b) Do you think that the surrogacy arrangements described in this case will lead to any harm to the future child? If so, make a list of the kind of harms that you anticipate. Do you think that any of these potential harms is serious enough to prompt Julie, Tom and Teresa to re-evaluate the ethical acceptability of their decision?

Professional Obligation and Personal Beliefs

A further objection to Julie's decision – one that was voiced by the midwife, Anne – might appeal to the idea that it is an attempt to defy the 'laws of nature' where the laws of nature mean 'the appropriate methods for procreation', namely heterosexual intercourse between a woman who becomes the genetic, gestational and nurturing mother of the child and a man who becomes the genetic and nurturing father. Because of her beliefs about the laws of nature in the area of procreation, Anne has concluded that surrogacy arrangements are a threat to the institutions of marriage and the family, and she believes that she must conscientiously object to facilitating such arrangements.

It could be argued that objections of the kind that Anne has voiced sweep too broadly and would disallow even minor adjustments to physical processes. If the line between the 'natural' and 'artificial' separates moral from immoral practices, then adherents of 'natural laws' should also forbid intravenous feeding, insulin injections, pacemakers, and so on. The claim that we ought not to interfere with the 'laws of nature' by adjusting the 'natural or standard physiology of reproduction' seems unable to defend with good reasons where this is permissible and where it is not.

However, even if we grant that Anne's concerns are well founded, there is the further issue of whether or not she is justified in withdrawing her care of Julie and her child. In our discussion of conscience and conscientious objection in Chapter 9, we suggested that nurses and midwives are not free to withdraw their care from patients based on any and all kinds of conflict they might have between their own personal beliefs and the beliefs of patients in their care. If all kinds of conflict were permitted to dictate what health-care professionals do, we would anticipate that there would be far fewer carers available for those who are in need of them.

Activity

a) What do you think of the midwife's concern that surrogacy arrangements are unnatural and, therefore, morally unacceptable? Take a few moments to reflect on whether or not you think appeals to nature help us to distinguish between morally acceptable and unacceptable practices.

b) Reread the section on conscience and conscientious objection in Chapter 9 and decide whether or not Anne Forde is justified in withdrawing her care from Julie in this instance.

RECONCEIVING FAMILIES

While in Case 12.1, the surrogate mother, Julie, is bearing a child, for altruistic reasons, for a couple with whom she is closely related, the following case throws light on the ethical challenges that arise when the surrogacy is commercial and the collaborating parties are strangers. Case 12.2 concerns an Irish couple and their three children.

Case 12.2: In the Name of the Fathers

Are we ready for the issue of same-sex parenting? Politicians and others voiced their opinions on the issue earlier this month, after an Irish gay couple arrived home from California with their six-week-old triplets, two boys and a girl. The couple met the surrogate mother through a Californian *in vitro* fertilisation agency. [. . .] Acting on a tip-off from a member of the public, gardaí called to the couple's home shortly after their arrival from the US, to check the validity of the children's papers. The authorities are satisfied the babies were brought into the Republic legally. But then the tabloids swooped. The media were probably the last thing on the new family's minds as they bonded with each other. But the couple's refusal to speak to the press and their endeavours to protect the children's privacy augurs well for their welfare, as well as the couple's commitment to parenting.

Dr Mary Henry, the independent senator, and Gay Mitchell TD have both spoken publicly on the issue. Mitchell believes the couple's sexuality is not his 'immediate concern', but says the issue 'deserves reflection and calm consideration'. Dr Deirdre Madden, a law lecturer at University College Cork, says: 'If this were a straight couple, we'd concentrate more on surrogacy and not the sexuality of the parents'. Her opinion is shared by Kieran Rose, co-chairman of the Gay and Lesbian Equality Network. He predicts the public will support the couple. 'It doesn't matter about the sexual orientation. It's the quality of the parenting and their relationship with the children that count', he says.

(Ger Philpott, *The Irish Times*, 20 August 2001)

Case 12.2 is similar to Case 12.1 in a number of ways. Like Teresa and Tom, the gay couple here – let's call them Mike and John – must deal with the fact that there is a shortage of children available for adoption. Mike and John also have great difficulty qualifying as adoptive parents. Like the couple in the first case, Mike and John's arrangement with the agency in California (where, as we have indicated, the intending couple are the legally designated parents) seems to have been their only hope of realising a good which is considered profoundly important to many people – giving individuals the chance to be born, and parents the chance to nurture children.

Case 12.2 also differs from Case 12.1 in a number of ways, but the following are key:

1. It involves commercial surrogacy;
2. The commissioning parents are both men.

The question arises in relation to each of these differences: are they morally relevant differences? In other words, do these differences make the surrogacy arrangements in this case any more or less morally acceptable than the surrogacy arrangements in Case 12.1? We will take each question in turn.

Commercial Surrogacy
While women like Julie undergo pregnancy and childbirth mainly for altruistic motives – to help infertile couples – many surrogacy arrangements,

such as those of Mike and John, are commercial transactions, facilitated by fertility clinics or surrogacy agencies. One ethical concern that arises in relation to commercial surrogacy is that the commercial (as opposed to the altruistic) nature of the arrangements will lead to harm. Some argue that commercial surrogacy 'substitutes market norms for some of the norms of parental love' and that, as a result, children suffer (Anderson 1993: 171).

> In this practice [surrogacy] the mother deliberately conceives a child with the intention of giving it up for material advantage. Her renunciation of parental responsibilities is done not for the child's sake, but for her own [. . .] One can question whether the sale of children is as harmless as proponents contend. Would it be any wonder if a child born of a surrogacy arrangement feared resale by parents who treated the ties between a mother and her children as properly loosened by monetary incentive? (Anderson 1993: 171–2)

Along similar lines, the following extract from the UK Brazier Committee Review on Surrogacy argues that any form of payment beyond expenses has to be regarded as a form of 'child purchase':

> It was argued by a number of respondents to our questionnaire that surrogacy need not be equated with 'baby-selling', because any fee paid to the surrogate can be regarded as payment for the pregnancy, i.e., payment for her services, not the baby [. . .] It is unimaginable that a commissioning couple should enter into a contract that required simply that the surrogate become pregnant and give birth. The contract would have to contain a requirement that in return for the fee the child was handed over to those contracting the pregnancy, with penalties for failure to fulfil this aspect of the agreement. (Brazier Committee Review 1998: 34)

The Committee ultimately recommends that payments to surrogate mothers should cover only 'reasonable' expenses and that agencies involved in establishing surrogate pregnancies should be required to register with the Department of Health and conform to a Code of Practice it would draw up.

However, some proponents of surrogacy, such as the UK organisation, Childlessness Overcome Through Surrogacy (COTS), argue that surrogate mothers should be financially rewarded for their labour, and deny that such reward means that these women are selling their babies. Supporting this view, ethical theorist, Laura Purdy, makes the following claim:

> If 'selling babies' is not the right description of what is occurring, then how are we to explain what happens when the birth mother hands the child over to others? One plausible suggestion is that she is giving up her parental right to have a relationship with the child. That it is wrong to do this for pay remains to be shown. (Purdy 2000: 108)

Basically Purdy argues that, rather than selling her baby, the surrogate mother is making a biological service available. This biological undertaking earns her a parental right (as opposed to a property right) over the child which, Purdy argues, the woman ought to be free to exchange for financial gain. She concludes by rejecting the idea that surrogacy is only morally acceptable if it is undertaken for altruistic reasons:

> People seem to feel much less strongly about the wrongness of such acts [as surrogacy] when motivated by altruism; refusing compensation is the only acceptable proof of such altruism. The act is, in any case, socially valuable. Why then must it be motivated by altruistic considerations? We do not frown upon those who provide other socially valuable services even when they do not have the 'right' motive. Nor do we require them to be unpaid. For instance, no one expects physicians, no matter what their motivation, to work for beans. They provide an important service; their motivation is important only to the extent that it affects quality. In general, workers are required to have appropriate skills, not particular motivations. Once again, it seems that there is a different standard for women and for men. (Purdy 2000: 108)

In Purdy's view, what makes surrogacy ethically acceptable is its social value and, as such, the motives of those who make it possible are not, directly, ethically relevant. She argues that what is unique about surrogacy is not the fact that the surrogate mother relinquishes the child, but rather the fact that she undertakes pregnancy and labour in order to fulfil the deep desire of another person to have a parental relationship with a child. Purdy compares the surrogacy situation with other situations in which conception is achieved:

> Considering the sorts of reasons why parents have children, it is hard to see why the idea that one was conceived in order to provide a desperately-wanted child to another is thought to be problematic. One might well prefer that to the idea that one was an 'accident', adopted, born because contraception or abortion were not available, conceived to cement a failing marriage, to continue a family line, to qualify for welfare aid, to sex-balance a family, or as an experiment in child-rearing. Surely what matters for a child's well-being in the end is whether it is being raised in a loving, intelligent environment. (Purdy 2000: 108–9)

Activity

a) Consider Purdy's arguments for, and Anderson's and the Brazier Committee's arguments against, the payment of surrogate mothers. Decide which of these positions is closest to your own.

b) We have argued that one of the ways in which Case 12.2 differs from Case 12.1 is in the fact that it is a commercial arrangement. Having considered some of the ethical questions that arise in relation to commercial surrogacy, do you think that it is, more or less, morally acceptable than Case 12.1? Jot down the kind of surrogacy arrangements (if any) that you think should be permitted.

Summary Learning Guide 12.1

Arguments For Commercial Surrogacy (Purdy):

- It is a socially valuable arrangement that meets the deep desire of individuals to have parental relationships with children;
- It is a biological service, not baby-selling;
- A woman is being paid for her gestational services, as are other professionals involved in the conception and birth of the child;
- Reasons for having a child are not as important to the child's welfare as the conditions in which the child is raised.

Arguments Against Commercial Surrogacy (Anderson and Brazier Committee):

- It loosens the natural ties between mother and child through financial incentive;
- It is, effectively, 'baby-selling' because any surrogacy contract would stipulate payment, not just for pregnancy and birth, but also for the eventual handing over of the baby;
- It substitutes market norms for the norms of parental love;
- It might make children fear resale.

Activity

In this chapter, we have been mainly concerned with the impact of surrogacy arrangements on the welfare and wellbeing of children. Do you think there are grounds for concern that surrogacy arrangements might also harm the surrogate mother? Can you think of any ways in which she might be harmed?

Gay Parents

Both the journalist and the commentators in Case 12.2 suggest that the sexual orientation of parents is ethically irrelevant and that any ethical concerns that arise in relation to Mike and John's situation pertain to the particular surrogacy arrangements that they have entered into, rather than their sexual orientation. According to this view, there is no ethically relevant difference between the situation of Teresa and Tom and that of Mike and John.

However, it could be argued that their gay orientation, while not ethically relevant in itself, might affect the quality of Mike and John's parenting in adverse ways (Knight and Garcia 1994; Clarke 2001a). For example, it could be objected that

- Mike and John's children will lack a mother and a female role model;
- The children will have more developmental difficulties than their heterosexually raised peers in relation to such things as gender identity, sexual preference and self-esteem.

Mothering

As we indicated in Chapter 11, the processes of assisted human reproduction touch on experiences – child bearing and rearing – that are considered core to human meaning, identity and purpose. Certainly the existence of gay and lesbian families such as that of Mike and John challenge the traditional understanding of 'family', understood as established through heterosexual intercourse and procreation (McCallum and Madden 2003: 70–71). In addition, the idea that children might have two parents of the same sex forces a rethink of what it might mean to 'mother' and 'father', and uncouples these roles from their traditional association with woman and man.

Concern that children have the opportunity to develop strong relationships with adults of both genders is expressed in the UK Human Fertilisation and Embryology Act (1990) which regulates the services provided by fertility clinics in the UK. Section 13 of the Act stipulates that the clinics should consider the welfare of any children who might be born following on treatment, including the child's need for a father. By implication, the welfare of children born of surrogacy arrangements such as those of Mike and John would also include the need for a mother.

Activity

a) How would you interpret this condition? Does the Act require that clinics treat only those who can provide a biological or a psychological father (or mother)? If we accept that children should, ideally, have a mother, do you think that it is possible that another member of Mike and John's family or circle of friends could fulfil this role?

b) Jot down your understanding of the key characteristics of the activity of mothering. Do you think it is possible for a man to take on a motherly role with his children?

c) Jot down your understanding of the key characteristics of the activity of fathering. Do you think it is possible for a woman to take on a fatherly role with her children?

d) Can one person be both mother and father to their children?

DEVELOPING

The question of whether or not the children of gay and lesbian parents do any better or worse than their heterosexually raised peers, from a developmental point of view, can be determined, to some extent, by empirical research. However, the research that exists at present is neither sufficiently representative nor comprehensive enough to provide a definitive answer. There is need for more research, particularly longitudinal studies, across a range of different social groups, of the children of gay, lesbian and heterosexual families before any answer can be compelling (Patterson 1992).

However, granted the dearth of research, various reviews of existing empirical studies suggest that there are no significant differences between both kinds of families with regard to various measures of adjustment (Cramer 1986; Bigner and Bozett 1990; Gottman 1990; Green and Bozett 1991; Patterson 1992; Barrett 1994; and Clarke 2001b). For example, Cramer (1986) reports that parent sexual orientation does not play an important role in the child's sexual development nor their adoption of an 'appropriate' gender role identity. Also, Patterson (1992) concludes that children of lesbian and gay parents were not at any greater risk than children of heterosexual parents on many different variables, including development of gender identity, role behaviour, sexual preference, risk for abuse, mental health, relationships and intelligence.

Activity

Reflect on the suggestion that the 'ideal circumstances' for parenting are those in which parents of children are married, heterosexual and young. What is your response to this?

CONCLUSION

This chapter has focused attention on a very old method of assisting human reproduction: surrogacy. What is a common ethical concern in relation to all AHR procedures, including surrogacy, is a concern that they might result in harm. As we have seen, responding to this concern involves an investigation into what kind of harm might be at stake in relation to any particular process.

Applying the harm principle, delineated in Chapter 11, some would argue that those who want to restrict the procreative autonomy of parents such as Teresa and Tom or Mike and John need to support their claim with empirical evidence that tangible harm is likely to occur. As we have seen, there is much debate as to the possible harm that might follow on commercial surrogacy, and concerns raised in relation to the welfare of future children have prompted many jurisdictions to regulate such arrangements. We also briefly considered whether or not the sexual orientation of Mike and John might eventually harm their children, from a mothering and developmental point of view. Here, we discussed the fact that the (limited) empirical research available suggested that sexual orientation was not directly relevant to quality of parenting.

Finally, we want to acknowledge that the way in which surrogacy arrangements reconceptualise 'family' life might be disconcerting and worrying for some people. For them, the idea that we need be concerned about harm only when it directly involves particular individuals or groups is deeply unsatisfactory. They might well reject Robertson's (1994) distinction between two kinds of harm, delineated in Chapter 11. To recap, Robertson distinguishes between harm to individuals and harm to ideas about what is a good society, and he argues that only concern for the first kind of harm, substantial and measurable harm, can, justifiably, limit procreative freedom. However, there are many who would reject Robertson's account of harm. For them, harm to conceptions and beliefs about what is good is genuine harm which can ultimately result in very tangible harm to future generations.

Activity

Are such claims about future harm purely speculative? Are they prompted by fears of the unknown? Even if there is little or no evidence to support such claims, can you think of any reasons why they should be taken seriously?

Companying the Chronically Ill and Dying

INTRODUCTION

This is the first of two chapters on moral challenges for nurses, family and clinicians surrounding the care of the chronically ill and terminally ill. Specifically in this chapter, we focus on the ethical queries that arise when care or treatment decisions are needed for **non-competent** individuals. In efforts to make decisions that respect the non-competent patient as much as possible, family and health professionals are 'companying the dying'. Without the voice of the non-competent person, we nevertheless can strive to keep to the forefront a focus on their particular values and life story.

To concretise our discussion, we introduce a case known informally as 'The Ward Case', which came to public knowledge in Ireland in 1995. The tragic happening to this patient alerts us to the importance of questioning:

1. Our view of what it means to be a 'person';
2. How these views impact on our moral judgements;
3. What standards or criteria can be used to make decisions about non-competent patients in care.

POWERS OF MEDICAL TECHNOLOGY

Death and dying are inevitable realities in any human life. In the words of Elisabeth Kübler-Ross:

> Since the dawn of humankind, the human mind has pondered death, searching for the answer to its mysteries. The key to the question of death unlocks the door of life. (Kübler-Ross 1975: 1)

In times past, people died from minor illnesses because science had not yet developed medical cures. Today, an impressive range of medical therapies and life-support technologies offers not only amelioration of disease but, at times, a considerable extension of good quality of life. In *The Patient as Person*, Paul Ramsey asks about our moral obligations to sustain life:

> Must a terminal cancer patient be urged to undergo major surgery for the sake of a few months' palliation? What of fragmented creatures in deep and prolonged coma from severe brain damage, whose spontaneous cerebral activities have been reduced to those arising from the brainstem but who can be maintained 'alive' for years by a combination of artificial activators and by nourishment? Is there no end to the doctor's vocation to maintain life until the matter is taken out of his hands? (Ramsey 1970: 115)

The rhetoric of 'the tyranny of technology' derives from anxiety about the possibility of living one's final days intubated, oxygenated and medicated, with diminished capacities for human communication. In this chapter, we explore the ways in which death and dying challenge our moral emotions and moral intuitions. Nurses are confronted with the reality of dying in acute-care hospitals, hospices, and homes. Their experiences sharpen the impact of topics such as:

1. What we mean by dignity in dying;
2. What is morally required of us in using technology to extend living for profoundly ill patients.

Moral Obligations to Use Life-Saving Technologies

Read the following case study about a young woman we call Liz, who lived in a near persistent vegetative state (PVS) for twenty-three years. As you read, you may wish to write down your first thoughts, responses and questions about the case and compare these with your thoughts at the end of the chapter.

Case 13.1 The story of Liz: Living in PVS

The 'ward' was born on 27 January 1950. On 26 April 1972, Liz was twenty-two years old. She underwent a minor gynaecological operation under general anaesthetic. During the procedure, she suffered three cardiac arrests, resulting in anoxic brain damage of a very serious nature. From that time, Liz was completely dependent on others, requiring total nursing care. She was spastic as a result of the brain damage. Both arms and hands were contracted. Both legs and feet were extended. Her jaws were clenched, and, because she had a tendency to bite the insides of her cheeks and her tongue, her back teeth were capped to prevent the front teeth from fully closing. She could not swallow. She could not speak. She was incontinent.

In the first five or six months after the catastrophe, there were minimal signs of recovery which unfortunately did not continue but faded with passing years. For some 20 years, she was fed through nasogastric tube. The family requested that

---

extreme measures to support life be resisted. The health facility could not agree to this request. Subsequently the hospital asked the courts to make Liz a **ward of court**.

In later years, Liz seemed to find the nasogastric feeding distressing and, in April 1992, a gastrostomy tube replaced the nasogastric tube. This required administration of a general anaesthetic. The tube became detached in December 1993 and a new tube was inserted which came out the next day. This had to be reinserted again under general anaesthetic. Assuming that Liz was adequately furnished with nutrition and hydration (nourishment), her digestive system operated normally as did her bodily functions, although bowel movements required some assistance.

If she continued to be nourished by tube, she could live for many years. She might also die in the short term if she developed some infection such as pneumonia, unless it was treated with antibiotics. The hospital chose to use antibiotics.

Liz had provided no record of her preferences about her 'dying' while she was alive. She had discussed it informally. In early 1995, the mother as legal representative for her daughter asked the Court for permission to discontinue use of the gastrostomy feeding tube. (Based on *Re a Ward of Court* 1995)

This Irish case of 1995 brings into sharp relief a number of ethical questions and concepts that are highly **contested**. To say that questions are contested means that there is not consensus among the various stakeholders on pertinent value questions involved in this case. Some of the main differences of ethical viewpoint are explained and offered for your discussion in this chapter. This chapter specifically focuses on ethical questions concerning non-competent patients, such as Liz who is a PVS patient. Who speaks for them? Are there standards or methods for decision making? Is there any way we can read a narrative of their best interests even if they are silent?

In reflecting on the case of Liz, give special attention to the facts of the case, since clinical facts of a patient's diagnosis and prognosis are very relevant to moral judgements. Two facts in particular need clarification – one of a clinical nature and the other about the legal status of the young woman in this case. We put these two points in question form:

1.   What does the concept of 'ward' mean?
2.   What are the clinical realities of Liz's condition of PVS?

The Status of 'Ward'

The young woman anonymised as Liz in this case is known in Irish law as the Ward of Court. The case name is 'Re a Ward of Court' and was heard in 1995. A **wardship** is a legal facility to enable consent to be given on behalf of an adult who lacks mental capacity (Office of Wards of Court 2003). The patient was made a ward of court and, by 1994, her mother was named the Committee for the Ward. In the case of a wardship, where a very serious decision regarding treatment decisions is being considered, the request of the Committee (in this case, the mother) for the Ward must go to the High

Court (Donnelly 2002). After the young woman's anaesthetic accident which left her seriously brain-damaged, the Ward had no capacity or way of voicing her own views on her treatment. Because of her injury, the Ward lacked all competence. On 14 March 1995, the Committee and family went to the High Court and sought discontinuation of the abdominal feeding tube.

Activity

a) Based on your nursing experience, are you aware of patients who were made wards of court in recent times? If so, what were the reasons for requesting the wardship?

b) The 'ward' decision was applied in Ireland in the early 1970s because of disagreements between the family and health workers about what life-support measures should be provided for Liz. Give reasons why you think that the hospital and clinicians felt they had to resort to this legal solution.

c) What alternative approaches would you suggest for today that could help in a variety of situations to avoid litigation procedures?

CHARACTERISATION OF PVS CONDITION

Bryan Jennett is an internationally renowned expert on the PVS condition. He offers this description of Liz's life:

> These patients have suffered severe brain damage that has resulted in the cerebral cortex being out of action. Without the thinking, feeling and motivating part of the brain these patients are unconscious, in the sense that they make no responses that indicate any meaningful interaction with their surroundings, and remain unaware of themselves or their environment. They never obey a command, nor speak a single word. More primitive parts of the brain that are responsible for periodic wakefulness and for a wide range of reflex activities are still functioning, giving the paradox of a patient who is at times awake but always unaware. When open, the eyes roam around but do not fix or follow for long, while the spastic paralysed limbs never move voluntarily or purposefully. They can, however, withdraw by reflex from a painful stimulus that may provoke a grimace and a groan – but there is no evidence that pain or suffering is experienced. Occasional yawning, smiling, weeping and sometimes laughing can occur but these are unrelated to appropriate stimuli. Reflex swallowing, chewing and gagging occur and breathing is normal with no need for a ventilator. (Jennett in Keown 1995: 171)

The heart and lungs of the Irish 'Ward of Court' functioned normally. Care for the Ward was extensive. It was noted in the records of the court hearing on the Ward case, that the nursing care was second to none in providing for the needs of the Ward. Each day for 22 years, she was washed, groomed, talked to and turned by nurses. Nurses explained in court that special relationships developed with Liz over the years.

Tracking, Caring and Relationships

In their caring, nursing staff commented especially on the psychological impact of 'tracking' in the Ward. 'Tracking' is a reflex tendency to 'follow objects' which the patient does, with eyes wide open; PVS patients follow sources of noises with their eyes and move their head to follow such noises or other bodily movements in and out of the room. According to the research on PVS, such 'tracking' activity by patients is without cognitive significance or meaning but is rather a reflex reaction (Jennett 2002).

Some of the nurses were emotionally moved by the 'tracking' because it seemed to them that the Ward was clearly aware of different staff coming on duty rotations. This 'tracking' feature of PVS patients can contribute to a sense of presence of the suffering individual and sometimes increases a kind of emotional bond with some of the health-care staff. Because of the time spent caring for multiple needs of PVS or comatose patients, health-care workers, and nurses in particular, can form a close emotional and caring relationship with the patient. In these circumstances, clinically speaking, there can be no 'conversation' from a patient in the condition of the Ward.

The 'relationship' with the young woman developed as staff responded to Liz's daily needs. It was her higher cortex that was thoroughly damaged. Her brainstem functioned and allowed her to breathe on her own. Her capacity to breathe on her own without ventilator assistance added to the felt presence of a human being who seemed responsive to changing nurse schedules.

The care relationship developed between nurses and the Ward over months – for some nurses, over years. Grimaces by the Ward added to the perception of significance and meaning and were interpreted by some as responses to different health-care staff. This emotional response of nurses and other carers to the Ward was relevant to nursing staff's moral response to the case decision. Nurses testified to their experience of Liz tracking them in and out of the room, seeming to grimace when some nurses arrived or smile when others appeared. It was largely nurses' testimony in court that brought a compromise change to the diagnosis to read: 'Near PVS'.

The role of human emotions of carers is not trivial in the nurse's evaluation of a patient. But it is not an easy inference to make from our emotional responses to any clear moral position. Emotions can signal strong revulsion, doubt, anxiety, fear or attraction to situations. This important question of how emotions relate to morality is developed in Chapter 18 where Traditional Moral Theories are explained (See Scott 2000).

High Court and Supreme Court Decisions 1995

The High Court case legally allowed the family to take their loved one to an alternative site for care. In 1995, the High Court and, on appeal, the Supreme Court in Ireland consented to the following:

1. It would be lawful to remove the feeding tube.
2. Cessation of treatment of infections or other conditions that might affect the Ward *unless* such treatments were believed necessary for palliative relief.
3. Out of respect for the ethical and religious perspectives of the hospice where the Ward was cared for at the time of the legal case, the Courts asked that the young woman be moved to a venue which did not have ethical objections to removing the feeding tube.

The family took the Ward to her family home in Dublin. Volunteer nurses and doctors assisted in removing the feeding tubes and giving comfort care. The woman died on 20 September 1995. The prayer card for the funeral reads as follows:

> **Ward's Name**
>
> 27 January 1950 – 26 April 1972 – 20 September 1995

Activity

Take a few moments to write down what you think the family wanted to convey by the prayer card.

a) What does the card suggest happened in 1972? And in 1995?

b) Compare your interpretations of the prayer card with those of your colleagues. If there are differing positions, try to get clear what is at the basis of the different interpretations.

A FAMILY'S NARRATIVE IN COMPANYING THEIR LOVED ONE

One interpretation of the prayer card is that the family felt that their loved one had died as a person in 1972 when the medical accident occurred and severe brain damage ensued. In 1995, the Ward also 'died in some sense', recognisable in medicine and law. She was then given a memorial ceremony. But can someone die twice? Do they die in two different senses? Let's look at one author who would say yes, an individual human might die twice: once as a 'person' and then in their 'bodily being'.

The family of the Ward had watched her day in and day out for over twenty years. Her mother explained that she knew that her daughter would never 'return', never be conscious and aware of who her family was, of who she herself was. As the mother realised that she was growing older with each passing year, she knew that a motherly responsibility urged her to stop a ceaseless 'life' that was not 'living'. It was only non-reflective, non-cognitional biological life – a life her daughter had said in various discussions that she would never wish to endure. The mother and siblings of the Ward felt confident that were their loved one able to voice her heart's hopes, she would ask please to be allowed to die naturally and, should she arrest or get an infection, that she would want not be rescued by any life-saving options, CPR or antibiotics. The prayer card is symbolic of many of the conversations had during those two decades of 'companying their daughter' in her silent state.

Biological and Biographical Life

> There is a deep difference between having a life and merely being alive. Being alive, in a **biological sense**, is [on its own] relatively unimportant. One's **biographical life**, by contrast, is immensely important; it is the sum of one's aspirations, decisions, activities, projects, and human relationships. In deciding questions of life and death, the crucial question is: Is a life, in the biographical sense, being destroyed or otherwise adversely affected? The concept of life is ambiguous in this way and so is the concept of the sanctity of life.
>
> The doctrine of the sanctity of life can be understood as placing value on things that are alive [only in the biological sense]. But it can also be understood as placing value on 'lives' and on the interests that some creatures, including ourselves, have in virtue of the fact that they are the subjects of lives. Very different moral views will result, depending on which interpretation one chooses . . . The sanctity of life ought to be interpreted as protecting lives in the biographical sense, and not merely in the biological sense. (Rachels 1986: 24–7)

James Rachels offers a distinction that suggests one interpretation of the prayer card for the Ward. The distinction is between an individual's **biological life** and their **biographical life**. Rachels claims that the concept of 'life' is ambiguous because included in that one term, 'life', are two meanings: 'biological life' and 'biographical life'. We have biology and biography.

Rachels would argue that an individual in the PVS condition lacks biographical life. Liz is no longer able to communicate, to choose, to have active interests, make plans and enter into relationships. In Rachels' account, the Ward is only biologically alive. But mere bodily existence without mental/affective functions is not sufficient to say that someone is a 'person'. So Rachels' view insists on the essential feature of awareness and consciousness in defining what it means to be a person.

Activity

a) Consider the consequences of Rachels' definition of what it means to be a 'person'. In what ways might his understanding impact on health-care decisions?

b) How is Rachels' distinction between 'having a life' and 'being alive' applicable to Liz? Is Liz alive biologically or biographically or both?

c) Using Rachels' distinction, how would you apply it to the family's recorded dates on the prayer card?

In reflecting on the ethics of dying patients and health-care obligations towards them, you will notice that writers offer different views about:

- What it means to be a person, and
- What it means to respect the dignity of persons in decisions about their dying – this most poignantly when, like Liz, they cannot participate in these decisions as competent patients.

Diminished Persons: An Alternative View

Read the following text from John Finnis who thinks that no matter how damaged the human being is, we should not separate body *and* biography in defining what it means to be 'person'. As you read, consider why Finnis thinks that this holistic idea of 'person' is so important to insist upon when describing a patient with PVS.

[1]   A being that once has human (and thus personal) life will remain a human person while that life (the dynamic principle for that being's integrated organic functioning) remains – i.e., until death. Where one's brain has not yet developed, or has been so damaged as to impair or even destroy one's capacity for intellectual acts, one is an immature or damaged human person. . .

[2]   In short, human bodily life is the life of a person and has the dignity of the person. Every human being is equal precisely in having that human life which is also humanity and personhood, and thus that dignity and intrinsic value. Human bodily life is not mere habitation, platform or instrument for the human person or spirit. Bodily life, therefore, is not merely an instrumental good. It is an intrinsic and basic human good.

[3]   In sustaining human bodily life, in howsoever an impaired condition, one is sustaining the person whose life it is. In the life of the person in an irreversible coma or irreversibly persistent vegetative state, the good of human life is really but very inadequately instantiated.

[4]   To preserve human solidarity with such people, and to respect rather than violate the one good in which they still participate – bodily life bereft of participation in other human goods such as knowledge and friendship – the care to be provided to them need not, I think be more than is provided to anyone and everyone for whom one has any respect and responsibility: the food, water and cleaning that one can provide at home (Finnis in Keown 1995: 31–3).

We have divided this text into four parts for your reflection since the author introduces a number of claims in the text to clarify the importance of this idea of 'person'. Finnis believes this discussion is not just about a concept. How we define 'person' has moral consequences for decision making.

The Finnis view of persons insists that both 'body' and 'biography' continue throughout one's life *even if* one is in a persistent vegetative state. Finnis interprets Rachels' position as a dualist view. A **dualist** view has a view of person that separates the individual's body-being from their mental, affective and spiritual existence but claims priority of value to the mental and affective. Thus, when mental capacities are irreversibly damaged, the body remains but no person.

Finnis rejects this dualism in favour of a holism that claims a PVS patient may lack consciousness and awareness but, in their diminished human condition, they should still be viewed as persons.

Activity

Reflect on Rachels and Finnis and try to clarify their differences especially regarding the notion of 'person'. As you focus on John Finnis's statement, consider the following:

a) Why does Finnis think that the Ward is still a 'person' even though she suffered the loss of all her cognitive and affective capacities?

b) From the passage above, what would Finnis concretely recommend about the continuation of gastrostomy feeding? Would he think it is morally required 'care' for a patient such as the Ward?

c) What does Finnis' idea of 'human solidarity' mean for you as a nurse who perhaps spends time in the company of the dying or unconscious?

THE MORAL SIGNIFICANCE OF 'PERSON' TALK

Let's briefly review the discussion on 'person'. Drawing the boundaries of what it means to be a 'person' may seem like semantic game-playing, but the task of spelling out criteria for 'being a person' has occupied moralists for centuries, because how you draw the boundaries around 'personhood' may have consequences concerning how we should behave towards non-persons. Some exploration stories narrate discovering indigenous peoples who looked, spoke and acted so differently from 'white explorers' that they thought they were not at all persons and perhaps not even human. We can almost hear an exclamation to the effect: 'They're not persons! So we can eat them or sacrifice them to the gods!' The caution about the value connotations of 'person' offers a note of vigilance for you to be alert to the fact that, in ethics, discussion about the concept of 'person' is not just a mental game of semantics.

Authors differ in their views about the consequences of calling someone a person or not. If someone can 'cease being a person', then one of the difficulties we face is where to draw the line in marking person features. What has to happen to someone for them to cease to be a person? How brain-damaged or dysfunctional does someone have to be to lose their personhood?

Authors like John Finnis voice concern that withholding the category of person because of severe brain damage or congenital diminution might make us less careful in according dignity or moral valuing of that individual (see also Iglesias 1995). Even if a patient is comatose or PVS, there is still moral expectation to try, to the best of our ability, to foster their wellbeing and protect the autonomy they once experienced. But how do we try to respect the previous autonomy of non-competent patients?

How you understood what it means to be a 'person' impacts on many areas of your life: professional and personal. You've read two philosophers here speak of their understanding of what 'person' means.

Summary Learning Guide 13.1

The view of James Rachels on the meaning of 'person' claims:

- That the body or one's **biology** is important but you are not a person if you have only biology or body;
- That to be a person, one must currently have the capacity for aspirations, projects and human relationships;
- That these capacities define one's **biographical life**;
- That the doctrine of the **sanctity of life** is wrong if it values biological life in the absence of biographical life.

John Finnis disagrees with James Rachels and offers the alternative view:

- Once a human being has a personal life (body and biography), that being remains a human person while the body functions;
- The PVS patient or the brain-damaged individual without any mental capacity is nevertheless an immature, damaged human person;
- There is 'moral' significance and there are moral consequences in one's understanding of person;
- The body too is an intrinsic, basic good not merely an instrument for mind;
- In sustaining human bodily life, one is sustaining a person, in whatever diminished state, through illness.

Incompetent Patients: Protecting Autonomy and Wellbeing

In Chapter 1, you read about respect for autonomy as a central value in ethical theory of recent decades. A substantial consensus is current that health-care decision making must recognise the centrality of respect for such autonomy. However, when a patient is not competent, as in the case of Liz, we need to look for criteria for decision making.

THREE SURROGATE DECISION STANDARDS

There are three main decision standards we want to discuss here:

- Best-Interests Standard
- Substituted Judgement
- Advance Directives: Transferred Autonomy.

Best-Interests Standard

Reflect on one element of what Justice Lynch said in delivering his judgement in the High Court of Ireland on 5 May 1995. Lynch appeals to what is called the **best interests test** in deciding how to respect the human dignity of the Ward. The 'best-interests' standard is designed to protect the wellbeing of the patient who is lacking all capacity for competent decision making.

> I take the view that the proper and most satisfactory test to be applied by the Court in this case is the **best interests test**, i.e., whether it is in the best interests of the Ward that her life, such as it is at present, should be prolonged by the continuation of the abnormal artificial means of nourishment or whether she should be allowed to slip away naturally by the withdrawal of such abnormal artificial means. According to the evidence given, this would happen within two weeks or so and without pain or distress. (High Court Judgement, 'Re a Ward of Court' 1995)

This approach for decision making appeals mainly to the principle of **beneficence.** The 'best-interests standard' is generally used with individuals who:

1. Have always been incompetent, or
2. Have been rendered non-competent by virtue of trauma or illness, and
3. In cases where no suitable surrogate can be found for a patient.

Applying the best-interests standard in the Ward of Court case allowed Justice Lynch to argue that continued use of ANH (artificial nutrition and hydration) was both ineffective in improving the young woman's condition and excessive given the condition of the Ward (Tomkin and McAuley 1995: 48).

The best-interests standard has an objective component and a subjective component. The standard requires an objective analysis and careful calculation of the harms and benefits that the use of different treatments might involve or, alternatively, the harms and benefits that withholding of treatments would involve. One way to ensure that a decision is as 'objective' as possible is to ask if it is one that the most reasonable persons would choose for themselves in similar circumstances. If we appeal to 'reasonable persons' preferences, this can be especially difficult when reasonable persons can and do disagree about the choice.

However, in making the judgement of 'best interests', we also see a judgement about quality of life that unavoidably utilises the subjective perspective of the decision maker. This subjective perspective is always with reference to the particular features of the patient's condition and likely prognosis.

Substituted Judgement

Another surrogate decision method used in the Ward case and thought better to value the known wishes of the patient is **substituted judgement**. One passage from Justice Lynch shows an appeal to substituted judgement:

While the best interests of the Ward is the acid test, I think that I can take into account what would be her own wishes if she could be granted a momentary lucid and articulate period in which to express them . . . I think it is highly probable, and I find the evidence of the family on this aspect of the case to be clear and convincing that the Ward would choose to refuse the continuance of the present regime to which she is subjected. (High Court Judgement, 'Re a Ward of Court' 1995)

The young woman did not have documented preferences or goals in relation to medical treatment, so the **substituted judgement** standard was applied. The substituted judgement standard involves a decision about accepting or refusing treatment in a way that is consistent with what the patient would decide if they were competent. To achieve this, the substituted judgement must be made by someone (or some persons) who knew the patient and shared an understanding of their personal values. In the Ward case of Liz, the 'evidence of the family' was taken into account. In conversations at home and with friends, Liz had said that she would never wish to live in a permanently non-aware state. In brief, the substituted judgement approach is helpful on two counts:

- In helping to arrive at decisions that are more in accordance with the patient's wishes;
- In making the psychological and emotional burdens easier for surrogates to carry and in facilitating their effective participation in decision making.

The goal in using this standard is to achieve, as accurately and sensitively as one can, a decision about how to proceed – a decision that is focussed on the particular patient of concern.

Narrative Model and Holistic Focus

This holistic focus is part of a **narrative model** of care. One begins by considering the life story of the patient and then tries to evaluate a particular option (life support or therapy) in terms of its 'fit' with the rest of the patient's life narrative. The **narrative model** relies on the idea that a person creates her or his sense of self or personal identity through their life story and journey of choices. In this view, the surrogate attempts to continue the story of the patient in a way that coheres with the patient's self-conception thus far. A nurse in conversation with the family of a PVS patient might elicit a substituted judgement from the mother of the patient by asking NOT: 'What do you now want us to do for your daughter?' but rather: 'You, of course, knew your daughter better than I did, so help us decide together what she would have wanted done for her now.' This approach to the right question allows the surrogate to sense that the decision will reflect the life story and values of their loved one rather than be a simple application of another's preferences (McCarthy 2001).

Summary Learning Guide 13.2

The Substituted Judgement is a surrogate decision method that had the following features when applied in the case of Liz:

- It is not an abstract standard but focuses on understanding and interpreting beliefs of a particular patient who is non-competent;
- It helps in the making of health-care decisions for a non-competent patient when no explicit statement is available from the once-competent patient;
- It facilitates making of treatment or life-support choices that are respectful of what the patient would decide if they were competent;
- It assumes the trustworthy evidence of spokespersons who have knowledge of the beliefs and values of the patient.

Advance Directives and Powers of Attorney

One method of trying to protect the autonomy of individuals is to provide for **advance directives (ADs)**. Such directives have been in use in North America for over twenty-five years and in Europe for many years. An **advance directive** is a document that enables a competent person to make decisions about his or her medical treatment in the event that they become incompetent and, therefore, lose the capacity to make decisions.

There are mainly two kinds of advance directive that are *more explicit* than the informal method of substituted judgement: **living wills** and a **durable power of attorney**:

1) A living will is a written directive that states the types of treatment an individual would wish to receive or forgo in specified circumstances of illness or degeneration. The AD document is a means to promote the ability of patients to determine the medical treatment they will have at the end of their lives – at a point where they would not be able to voice their preferences. Often the document refers to the withholding or withdrawing of life-sustaining procedures in the event of a terminal condition. Some persons, such as the Jehovah's Witnesses might, for religious reasons, specify a refusal of transfusions and a request for alternatives to blood products. (For sample ADs, see Appendix 3).

2) A **durable power of attorney (DPOA)** for health care refers to a person who is legally designated by an individual to make decisions on behalf of that person when they cannot choose for themselves. Some individuals draw up advance directives that combine living wills and also naming someone trusted as a durable power of attorney (DPOA). The DPOA can assist very much by helping to interpret the living will on the basis of knowing the patient. This would be important if differences of interpretation were to arise about the living will.

Notice the values that support or justify Advance Directives. They are narrative instruments or tools that facilitate the inclusion of the patient and the family in the process of decision making at the end of life. ADs are supported socially and through legislation in countries where patient autonomy and the principle of informed consent are privileged over medical paternalism. The Irish Powers of Attorney Act 1996 in Ireland permits a person to appoint another as decision maker in the event of that person becoming incompetent. However, it is noteworthy that the 1996 Act intentionally omits health-care decisions of the kind discussed here in the Ward case.

Activity

Compare your responses to these questions with those of your colleagues and friends and see whether your views diverge much from theirs.

a) Why, do you think, are there very few people drawing up Advance Directives in Ireland?

b) Have you met with cases in your nursing practice where a patient had a living will or AD? How was it made known? By the patient or family?

c) Why do you suppose the Powers of Attorney Act, 1996, intentionally omits serious health-care decisions from its application?

d) Would you consider having an AD for yourself?

PROBLEMS OF INTERPRETATION OF ADVANCE DIRECTIVES

There are some problems of interpretation of advance directives and not all writers are persuaded of their value. Consider the following questions and challenges about ADs as instruments for facilitating respect for individual autonomy:

1. ADs contain judgements about situations in the future that one cannot really know.
2. Persons might be denying themselves the benefit of medical advances.
3. Is the individual who is no longer competent the 'same person' as the one who made out the AD?
4. How can a former wish be balanced against the pleasures that a person might experience while in a state of incompetence? The case of an Alzheimer's patient is an example.

Some critics think that rather than solving problems of protecting autonomy, ADs actually introduce difficult new ones of interpretation. Some clinicians also prefer not to be constrained in their medical decision making by documents of the once-competent patient. The questions remain for you to consider: Why have ADs not been a subject of public discussion and debate in Ireland? Is our health-care system sufficiently different from other countries in North America and Continental Europe to explain why the option is not legally recognised in Ireland?

CONCLUSION

In this chapter, we focused on the moral questions that challenge us with cases of non-competent severely brain-damaged patients who were once fully competent. The Irish story of Liz in 'Re a Ward of Court', whose condition and consistent care allowed her to survive without consciousness for twenty-three years, raised a cluster of serious moral issues. We focused in on two main ideas that will be necessary in proceeding to Chapter 14.

Firstly, the texts of James Rachels and John Finnis opened up the question of what it means to be a 'person'. These texts help us to tease out our beliefs about what *we* mean by 'person' and whether it makes any difference! If you take Finnis and Rachels seriously, it seems that the task of probing meanings of 'person' is not just an academic exercise about words. Rather, such understandings of 'person' might have consequences for human living and dying.

The second idea in focus here looked at three main surrogate decision standards used in adjudicating how health-care professionals can best make decisions of care for non-competent patients: best interests; substituted judgement; and Advance Directives.

The following terms are explained in the glossary:

advance directive
best-interest standard
biological v biographical life
contested concepts
dualist
durable power of attorney

narrative model of ethics
person
PVS (persistent vegetative state)
substituted judgement
surrogate decision standards
ward of court

– 14 –

Falling Down the Slippery Slope

Objectives

At the end of this chapter, you should be able to:

- Discuss moral differences between withholding and withdrawing treatments;
- Analyse the **principle of proportionality** and how it applies to decisions on prolonging life;
- Offer your evaluation of who should participate in end-of-life decisions;
- Argue the pros and cons of a requirement to provide feeding;
- Explain and evaluate the challenges of the **slippery slope**.

This chapter continues discussion on the ethics of decisions at the end of life. Here we take a closer look at the question of what principles and moral values support non-use of life-saving therapies. How does the patient give their voice to such decision making?

The power of medical technology today has produced profound ethical challenges. The Ward case of a non-competent patient is carried forward for analysis applying the moral principles of decision making offered for discussion and critique. The moral principles included in this chapter cover a range of patients: non-competent and competent. With that in mind, we also offer here the case of Katherine who is competent but wishes to be allowed to forego further use of life supports and to die. Unlike Liz in the Ward case, Katherine's voice is concretely present and audible. What do justice, beneficence, compassion and respect for autonomy require?

Case 14.1: When a Competent Person Refuses Treatment

Katherine Lewis is an intelligent, single, forty-year-old woman suffering from Guillain Barre's syndrome, a painful neurological illness that leaves its sufferers paralysed for unpredictable lengths of time. Many people recover from the syndrome more or less completely and live long, relatively healthy, lives. However, Katherine has been paralysed for three years. Ten months ago, it was recognised that she was unlikely to be able to move or breathe on her own again because of the extent of damage to her nerves and muscles; she now needs a ventilator to help her to breathe. As the nurse in the neurological unit, you and the clinician explained this to Katherine in a gentle but clear manner.

> Last week, Katherine asked to speak with you privately. A relationship of trust had developed between yourself and Katherine and she had confided in you earlier about her pain and realisation that it was difficult to get adequate pain control. You suggested that she speak with Dr O'Shaughnessy from the nearby hospice who has helped many patients with pain relief, comfort and understanding.
>
> Nevertheless, Katherine tells you that she has considered her options and decided that she no longer wants to live. She reminds the staff that she had drawn up an Advance Directive some ten years earlier and says that her wishes there should be seen as her values that she still holds. She tells you that her life holds no value for her if it means being in constant pain and without the freedom to move or even breathe on her own. She also tells you that she has discussed this with her family and they have accepted her wishes to have the ventilator removed.

The cases of Katherine and Liz (Ward of Court) raise moral questions about justifications for *withdrawing* treatments. In health care, there are circumstances where treatments are withheld – not started – and treatments which, once begun, are discontinued. The right of competent patients to forgo life-sustaining treatments is generally accepted by ethicists under respect for autonomy (see Chapter 1). This respect for patient autonomy does not diminish even when the likely result of withholding or withdrawing treatment is the patient's death. Even so, it is true that psychologically it may prove stressful or cause unease for health-care professionals to respect the patient's autonomy, especially if death follows their choice.

Unlike Liz in the previous chapter, Katherine Lewis seems competent and autonomous in every substantive sense explained in Chapter 1. Given Katherine's clarity and competence, should her request perhaps be granted and let that be the end of it?

Activity

a) Even if Katherine is competent, given the seriousness of this request, would you consider her request as uncomplicated and to be respected without further discussion?

b) Explain what quality of information and understanding you would provide for Katherine considering her request. Since she has approached you about this desire of hers to discontinue all treatments, what kind of conversation would you have with her?

c) Who should participate in this decision? Hospice? Entire clinical team? The ethics committee of the hospital? Any others omitted here? Why would you argue for certain participants?

SUGGESTED GUIDELINES: DECISION PRINCIPLES AND PRACTICE

Difficult decisions often have to be made: should treatment begin? How long should treatment continue? And, on what basis should we conclude that a particular treatment should be discontinued? These questions are more difficult if the patient is a minor or, as in Liz's case, is not competent, or has not given explicit voice (by way of Advance Directives or Durable Power of Attorney) for their preferences.

In Ireland, the numbers who have made advance directives is unknown and, to date, only one case has come before the Irish courts in relation to them (*JM* v. *Board of Management of St Vincent's Hospital*, 2003). The use of ADs in Ireland has not yet been publicly debated and it not widely encouraged or facilitated in the health-care setting. In addition, where consultation with the patient or family is not common procedure, it is often hospital practice to have consultants responsible for issuing DNRs ('Do not resuscitate' orders) but without always looking for consent from competent patients or without consultation with families (Sheikh 2001).

While nurses do not issue DNR orders, they are often given the responsibility to carry out DNR orders. Nurses are familiar with being told to 'walk slowly' if a patient should have cardiac arrest even though they have not witnessed a signed DNR order by a clinician. There are ongoing efforts among nurses and clinicians to try to spell out some guidelines on the process of decision making near dying. Consider the following such guidelines from UK health-care colleagues. They come from the British Medical Association, the Resuscitation Council (UK) and the Royal College of Nursing (2001):

Principles:
- Timely support for patients and people close to them, and effective, sensitive communication are essential.
- Decisions must be based on the individual patient's circumstances and reviewed regularly.
- Sensitive advance discussion should always be encouraged, but not forced.
- Information about Cardiopulmonary Resuscitation (CPR) and the chances of a successful outcome need to be realistic.

Practical Matters:
- Information about CPR policies should be displayed for patients and staff.
- Leaflets should be available for patients and people close to them explaining about CPR, how decisions are made and their involvement in decisions.
- Decisions about attempting CPR must be communicated effectively to relevant health professionals.

In Emergencies:
- If no advance decision has been made or is known, CPR should be attempted unless:
  a) The patient has refused CPR;
  b) The patient is clearly in the terminal phase of illness; or
  c) The burdens of the treatment outweigh the benefits (Sheikh 2001: 7).

Activity

Consider these values from the Joint Statement 2001 and see if they are applicable in the Irish health-care context.

a) Does discussion or publicity about CPR frighten patients needlessly? Do patients need to know these principles and policies as part of an acute-care or hospice setting?

b) As a health-care professional, would it help you if you knew clearly what the policies about CPR are in your workplace? Have problems arisen because you did not know?

c) Based on your experience, would these guidelines be positively welcomed in Ireland? In many diverse cultures? (Rumbold 1999: 27–45).

STARTING AND STOPPING TREATMENTS: A MORAL DIFFERENCE?

If you decide that a certain treatment or life support like CPR should not be used or should not be further administered for a particular patient, on what basis do you do this? Doctors and nurses sometimes claim they are morally very uneasy about stopping a treatment that has already been started because doing so seems to them to count as 'killing' the patient. In contrast, not starting a treatment or therapy seems more acceptable, apparently because it involves an omission rather than an action. Based on your own nursing experience, consider the following position given on withholding versus withdrawing treatment:

> If we adopt the view that treatment, once started, cannot be stopped, or that stopping requires much greater justification than not starting, then it is likely this view will have serious adverse consequences. Treatment might be continued for longer than is optimal for the patient, even to the point where it is causing positive harm with little or no compensating benefit. An even more troubling wrong occurs when a treatment that might save life or improve health is not started because the health care personnel are afraid that they will find it very difficult to stop the treatment if, as is fairly likely, it proves to be of little benefit and greatly burdens the patient. Fear of being unable to stop treatment can lead to failure to treat. Ironically, if there is any call to draw a moral distinction between withholding and withdrawing, it generally cuts the opposite way from the usual formulation: greater justification ought to be required to withhold than to withdraw treatment. (President's Commission (US) 1983: 75–6)

This view holds that it is often more serious, morally speaking, to withhold than to withdraw treatments. The reason given is that by deciding not to start a treatment or life support for a particular patient, we are not giving ourselves the opportunity to see the evidence coming from the treatment: Does the person respond to treatment? If we decide not to apply a treatment or therapy are we sure – in all likelihood – that the patient would not respond or improve with the therapy? The authors of the report put it this way:

> Whether a particular treatment will have positive effects is often highly uncertain before the therapy has been tried. If a trial of therapy makes clear that it is not helpful to the patient, this is actual evidence (rather than mere surmise) to support stopping because the therapeutic benefit that earlier was a possibility has been found to be clearly unobtainable. (President's Commission 1983: 76)

If we do apply a therapy or life-support provision and find that there is little or no response or improvement of benefit in the patient's condition, the discontinuing treatment is not an act of 'killing'. Rather, the authors in the text above would argue that beneficence does not require continuation of a therapy if it does not offer any benefit to the patient or if it might more clearly cause distress or harm to them.

Unless all of the clinical facts of the diagnosis and prognosis are crystal clear and quite certain (which is not often the case), beneficence and concern for wellbeing of the patient would seem to oblige us morally to apply the treatment *even if, on the basis of further observation and evidence, we might have to decide to discontinue.* Our motive for discontinuing a treatment with a particular patient is to opt for another treatment effort or, with seriously ill patients suffering extreme brain damage, to allow the process of dying to take its course with all the comfort care and pain alleviation available.

Benefit and Burden of Treatments Sustaining Life
Before evaluating the means to prolong life as morally obligatory or not in the ethical sense, *one must consider the precise and particular condition of the patient.* Letting die, when therapy will not benefit the patient, is generally viewed as ethically justifiable. A **principle of proportionality** is the value basis for deciding:

> It needs to be determined whether the means of treatment offered are proportionate to the prospects for patient improvement. To forego disproportionate means is not equivalent to suicide or euthanasia: it rather expresses acceptance of the human condition in the face of death. (Ashley 1997: 419)

The important consideration stressed here is that the judgement about providing or withdrawing treatments including Artificial Nutrition and Hydration (ANH) is patient-specific. Abstract principles alone will not be sufficient. Writing of patients in a permanent vegetative state, the United States President's Commission for the Study of Ethical Problems in Medicine writes:

> Since permanently unconscious patients will never be aware of nutrition, the only benefit to the patient of providing such increasingly burdensome interventions is sustaining the body to allow for a remote possibility of recovery. The sensitivities of the family and of care-giving professionals ought to determine whether such interventions are made. (President's Commission 1983: 190)

Activity

The language of 'benefit and burden' is central in many discussions of ethics and the end of life. But are benefits and burdens transparent in their meaning and application to individual patients?

a) What do the authors cited above mean when they say that a decision should be taken about withdrawal of treatment on the basis of 'benefits' and 'burdens' of the treatment for the particular patient?

b) What was the 'burden' of feeding for the PVS patient, Liz?

c) Consider Katherine who asks that she be given comfort care but sedated and not provided with food. Would this course provide 'benefits' for Katherine or 'burdens'?

Summary Learning Guide 14.1

The morally relevant points to consider when reflecting on the moral differences between withdrawing or withholding treatments are:

- Whether a particular treatment is effective in improving the prognosis of a patient.
- By withholding treatment we may not be able to get evidence about whether or not it will benefit a patient.
- Based on the above points, it is morally preferable to start a treatment, determine its efficacy and then decide whether to discontinue the treatment.
- The belief that stopping a treatment is morally more serious than omission can lead to failure to treat.
- Therefore, greater moral justification ought to be required when omitting or withholding treatment than when withdrawing treatment.

Nutrition and Hydration: The Debate

There are two positions on the moral necessity to provide food. We ask: Is the withdrawal of nutrition-hydration (ANH) morally justified? One view, for example, claims that yes, it is morally justified to discontinue food if the patient competently and with lucidity refuses food. According to this view, Katherine's refusal of further food would seem justified.

But ethicists disagree about ANH for non-competent and unconscious patients such as Liz. Those who argue strenuously that feeding is always required might consider the Ward of Court case and believe that the Supreme Court Judgement was the top of a '**slippery slope**'.

The slippery-slope concern applies to many areas of decision making. The form of the concern is this: If we take a particular decision – even if it is a good decision – is it likely to lead to another decision which we would not desire or think good? So, slippery-slope concerns in allowing competent patients to decline all life supports would be that we might slowly come to think it justified to discontinue all life supports for non-competent patients who seem to us to lack a good quality of life. Likewise, withdrawing feeding as in the case of the Ward is judged by some to be the top of the slippery slope to a policy allowing for involuntary euthanasia. One of the difficulties with slippery-slope worries and concerns is that they often frustrate very good decisions out of fear that less desirable results will follow (Lamb 1988).

While the report from the US President's Commission believes feeding is like any other life support and should be decided by the same reasoning of benefit versus burden, Gilbert Meilaender believes that we are poised at the top of the slippery slope if we do not view the provision of food as a universal obligation.

Meilaender states the position *against removal* of ANH this way:

> For many people the uselessness of feeding the permanently unconscious seems self-evident. Why? Probably because they suppose that the nourishment we provide is doing no more than 'sustaining the body'. But we should pause before separating personhood and body so decisively. We can know people, of all ranges of cognitive capacity – only as they are embodied; there is no other 'person' for whom we might care. Such care is not useless if it 'only' preserves bodily life but does not restore cognitive capacities. Even if it is less than we wish could be accomplished, it remains care for the embodied person. (Meilaender 1984: 12; See also: Iglesias 1995; Derr 1986.)

In rereading Meilaender, you may see the similarity with the discussion on 'person' from John Finnis and James Rachels in Chapter 13. Meilaender thinks that the benefits of feeding far exceed 'burdens' for the person. To him it is not clear that it is useless or 'without benefit' to feed the permanently unconscious.

Below we review the arguments **for** a universal requirement to provide food (ANH), and arguments that would, in precise circumstances, morally allow withholding or withdrawing of food.

Activity

Do you think that there are some arguments that should be listed but are omitted? Write in your additional arguments for discussion in seminar.

Arguments for the Universal Moral Obligation to Provide Food
The argument for a universal requirement always to provide feeding for patients following on Meilaender's quote can be summarised like this:

- Out of respect for patient autonomy, if a patient who is conscious and competent requests continued nutrition and it is not clearly harmful to the patient, the patient's request should be granted.

- For most patients, ANH is not burdensome and the patient given this nourishment does derive a benefit in that their life is sustained.

- Feeding remains 'care' for the embodied person and it is dualistic to think otherwise.

- If a patient is in a PVS condition, they are not 'terminally ill' and the denial of food and water will inevitably guarantee and cause a preventable death (See McCormick 1989: 378, for proponents of these arguments).

- Withdrawal of nourishment from PVS patients involves us in 'aiming at their deaths'. It is tantamount to 'killing' the patient.

- ??

- ??

Arguments for Allowing Withdrawal of ANH Under Precise Circumstances

- If a patient is conscious and competent or has left a living will documenting their preference to cease ANH under specified circumstances, this request should be given priority in decision making.

- ANH is to be evaluated in terms of its burdens and benefits to the particular patient. The ideas of 'benefits' and 'burdens' need to be understood in a holistic and person-focused manner to embrace dimensions of existence that are psychological, spiritual, emotional and physical.

- Where the burden of extending life support of food exceeds benefits, ANH can be justifiably discontinued. The burden is the reality of being subjected to the indignity of being sustained for many years in the condition of non-consciousness (McCormick 1989: 376–7; Lynn 1989: 51–3).

- There is no benefit for an individual human person if ANH merely sustains biological human life or indeed proves too stressful for the human system in its last stages of living. If there is distress of this sort or if there is no realistic hope of a return to a cognitive, sapient state, then there is no benefit. Comfort care and human presence become the priorities.

- Discontinuing treatment is not equivalent to killing the patient but is rather to be understood as offering to company with them in their process of dying.

- ??

- ??

Irish Medical Council and Irish Nursing Board

In August 1995, shortly after the Supreme Court decision in the Ward Case, the Irish Medical Council and the Irish Nursing Board, An Bord Altranais issued their statements on the question of withdrawing ANH as decided in the Court judgement. The short form of the Irish Medical Council Guide was issued on 4 August 1995 and stated:

> It is the view of the Council that access to nutrition and hydration is one of the basic needs of human beings. This remains so even when, from time to time, this need can only be fulfilled by means of long established methods such as naso-gastric and gastrostomy tube feeding. The Council sees no need to alter its Ethical Guide. (For full statement, see Appendix 4a.)

The Irish Nursing Board, An Bord Altranais, acknowledged the Supreme Court judgement in the Ward case but reaffirmed its principle as follows:

> . . . so long as there remains a means of nutrition and hydration of this patient, it is the duty of the nurse to act in accordance with the Code and to provide nutrition and hydration. (An Bord Altranais, 18 August 1995. See summary learning guide below and full statement in Appendix 4b.)

These guidelines from the Medical Council and the Nursing Board make clear that the classification of food and hydration is a contentious one. The Medical Council and Nursing Board take the stand that access to hydration and nutrition is *one of the basic needs of human beings and remains so even if feeding requires a gastrostomy tube.* But the High Court and Supreme Court, in 1995, after taking advice from numerous ethicists and theologians, decided the contrary.

Denis Cusack explains the possible clash that could occur because of the divergence between the legal decision in the Ward Case and the guidelines from the Medical and Nursing bodies:

> A serious clash of medical law and medical ethics would occur if the Medical Council or An Bord Altranais were to decide to sanction any doctor or nurse who carried out a lawful act in accordance with their conscience but contrary to the ethical guidelines of their statutory profession registration bodies. Would the court declare that it was proper to make such a decision or would it cancel the decision? (Cusack 1995: 44)

Summary Learning Guide 14.2

The Irish Ward of Court Case of (1995) allowed health-care organisations to consider the ethics of removal of feeding tubes in permanent vegetative state patients. In the weeks following the Supreme Court judgement, An Bord Altranais (Irish Nursing Board) issued these guidelines (full statement in Appendix 4):

An Bord Altranais (18 August 1995):

- Reiterates its role of giving guidance to the nursing professional on all matters of ethical conduct;
- Claims it finds no reason to change any of the fundamentals of its Code following the Ward decision;

- Reaffirms the underlying guideline: *The nurse must at all times maintain the principle that every effort should be made to preserve human life both born and unborn*;
- States that the ethical principle requires that it is the duty of the nurse to provide nutrition and hydration;
- States that, in this specific case, a nurse may not participate in the withdrawal and termination of the means of nutrition and hydration by tube;
- Advises that, in the event of withdrawal and termination of the means of nutrition and hydration by tube, the nurse's role will be to provide all nursing care.

Comment: A challenge for nurses is that the nursing ethical guidelines from An Bord Altranais conflict with the Supreme Court legal decision to allow discontinuation of the gastrostomy tube. One would be justified in drawing the conclusion that there may be an uneasy relationship between law and morality, between law and professional organisations' codes of conduct.

Public Policy and Personal Autonomy

The issues raised about death and dying come from a background of diverse cultural, religious and moral views about the meaning of 'valuing human life'. Dan Brock and Joanne Lynn, in the following view on the nature and valuing of life, emphasise the value of personal autonomy for competent patients such as Katherine Lewis to decide questions of their dying:

- We believe that public policies should not depend upon any single understanding of the nature of life or of the good life. Instead, autonomous persons must be free to affirm some such conception for themselves.
- These are ultimately and properly matters of personal choice, all the more so in a society that values religious freedom and is pluralistic in the classical liberal sense of not enforcing one single conception of the good life, but of ensuring conditions in which persons can pursue their different and sometimes conflicting views of the good life.
- Thus, even if deliberate choice to forgo food and water may be seen as an affront by holders of some particular conception of the nature or meaning of life or of the good life, public policy should not prohibit that choice to persons who do not share that conception of life. (Joanne Lynn 1989: 210).

Activity

a) Do Lynn and Brock provide any helpful perspective on the questions raised about Katherine's choice to die?

b) Consider their perspective in the light of the request from the Ward's family to allow their loved one to die.

c) Can you formulate your response to these two authors: agreement, disagreement, and qualifications on the view?

CONCLUSION

As technology offers more opportunities to survive dying, the discussions continue about our moral obligations at the end of life. They raise questions about whether dying has become medicalised to the detriment of the values many would hold about a 'good life'. The arguments given above for the diverse views offer a basis for an informed judgement about the Ward case and many other situations of critical care.

We argued in this chapter that, unless strong reasons prevail, a patient's competent decision should be respected about continuing life supports. Conversations would be essential to ensure the patient's understanding of what can be done, what alleviation of suffering is possible and what hospice might offer.

In the light of many cases of PVS, the question of withdrawing feeding poses special moral difficulties. While it is a value priority initially to give respect to the competent, conscious patient's preferences on these questions, cultural practices and differences also need to be taken into account. Positions from the diverse sides of this ongoing debate were presented in this chapter. Conscience judgements can only follow evaluation of the positions.

The following terms are explained in the glossary:

An Bord Altranais	narrative model of ethics
ANH	principle of proportionality
CPR	slippery slope argument
DNR	

Section Three:
Resources, Justice and
Accountability

A fundamental issue of distributive justice is how a country allocates its health-care resources. These decisions inter-relate at several levels: the micro, meso and macro. Nurses traditionally felt the impact of distribution decisions only at the micro level but increasingly are engaged at all levels. While the idea of justice seems vague and imprecise, Chapter 15 explains that it is more accurate to see it as a multi-dimensioned reality. The many dimensions are clarified in the three main theories of distributive justice. The discussion of case studies reveals that no one theory is agreed to be universally correct in all situations.

Several criteria are seen as central in health-resource allocations. Using a case study of a liver-transplant patient who is addicted to drugs, medical criteria of outcome and benefit are scrutinised. Such criteria often camouflage moral and social evaluations when applied uncritically. The result is that fairness is jeopardised in the name of medical expertise. The case study also exposes dubious assumptions involved in saying that some individuals are 'undeserving' of health resources because of their lifestyle choices. The uncritical assumption is addressed. Are some of us completely autonomous and free in our lifestyle choices?

The justice and equality of a health-care system can be threatened if it operates as a two-tier system. Two positions are explained about the two-tier system of health care in Ireland. One view claims that it is unjust to offer better care and access to those who can pay. A second view claims that a two-tier system is compatible with the just provision of a basic standard of health care. One model of a just health-care system is offered for reflection and evaluation.

Chapters 16 and 17 extend the discussion of justice with a discussion of the expanding accountability of nurses to effect improvements in the delivery of health care. Two mechanisms for change are discussed: whistle-blowing and strike action. Using these strategies, nurses cross over the micro, meso and macro levels of decision making.

Whistle-blowing, an action of dissent and accusation, makes public the behaviour of another that is potentially harmful to patients and staff alike. Diverse moral judgments on whistle-blowing are detailed. One viewpoint sees it is a betrayal of loyalty to friends or colleagues. A second perspective interprets whistle-blowing as an act of advocacy that reflects positively on the integrity and courage of the nurse revealing the behavioural threats to the wellbeing of patients and health-care staff.

Strike action is the second strategy for change. Three diverse positions on strike action are explained. Each reveals an underlying philosophy of nursing that motivates the strike action. A 'strong position' on strike action views nursing as a special vocation and so prohibits strike action categorically, with the argument that a nurse's vocation cannot compromise on the commitment to optimal patient care. A 'weak position' on strike action claims that nurses are different from many workers but do not enjoy a 'special vocation' that prohibits collective bargaining. Strike action is justified if the reasons for the strike action are sufficiently serious and the expected adjustments in patient care are minimally disruptive. A third perspective, 'the no difference thesis', claims that nurses are no different from any other worker and are entitled to take action for better working conditions that ultimately improve patient care.

Allocating Scarce Health Resources

INTRODUCTION

The question of how a country should distribute health-care resources is one of the most pressing debates in health-care ethics today. It is fundamentally a question that has consequences for every citizen in a state. The reality is that no country has an unlimited amount of monies for health-care needs. When resources are limited in any context, and when desire and need exceed the resources available, difficult decisions must be made. These decisions are never value-free. This is especially so in the health-care sector. Criteria of decision making are used, whether or not these criteria have been consciously formulated and examined. The issues in distribution decisions are not simply the cost in terms of euro and cent – they may be costs in terms of demands on nurse time, primary-care services, and adequate levels of health-care personnel, beds, human organs, and technology. The central ethical questions about health-care allocations are: by what values and priorities are the decisions made; and by whom are the decisions made?

Activity

We begin by asking you to identify two recently publicised disputes about health resources in Ireland. The examples you choose may be in something like the following: resource wastage as a result of hospitals that are built but not furnished and so standing unused; nurse shortages, Health Department failure to observe contract promises, gerontology units, breast-screening facilities, or any other dispute of which you are aware. Use the questions below to clarify the elements of the situations that you have selected. Draw on your experience of the health-care sector in Ireland and your creative imagination to see if you can suggest negotiated resolutions in the disputes you identify.

a) What was the case about?
b) Who were parties to it? (unions, nurses, GPs, clinicians, patients, families of patients, etc.)
c) What kind of conflict resulted?
d) Were nurses centrally affected by the dispute?
e) Has it been a recurring dispute?
f) Why has it not been resolved?
g) As Minister for a day, what solutions would you suggest?

THREE LEVELS OF DECISION MAKING

Consider the situations you identified above. Where was the problem located? Was it at hospital ward level? With hospital administration? With nursing personnel? At the Department of Health? The Department of Finance? It helps, if possible, to locate the centre of any difficulty.

We can distinguish three levels of decision making: **micro**, **meso** and **macro** levels. At each of these levels, ethical questions arise. The three levels are interconnected and yet each is distinct. The distinction among levels of decision making should help you to clarify:

- Where responsibility and accountability can be located for resource decisions;
- Where injustices arise in the distribution process;
- Whether nurses have a role to play at the various levels spelled out below.

Macro Level: These decisions concern the amount of monies allocated to health care by a government. **Macro-level** ethics is about the politics and economics of a state's national health service. Total government budgets have to look out for education, defence, social welfare, and housing. Of this resource cake, how much should be allocated to health care? On what basis are the decisions made? When macro-level decisions are being decided, it is debatable whether, for example, infertility treatments and reproductive technologies should receive resources from the state kitty. The question arises as to whether other essential services are more worthy and fertility treatment less essential.

Meso Level: This is the level of internal management of health-care institutions. The meso level involves the ethics of managing nursing services, such as human resources management, employment policies, work allocation schedules, grievances, corporate ethical standards and quality assurance (Thompson, Melia and Boyd 2000: 101).

Micro Level: This level pertains to the one-to-one nurse–patient relationships. The ethical issues at this level arise in departments within a hospital or in specialty units where, for the most part, clinicians have to make choices about individual patients. Which patients will get particular services or treatments where only a limited quantity is available? This might involve deciding who should have priority in an accident or emergency department, who should get the last bed in an intensive care unit or hospice or who should get a kidney when three patients are seriously in need. Even when it is the medical staff who must make these micro-allocation decisions, nursing staff must live with and try to adapt to the consequences.

These levels of decision making interact dynamically and cannot be kept neatly separated. Decisions made at the **micro** level can be facilitated or frustrated by the **meso** and **macro** levels. Similarly, judgments made at the micro level can be observed by hospital management at the **meso** level and have repercussions on further allocations at the micro level. But should nurses assume some responsibility for decisions about health-care resources whether at the **micro, meso** or **macro** level?

Should Nurses Be Involved in Management of Health-Care Resources?

Are strategies to improve or change health resources and health-care practices activities that do or should involve nurses? It is widely recognised that resource decisions and establishing priorities have traditionally been the domain of hospital administrators, health boards (or centralised Health Executive Groups) economists and the Department of Health. By and large, nurses are viewed as dedicated carers for patients in health-care institutions and outside the circle of decision making on health-resource questions. Wilmot discusses this assumption of the nurse's negligible role:

> Nurses have had less involvement than other groups in making rationing decisions during the years when it has been part of the agenda in National Health Service organisations. There are many individual exceptions to this, but those exceptions do not seem to have percolated into the common arena of professional thinking in nursing.
>
> Nursing as a profession seems still to be relatively uncontaminated by the rationing experience [. . .] Rationing is alien to the ethics of nursing. The code of professional conduct says nothing about the fair distribution of resources, whereas it emphasises strongly the individual nurse's commitment to the well-being and autonomy of the individual patients. (Wilmot 2003: 135–7)

Activity

Consider several assumptions that Wilmot makes in the above passage. Do you agree with his view of the conflicts between resource decisions and the nurse's role? Let's take up a few of Wilmot's points and think through the assumptions here:

a) Nursing is still relatively uncontaminated by the rationing experience. But what is 'contaminating' about rationing decisions?

b) Rationing is alien to the ethics of nursing. Why? What is Wilmot's view of nursing that makes him think that 'rationing' decisions are so antithetical to an ethic of nursing?

'Rationing' has become a negative term associated with denying health resources to individuals who are legitimately entitled to them. To soften the blow of hardship on patients, associated with 'rationing', the language of 'priority setting' or 'allocation of scare resources' is more commonly used. But whatever language is used, ranking decisions among areas of health care and ranking priorities in relation to which patients to treat are decisions that seem inevitable in a situation of scarcity.

Wilmot argues that nurses find rationing decisions 'contaminating' because a nurse's primary duty is to the individual patient. Each patient counts as important in his or her own right. To be expected to make resource decisions is to be asked to engage in trading off the benefits of one patient against the benefits of another. In this way, the goals of nursing, understood as including a primary commitment to each individual patient, seem contaminated by the need to choose one patient over another in prioritising distributions (see Case 15.1 below).

Justice as Fairness
How do we know if a society's health-care system is 'just'? The term, *justice*, comes under the conceptual umbrella of morality and is considered basic to any discussion of what constitutes a good society. Justice is a concept dating back to Plato, who understood it as a name given to virtue in our relations with others. It is often made synonymous with 'fairness' in dealing with other people. Social justice is about *how* a society ought to be organised, so fairness operates in all or any of the distributions (property, health, education, welfare, etc.)

Distributive and Corrective Justice
There are two forms of 'justice': **corrective justice** and **distributive justice**. Corrective justice is concerned with punishments given out for offences committed within a society. A society's sanctions for a range of offences from tax evasion to theft and murder come under corrective justice.

Distributive justice is traditionally explained as being concerned with sharing good and bad things, burdens and benefits among members of society. Examples of burdens are taxes and jury duty; examples of benefits are 'children's allowance' and old-age pension. Questions about justice in health care are about distributive justice in relation to what is universally regarded as a good thing: health.

Scarcity and Changing Expectations

Problems of distributive justice arise when there is a scarcity or shortage of goods within a society. If it were possible to provide every person who needed it with a hip replacement, cancer therapy or treatment for Parkinson's disease, many of the challenging questions about whom to treat and how to divide the health monies simply would not arise.

One factor that has altered perceptions of 'justice' or 'fairness' in health-resource distribution is the changing expectations of people in diverse societies. Life-enhancing technologies and life-saving therapies that were utopian even ten years ago can now be used to enhance quality of life, diagnose illnesses with great accuracy and extend life for patients with conditions formerly seen as untreatable. Reproductive technologies now available have altered expectations of individuals about their prospects for bearing children. The successes of modern health technologies raise expectations that result in ever-increasing demands on the health allocation of a state's budget. These increased expectations can elicit allegations of injustice if the technologies are not made available to all who might benefit from them. The level of citizen expectations about health-care resources in any country varies considerably. Citizens of developing countries may expect services of a family doctor but not the technological provisions for cosmetic surgery or assisted reproduction clinics. The level of expectations putting demands on distribution correlates with the overall affluence of citizens in a country and the level of citizen knowledge about what is available in health care.

Activity

Consider at least two ways in which you think that changing expectations in your society have altered beliefs about the justice and fairness of the health-care system.

a) Are these expectations about reproductive options? Cosmetic surgery? Mental-health expectations requiring stays at 'health farms'? Others?

b) Should a health-care system be obligated to respond to changing expectations in health care of this nature?

c) Can you think of any problems in arguing that changing expectations (without any qualification) oblige a state to respond with appropriate provision? For example, it might be proposed that cosmetic surgery should be provided out of tax payers' money. Alternatively, some might argue that fertility treatment should not be funded out of public monies. They might suggest that the desire to reproduce is not a 'health need'. Ask yourself: are there limits to the obligations of a society to provide for changing medical possibilities and individual expectations that are not 'basic' health provisions?

NURSE TIME AS A SCARCE RESOURCE

One resource over which individual nurses might seem to have some control is the distribution of their own time and nursing-care skills at the **micro** level. Nurses generally do not have the luxury of devoting themselves to a single patient – no matter how needy that patient. In the intensive care units, for example, any single patient might be served by several practitioners throughout their stay. Given the growing demands on the health-care services, nurse time is becoming one of the more scarce resources in the Irish health-care system (Dickenson 1994).

The following case study gives you an opportunity to consider how ward tensions and ethical unease may be experienced when decisions have to be made about distributing time for a number of patients.

Case 15:1: Nurse Allocation of Time to Patients

Thomas Farrell has been working in the paediatric intensive care unit of a public hospital since he completed his nursing studies five years ago. Two nurses usually staff the unit, but on this particular shift, his colleague has gone home ill and there are no critical-care nurses available for relief. The unit is currently at maximum capacity with three children:

Oliver: an infant of five months with profound physical and mental disability, awaiting transfer to a specialty hospital for cardiac surgery;

Sinead: a three-year-old trauma victim admitted the previous day, on a ventilator and requiring constant care; she is not expected to survive;

Ansari: a five-year-old who is post-surgery, ready for the step-down unit as soon as a bed becomes available. He is extremely anxious about leaving the protective environment of the unit.

Thomas is struggling with the imminent decisions needed about how he should distribute his limited time and care among the three patients. (Variation on a case from Yeo, Moorhouse and Donner, Yeo and Moorhouse 1996: 251–2)

The case provides an exercise in specifying some of the values or principles that you might use when trying to distribute your pressured or scarce time. The stark challenge in making decisions on time allocation is that to decide in favour of one child is at the same time to decide against another. There is an **opportunity cost** involved when we decide for patient x, but in doing so forego time for patient y. Whatever comfort Thomas takes from being able to care for the child to whom he gives the larger share of his time will also have a bitter element in the painful knowledge that this will be at the expense of one or both of the other children. Who will be the loser in this decision? Whether or not Thomas is conscious of explicit grounds for making his decisions, he will be using some criteria as he proceeds here.

Before you focus more closely on this case of distributing 'nurse time', we look at a range of often-cited values and principles of justice for apportioning health benefits – including nurse time.

Apportioning Benefits Justly

The following are three main theory-alternatives for deciding how resources should be allocated (see Veatch and Fry 1987: 81–3).

1. **Classic Utilitarian View of John Stuart Mill:** Allocate benefits by using the principles of beneficence and nonmaleficence. We calculate benefits and harms. The decision makers are morally obliged to choose the course that produces the most benefit or good, the standard method of utilitarian reasoning. In previous chapters, we saw some of the challenges in deciding what is the 'most beneficial' or 'the greatest good'. These challenges to utilitarian reasoning still exist when applied to health care.

2. **Libertarian View:** This theory holds that the principle of **autonomy** or liberty provides an important counterbalance to utilitarian reasoning. The argument claims that resources should be allocated according to the free choices of individuals who 'own' them, who have bought the services. According to this view, if health care is provided for those in **need**, it is not because it is their natural right. Rather, they have negotiated with a health provider to give the care.

Anarchy, State and Utopia, a study by the late Robert Nozick, explains this libertarian theory. It is most pertinent to a country with a capitalist, free market economy that prizes the liberty and autonomy of individuals and chooses to minimise state interventions in service provision.

3. **Egalitarian View:** Proponents of this view claim that justice is a principle that should be paramount, and justice requires producing equality wherever possible. John Rawls in his volume, *A Theory of Justice*, argues that equality is a basic ethical requirement of practices in the health-care sphere. But Rawls' theory qualifies this equality rule: It is just to sacrifice equality in the name of justice whenever it benefits the least well off to do so. **Deontologists** would largely sympathise with the egalitarian position but stress that health care should be an entitlement or right insofar as it is one of the basic human goods for any society.

If we review the larger theories just explained, we can see specific values for decision making that emerge in various ways from these theories.

One formulation of the values is the following:

1. To each person **equally**.
2. To each person according to need. The more needy get priority in the distribution of the precise goods they lack.
3. To each according to likely outcome or potential for benefit.
4. To each person according to their autonomy or liberty.
5. To each according to individual merit (position in a community, employment status, moral character, etc.)

Activity

Before we tease out these criteria, reread the case of Nurse Thomas Farrell and his three patients. Reflect on the five principles just stated and write initial remarks you would make about the use of these criteria in the allocation of Thomas's time.

a) Are some of these criteria more helpful than others?

b) Do some of the above criteria seem irrelevant?

c) Try to justify (give reasons for) your choice of some of the criteria over others.

d) Would you want to mention other criteria that you might use if in this situation?

Teasing Out the Principles

No single principle works in enough circumstances to argue that it is the *one* principle of decision making for achieving distributive justice in health care (Dooley 1996: 281–4). If we look more closely at the value principles, they seem legitimate on first reading, but then, on examination, we recognise problems.

1. **Equality:** Many theorists follow the ancient Greek philosopher, Aristotle, who deploys a formal principle of justice, referred to as the principle of equality of consideration. This principle means that equality is fundamental. However, equality does not mean that everyone is the same and ought to be treated the same. The principle of equality claims that *we treat similar cases alike except where there is some relevant difference.* This principle of justice emphasises the elements of impartiality in justice decisions. Differences in how we treat individuals are justified only if cases can be shown not to be alike. Injustice occurs when like cases are not treated alike.

But we need to ask: when are cases alike? How do we decide which characteristics are relevant in judging individuals as equals? One way of deciding which characteristics of individuals are relevant is to determine which characteristics do not count. Most would claim that a person's ethnic background, religion, gender or employment status should be ignored when resources like hospital beds are to be distributed among members of a society (Fletcher and Holt 1995: 85). On the other hand, some features or considerations are likely to be much more morally significant, factors such as: medical need, likely outcome, cost of treatment or age.

2. **Need:** Providing health care to those who need it seems to be the simplest way of allocating scarce resources. According to this view, every citizen has the right to get health care on the basis of clinical need. The aim is to provide equal access to health care for those in equal need.

So much seems obvious that nurses working in the health-care system might well consider 'need' the most important criterion for access to care. But the meaning of need is far from clear as Newdick explains in the following three points:

> If a very broad definition of need is adopted – for example, that a person can be said to need something if without it s/he will be harmed or detrimentally affected, then the term is so expansive that it becomes difficult to distinguish need from desire, demand or mere wants.
>
> Just as perceptions of illness, health and disease (which are subjective concepts) vary from person to person and time to time, so too are our perceptions of need culturally and socially determined.
>
> It is not surprising then that there has been little agreement to date on a set of consistent and objective principles that can be used to assess the basis of need. (Newdick 1995: 16)

The task of defining need is made no easier if the state's role is limited to satisfying people's basic health needs. This raises the question as to what counts as 'basic'? Many would not accept that only life-threatening conditions should be included. But how do you draw the line. Would 'basic needs' include treatment for conditions like hip replacement which, while not life-threatening, can greatly improve 'quality of life'? Raanan Gillon phrases the most challenging problem of justice in the needs-based approach:

> What happens when there are too many 'needy' patients chasing the same scarce resource? How should choices be made between these competing patients – agreed to be in need? Who should get priority? This question almost brings us back to where we began. (Gillon 1985: 96)

3. Benefit or Likely Outcome of Treatment: This criterion requires that we allocate resources according to the likelihood of medical success. This criterion is frequently combined with need since patients might be said to 'need' treatment if it will benefit them. How is 'medical success' determined or measured? There seems no objective way of determining effectiveness of treatment given the different perceptions people have of illness and health (Newdick 1995). Some claim that likely outcome is defined in terms of go-home rates, complications, mortality, likely re-admissions or even cost and efficiency. Increasingly the concept of 'outcome' is more broadly defined to embrace 'quality of life measures', such as wellbeing, social adjustment, emotional health, and so on. 'Outcome' is clearly a value-laden and relative term that cannot be defined with objective certainty.

4. Liberty or Autonomy: This criterion needs to be discussed because it is central in some theories of distributive justice. Liberty or autonomy as a criterion for distribution of health care means that if patients are free and able by financial means to get some medical treatment, they should be entitled to exercise their liberty in that way. We saw that Robert Nozick (discussed above) argues that such liberty should be acknowledged.

However, ability to pay and the freedoms that come with that ability seem to violate principles of justice and impartiality. The ability to pay is an advantage that is not available to all citizens in a society. A capitalist culture relies on many citizens paying for health care, but it may be antagonistic to forming a just society to require patients to pay for health, a most basic of all human goods.

5. **Merit** (position in community, employment status, talent, moral character, etc.): While merit can justly be used to award scholarships or prizes in a ploughing championship, the *principle of equality of consideration* would challenge merit as a criterion promoting justice. Merit as specified above seems a most dubious *morally relevant difference* among peoples in a society when it comes to receiving health care. Exactly what difference does one's employment or social position make to one's worthiness as a human being to receive health care?

Nurse Time Revisited

The critical discussion of the criteria for distribution of resources shows not that it is hopeless to make decisions on distribution, but that we need to weigh carefully the many different factors that could be thought simple and straightforward as the 'right' criteria. Darren Shickle explains that *where prioritisation is done, justice is an essentially contested concept. Agreement is required on which inequalities are relevant and must be addressed* (Shickle 1998: 872). Recognising where the challenges lie also helps us to strengthen our own reasoning in the matter of just distributions.

Activity

Now we return to the case of Thomas and his three needy patients. After further examination of the values and criteria, how would you decide for Thomas? Consider the values of need, benefit and equality.

a) If Thomas decides to give time according to the *need* of each patient, how would you advise him on the degree of need of the three patients here?

b) If Thomas gives time depending on how much the patients will benefit, how do you determine benefit? How anticipate benefit?

c) Would equal division of time be the most fair or just method of giving time? Can you cite one or two problems in adopting equal distribution as a valuable method?

d) You may think other criteria should be included here. If so, list them for further discussion.

Aiming Towards Being Just

1. Thomas might divide his time and care evenly or equally among the three children. Doing this, he might feel justified that he has been 'fair' to them and not judged one more worthy of his time than another. But the three children have unequal needs. Therefore the option of distributing time equally is in conflict with considerations of need and benefit and may not even be effective in promoting equality.

2. A second option is to consider which of the patients is most in need.

3.   A third option for Thomas would be to prioritise the three children in terms of the prospects for benefit. In effect, this means that Thomas would choose between the three children. This choosing will be done in terms of a range of considerations and values.

Sinead is clearly the sickest of the three. She needs the greatest amount of attention and would likely benefit most in the short term. But, in the long term, it would probably not make much difference. If Thomas gives Sinead less time, she might die sooner than she otherwise would if given more attention and care. But, even if Thomas can't provide Sinead lasting benefit, what can he do? Can Thomas make Sinead's dying easier? If so, how?

Ansari is on the road to recovery and requires little 'critical care'. Being very anxious, he could benefit from attention, emotional support and reassurance about leaving the unit's protective environment. Thomas's attention to Ansari would probably make a difference to him in the long run as he adapts to recovery elsewhere.

Oliver's needs are very great but there are many questions about what benefits can be expected down the road. What 'quality of life' can he expect? If Thomas decides to give Oliver the lowest priority, it seems that he is making a 'quality of life' judgement and communicating to Oliver's family that his life is less valuable than that of the other children in his care.

Are these the only options available to Thomas or can other options be explored? Thomas might refuse to operate his shift on his own because of concerns about client safety. He could insist on relief trained nurses from an agency or ask that one or more of the children be transferred to another critical care unit.

Or Ansari could be helped by someone with less training than Thomas, even a parent or volunteer. It might also be feasible to secure one or more staff nurses who may not have specialist training but who could provide basic nursing care under Thomas's supervision. The team of nurses could also decide to utilise a patient dependency scale to calculate the level of need of each of the three children.

At the very least, Thomas should receive emotional support and counsel from colleagues and his supervisor in the unit.

TREATING PEOPLE AS EQUALS

Most people would like to think that, as citizens, they are equally entitled to the protection and care of the state. This care is dramatically shown in a state's public institutions, such as those involved in the provision of health care. When people come into contact with health-care services, they expect to be treated on an equal basis because they believe they have a common need for health care. Would a 'just' or 'fair' society tolerate setting up a hospital that treats only white men under the age of sixty? (Fletcher and Holt 1995) If a justice ethic were given priority, it would be a universal practice that persons are entitled to health care because of their needs and would not have to rely on the generosity of nurses, physicians, philanthropists or charitable organisations.

A justice ethic would ideally require comprehensive, equitable health care for all groups within a society. Under a justice ethic, if a society restricts or refuses access to health care for any group of people, an explanation is necessary as to why some individuals living in the society have no entitlement to health care. Such explanations of restrictions might be necessary with regard to asylum seekers, 'resident aliens' or Travellers.

Summary Learning Guide 15.1

Distributive Justice (DJ):

- Is defined as sharing the goods, burdens and benefits among members of society in a manner that is fair;
- Requires relying on the principle of equality of consideration which means that
  - §   we act justly when we treat *similar* cases alike;
  - §   we can justly treat persons unequally or differently (not the same) *only if* there is some morally relevant difference between them;
  - §   features of individuals that would not be judged 'morally relevant' include: gender, race, religion, income, social status.

Theories of DJ are mainly three:

1. **Classic Utilitarian View** of J. S. Mill: the best distribution achieves the 'greatest good' in society.
2. **The Libertarian View** of Robert Nozick: let citizens make free choices to spend their income on the health resources they judge that they need or desire.
3. **The Egalitarian (deontological) view:** health care is an entitlement or right as a basic human good for any society. Equality can justly be sacrificed to benefit the least well off.

INSTITUTIONALISED INEQUALITY

There is another level of inequality that nurses encounter and patients suffer: institutionalised inequality. This refers to that inequity of discrimination that occurs in an institution by virtue of the way it is organised, structured, and financed. Maev-Ann Wren assesses the institutional health-care system in Ireland and finds not an ethic of justice but structured inequality throughout the Irish health-care services.

> Irish society today faces two major challenges: to fund the health care system adequately; and, within that system, whatever its level of funding, to deliver care equitably, giving priority to those in greater need . . . At the heart of the health care system, in Irish hospitals, there is a discrimination between patients that other European states would not tolerate. In public hospitals, there are two forms of apartheid: two-tier access and two-tier care. The reality of two-tier access is not in dispute. It exists, it is institutionalised and it has been getting worse. This is a system in which patients are treated according to income rather than need.

Private patient care is delivered promptly and, generally, by consultants in person. Public patient care comes tardily and is frequently delivered by doctors in training. Public patients may wait so long for care that they are effectively denied it. Death may intervene. Only in the accident and emergency departments of public hospitals is there a levelling, so that the insured and uninsured alike find themselves confronted by the chaotic, inadequate face of Irish public health care. That many patients yet emerge from hospital cured and happy is testimony to the efforts of the many medical, nursing and other staff, who work long hours with competence and dedication in difficult circumstances in under-resourced hospitals. Some of the most vocal critics of the two-tier care are among those who must deliver it. (Wren 2003: 139–40)

FAIRNESS AND 'TIERED' SYSTEMS

Maev-Ann Wren raises a fundamental ethical question: *How equal must our rights to health care be?* Wren argues that, at present, rights to health care are based on financial merit or 'ability to pay' for private health insurance.

Professor Dermot Walsh, Inspector of Mental Hospitals in Ireland, claims (not for the first time) that

the conditions in some public mental hospitals remain Victorian, while private psychiatric facilities are state-of-the-art. The stark inequalities between public and private services are unacceptable. The number of modern outreach and home-based psychiatric services, a central plank of the Government's stated mental health strategy – are also inadequate. (O'Keeffe and O'Farrell 2004: 1)

IS FAIRNESS COMPATIBLE WITH A TIERED SYSTEM?

But must everyone receive exactly the same kinds of health-care services and coverage, or is fairness compatible with a tiered system? Countries around the world that offer universal health insurance differ in their answers to this question. Norman Daniels explains that in Norway and Canada no supplementary insurance is allowed. All people are serviced solely by the national health-insurance schemes. So there is no 'tiering' in Canada and Norway. In the UK, supplementary insurance gives approximately 10–15 per cent of the population quicker access to services where there is lengthy queuing in the public system. There is a minimal form of tiering but, by and large, equality of opportunity is protected.

Norman Daniels argues that 'the primary social obligation is to assure everyone access to a tier of services that effectively promotes normal functioning and so protects equality of opportunity' (Daniels 2001: 323). Democratic decisions are made about how much of macro resources to invest in health care as distinct from education or job training, and so on. All individuals receive free the basic good of health care under equality of opportunity. But there will be some beneficial medical services that are very expensive relative to other needs of the society. In this case, it will be reasonable not to provide more expensive medical services in the basic tier.

PROTECTING LIBERTY AND EQUALITY OF THE BASIC TIER

Daniels endorses the principle of liberty or autonomy along with equality of opportunity. If a society permits significant income differences, why not let people buy coverage for additional services? We allow people to use their monies to pursue the 'quality of life' and opportunities they prefer in other areas (education, housing, etc.) Why not allow them to buy supplementary health care for their kin? If a supplementary tier undermines the basic tier, priority must be given to protecting the basic tier.

Daniels believes that it would be possible to design a system where the supplementary tier does not undercut the basic one. He wants to protect both the principle of liberty or autonomy and a basic equality. He argues that a system that permits tiering avoids restricting liberty in ways that some may find seriously objectionable.

Activity

a) Compare the accounts of Wren and Daniels. Can you reconcile Daniels' legitimation of a two-tier system with Wren's criticisms of two-tier care?

b) Drawing on your experience as a nurse, would the financing of the health-care sector be possible, be changed, or be improved if the government had to fund all citizens in Ireland?

ARE SOME PATIENTS UNDESERVING OF HEALTH RESOURCES?

Nurses often say that they distribute their care in response to human need. This need is usually met irrespective of people's social or economic status or other personal attributes. But is that always the case in practice? Consider the following story about Carol who might be viewed as bringing on her own illness. Could you defend a refusal of a transplant for her?

Case 15.2: A Patient's Lifestyle Causes Liver Failure

Just four weeks ago, Carol, a sixteen-year-old drug addict took an ecstasy tablet and had a severe reaction to it. Without a liver transplant, she will die, and yet doctors refuse to consider her for one. Maureen, a nurse working in the transplant unit, thinks this is very unfair. She thinks that Carol is being discriminated against because of her drug habit. Maureen also believes that other elements are coming into play in the decision not to transplant: Carol's lack of social importance or recognition and her status as a public patient unable to pay for the transplant. According to Maureen's reasoning, many less-'deserving' patients get transplants. There was Felix, for example – a famous and wealthy rugby player with a history of alcohol abuse who received two transplants in his forties. Maureen also believes that, given her age, Carol should at least be given a chance to live. (Variation on a case given by Hendrick 2000: 118)

Activity

a) What if a patient is the author of their own misfortune? What if a person is a drug user, obese, a heavy smoker or binge drinker?

b) Should a publicly funded health-care system be expected to provide a liver transplant or cardiac bypass surgery if a patient's lifestyle contributes to this need?

c) Can an institution justify treating one patient because they can pay, and refusing another, like Carol, because she does not have the resources? In reflecting here, consider as an example the fact that some London boroughs pay for Interferon treatment – why not the same for transplants for those without resources?

DECIDING SCARCE RESOURCES: A VARIETY OF CRITERIA

If we were to limit our considerations to clinical grounds alone for a decision, there might be justification for not proceeding in the case of Carol, but the same clinical grounds would also provide justification for not treating Felix. The argument would be that the medical benefit of the liver transplant simply could not be achieved because of the recidivist behaviour of both patients. On medical grounds, then, refusing Felix and Carol liver transplants might be justified where there are other patients who have developed liver failure through no fault of their own. The following three points might be considered as grounds to refuse the transplants to Carol and Felix, judging them to be 'undeserving patients':

1.   It is fair to hold people responsible for their own actions and decisions;

2.   Based on 1, we might require that persons seek effective treatment before it is too late;

3.   If effective transplant programmes require public support, this would be greatly reduced if patients with drug or alcohol addictions got equal treatment before children born with liver defects (Hendrick 2000: 138).

Both patients, Carol and Felix, *need* liver transplants. They may be *equal* in needing the liver. Both would *benefit* if they had a new, healthy liver, but perhaps they would benefit less than a child born with liver defects and lacking lifestyle impediments. So there is a morally relevant difference between Carol, Felix and a newborn child: a likely prognosis is that both Carol and Felix will revert to their earlier lifestyle, risking the efficacy of the transplant. So, according to Hendrick's argument above, perhaps they do not *deserve* or *merit* a transplant

Activity

a) Evaluate Maureen's reasoning in this case.

b) Enumerate the objections she offers to the clinical decision.

c) On what grounds might you decide not to give a liver to either of these patients?

ARE THESE UNDESERVING PATIENTS?

Can we successfully separate out the clinical reasons for the decision from social, judgemental or discriminatory reasons? Many of us expose ourselves to risk by bungee-jumping, driving fast cars, abseiling, playing rugby or being a pillion passenger on a motorbike. Some doctors in the United States fall into the high-risk group for insurance because of regular risks taken in the course of their duties. Medical criteria may not be as objective as sometimes claimed. Should health professionals be free to refuse to care for patients who are admitted to hospital from accidents in any of these voluntary activities, each containing considerable risk? Similarly, should they be free to refuse treatment to high-stress professionals: lawyers, accountants, secondary teachers or indeed non-consultant hospital doctors or nurses on long shifts? We could argue that these individuals choose to work under conditions of great stress and so expose themselves to risk of high blood pressure, or cardiac problems.

Is there a false assumption operating that individuals are wholly to blame for self-inflicted conditions they suffer or unhealthy lifestyles they lead? We can justify withholding health care from those who take risks voluntarily *only if* they are fully autonomous and are aware of the risks and accept them.

Is it more accurate to say that many of us have no real choice in exposing ourselves to danger? Should people be penalised with refusal of health care for participation in activities that they are not truly free to stop? If we say that health care should be saved for use with those who do not incur their own illnesses, would we have any patients at all? Can we accurately judge who has played a part in their own illness? Before answering the question, consider the following list of patients' behaviours which provide further challenge to the idea of 'undeserving' persons:

- Lung disease or heart disease in someone who smokes
- Liver failure in someone who drinks large amounts of alcohol
- Lower-back problems caused by work in a sedentary job for many years
- High risk to nurses who lift .3 tonnes per week on gerontology units
- Reversal of sterilisation
- Soft-tissue injury from sport
- Accident in someone engaging in risky behaviour, such as hang-gliding, or cycling along a busy road
- Accident caused by a person's careless driving
- Heart disease in obese persons
- Respiratory infection in someone who travelled in a crowded train or airplane
- Renal disease in someone with diabetes who has not controlled his diabetes carefully (from Hope, Savalescu and Hendrick 2003: 184).

The conclusion, based on the summary list above, is that if some risk-takers are undeserving, then perhaps all are undeserving. Either most of us are 'undeserving' of health care or none of us are undeserving!

ONE FRAMEWORK FOR A JUST SYSTEM OF HEALTH-PROVISION

A basic framework for a just system of health-care provision could consist of several core principles or values. Consider the following and see if you would add to or subtract from this list:

- Accepting that the only basis for discrimination is the degree of need for health care;
- In trying to put different needs into some order of priority, paying particular attention to the disadvantaged, since their liberty to improve their own health is likely to be most limited;
- Providing an **ethnic monitor** to gather data on how cultural minorities in a state experience the health-care system. On the basis of the data, assessing and trying to remedy where inequities in health provisions are most severe (Holland 2004: 5);
- When society has decided that a health-care need should be met, treating all those with that need equally;
- Defining a minimum entitlement to health care and applying it without discrimination (Campbell et al. 1997: 193).
- ??
- ??

As you read these justice provisions, see if you wish to add other features that you think are necessary to achieve a 'just health-care system'. Whether this framework leads to the fairest distribution of resources is debatable, but some system and set of criteria for deciding will be used anyway. If we cannot find the perfect set of value criteria, perhaps it is better to search for a less-than-perfect best.

WHO SHOULD DECIDE?

Recent work in distributive justice in health care does not stress theories of justice but focuses instead on the process by which decisions are made. Key questions that are addressed include: who should be involved in decision making and what methods should they use? Norman Daniels cites the following four conditions of 'accountability for reasonableness' in allocation decisions:

1. **Publicity:** Decisions and their rationales must be publicly accessible.
2. **Reasonableness:** The rationales for decisions should aim to provide a reasonable construal of how the organisation should provide 'value for money' in meeting the varied health needs of a defined population.
3. **Appeals:** There is a mechanism for challenge and dispute resolution regarding decisions that set limits on health provision. This appeal process includes the opportunity for revising decisions in light of further evidence or arguments.

4. Enforcement: There is either voluntary or public regulation of the process to ensure that conditions 1–3 are met. (Daniels cited in Hope, Savulescu and Hendrick, 2003: 187)

Nurses sometimes claim that they are out of the loop in terms of decision making about resources. The feeling goes deeper to form the belief that, in the last analysis, the health-resource decisions are purely political and based on sectional interests and pressure groups. However, increasingly writers argue that the procedures given by Daniels above require the setting up of a group of people from a variety of backgrounds, to decide issues of resource allocation. An example would be Community Health Councils in the UK. However, for such a group to be truly representative, individuals would have to include the marginalised, homeless people with infectious diseases or mental health needs. A challenge to Daniels' suggestion would be choosing the criteria for selection of people as representatives. What mechanisms would be used to be fair in the selection of a genuine diversity of individuals?

Activity

a) Earlier in this chapter, we considered the institutionalised inequality in the Irish health-care two-tier system. If the public were involved as decision makers about health resources, would you envisage that public participation would change the existence of the two-tier system?

b) Critically consider the following two reasons for involving the public in resource decision making:

- In most health-care systems, public money in the form of taxation or further levies provides a substantial portion of the resources.
- The purpose of health care is to help patients. The public are the patients of the future and, as a result, their perspectives are important.

CONCLUSION

In this chapter, we saw that resource-allocation decisions occur and inter-relate at several levels – micro, meso and macro. We argued that 'justice' seems to be inherently confused or unclear or at least irreducibly pluriform – multi-dimensioned. This is to acknowledge the challenges in efforts to approximate a just and equal distribution of health care.

Several main theories of justice were reviewed but no one theory was found to be universally agreed as the decisive and absolutely correct one for distributing resources.

Two case studies – nurse time and allocation of organs – were focal points in the chapter for discussing the issues of justice and equality. We examined a list of principles as a basis for distribution decisions. Criteria that seemed straightforward and easy to apply were nevertheless questioned for their fairness. Through analysis of the case study of a liver-transplant patient, we found that, too readily, medical criteria of outcome and benefit shade into social and moral evaluations, and so jeopardise the fairness of using those criteria uncritically. Judgements that some patients are 'undeserving' of health revealed dubious assumptions about individual freedom to choose lifestyle factors that greatly influence health and mortality.

The two-tier system of health care in Ireland came under scrutiny and we questioned the extent to which it is a source of inequality and injustice. The discussion offered an alternative view by Norman Daniels, claiming that a two-tier system need not be incompatible with justice and equality as long as a basic standard of care is supplied to all citizens in a state. We concluded by suggesting for consideration one model of a just health-care system, and indicated who might be involved in decisions related to resource allocation.

A key theme in this chapter has been the pivotal role of nurses in decision making at all levels of resource allocation. The role responsibilities of nurses are further explored in the following chapter where they are firmly placed in the public domain.

The following terms are explained in the glossary:

corrective justice
distributive justice
ethnic monitor
justice ethics

opportunity cost
principle of equality of consideration
two-tier health system

Accountability
and Whistle-blowing

Objectives

At the end of this chapter, you should be able to:

- Discuss views on nurse accountability for effecting changes in health care;
- Define and discuss key features of whistle-blowing: dissent, accusation and loyalty;
- Distinguish between levels of incompetence and degrees of ethical misconduct;
- Consider some of the personal and professional challenges that arise in relation to whistle-blowing, such as fear of consequences and personal motive.

INTRODUCTION

Being called to account simply means being asked to give reasons for your actions. This is often part of everyday life. In various circumstances, we are called to account for our actions or failures to act in a moral, legal or completely neutral capacity (Fletcher and Holt 1995: 107). The concept of **accountability** in this chapter relates to the role of nurses in exercising strategies for change, improvement or correction in some context of nursing practice.

Nurses have been most concerned and vocal about the resource needs at the **micro** level, that level where patient–nurse care is most concentrated in acute-care hospitals, nursing homes or the community. Consider your response to the text that follows, articulating a view that uses the language of 'obligation' for nurses to take part in decision making at the three levels of **micro**, **meso** and **macro**. What response would you take to this characterisation of nursing?

> At all levels of resource allocation, nurses have an obligation to become more involved. At the micro-level, the development of genuinely open and participatory health teams will facilitate this. At the meso-level, nurses can express their concerns about justice by becoming more administratively and politically involved in the affairs of the institutions in which they work. At the broader macro-level, nurses, as informed and concerned health professionals and citizens, can make valuable contribution to the process of forming public policy. (Yeo and Moorhouse 1996: 242; see also Thompson, Media and Boyd 2000; Fletcher and Holt 1995.)

The two strategies discussed in this chapter and in Chapter 17 are ones that, for better or worse, influence events across all three levels – micro, meso and macro. They are: **whistle-blowing** and **strike action**. These measures are most often undertaken to improve practice by addressing problems, be they personnel, work conditions or resource decisions. They are controversial and frequently very emotive decisions to effect change. These measures are often defended by nurses as chosen out of concern that patient care, professional trustworthiness or their own personal integrity are under threat. Where this is the case, whistle-blowing and strike action can be understood as part of a nurse's **advocacy** role discussed in Chapter 4.

Strike action and whistle-blowing often bring nurses into conflict with nurse and medical colleagues, hospital management, and the State's Department of Health. As such, they are often decisions taken with considerable conscience conflict. Where this is the case, these two actions can challenge a nurse's sense of **integrity** (See Chapter 4). Having decided on a course of action, the nurse should be able to give reasons for choosing to act in this way rather than selecting another course of action (Fletcher and Holt 1995: 107). Because whistle-blowing and strike action most often have consequences for the wellbeing and sometimes professional reputation of others, these chosen measures for change also have moral consequences.

CHOOSING TO 'BLOW THE WHISTLE'

We begin our discussion on nurse accountability with a study of the strategy for change that is popularly known as 'whistle-blowing'. In May 2004, the Irish Nurses' Organisation (INO) at its annual delegate conference passed a motion to formulate a 'whistle-blower policy'. Such a policy would enable nurses to report practices in their health-care context that they felt were of concern, without having any fear of retribution. According to the INO, nurses need to feel safe to report to management concerns they have about the way colleagues (peer nurses, other professionals and students) are treating patients. Presumably, a whistle-blowing policy would empower nurses to come forward and report incidents (*The Irish Times*, 4 May 2004: 5).

Blowing the whistle is an attempt by an employee, a former employee or a patient to bring a wrongful practice to the attention of those who one believes have power to remedy the situation. It is defined by Chadwick and Tadd in the following way:

> Blowing the whistle refers to the act of calling to public attention abuses or dangers that jeopardise public safety and that would not otherwise be publicised. In health care, this may involve informing on the incompetent, unethical or negligent practices of colleagues. But there are powerful influences that make this much easier to discuss than to do in practice. (Chadwick and Tadd 1992: 54)

Though not explicitly describing it as whistle-blowing, the Code of Professional Conduct of the Irish Nursing Board, An Bord Altranais, states in the following two paragraphs that nurses have a duty to protect patients (and colleagues) from unsafe, harmful and abusive practices:

The aim of the nursing profession is to give the highest standard of care possible to patients. Any circumstances which could place patients/clients in jeopardy or which militate against safe standards of practice should be made known to appropriate persons or authorities . . . The nurse shares the responsibility of care with colleagues and must have regard to the workload of and the pressure on, professional colleagues and subordinates and take appropriate action if these are seen to be such as to constitute abuse of the individual practitioner and/or jeopardise safe standards of practice. (An Bord Altranais 2000)

However, in spite of the fact that protecting patients and colleagues is a professional obligation, the labels often associated with this action give a clear indication of how it often elicits disapproval not popularity for the person informing. The use of such negative valuation labels as 'snitch', 'grass', 'squealer' and 'tell-tale' communicates social pressure to conform to the presumed demands of silence. In any country, like Ireland, where colonisation by a foreign power has been an historical experience for centuries, these pejorative terms resonate with many citizens even today. Their emotive force needs scrutiny since the pressure of these labels may deter a nurse from taking action that might be required by conscience.

FEATURES OF WHISTLE-BLOWING

Sissela Bok characterises whistle-blowing as having three features. Each requires considerable thought on the part of one deliberating about blowing the whistle. The three features are: dissent, accusation and breach of loyalty. We explain each in turn and focus in greater detail on the third.

1. **Dissent:** involves calling attention to an irregularity in order to safeguard patients or the public from harm. Based on their learned views about expectations of responsible nurse care, a nurse disagrees with or dissents from the action that they are reporting. Bok makes clear a proviso about the accusations made in dissent:

> Before declaring one's dissent it is essential that the circumstances and facts surrounding the alleged abuse are accurate, as hearsay and intuition are inadequate grounds. (Bok 1980: 2–10)

Examples of practices that underline the dissenting nature of whistle-blowing are those unquestioned and habituated practices in care settings that prioritise efficiency over holistic and individualised care. Staff in a facility that cares for people with serious learning disabilities, for example, might share clothes among the residents rather than allow individuals to have their own wardrobes. In this case, for whatever reasons, there is a practice in place that is endorsed by the staff and the institution, which does not preserve the dignity of the residents concerned. A new member of staff or a student nurse, coming to the facility with a fresh perspective, might feel uncomfortable with the practice, especially given that the individuals in the situation may not be able to speak for themselves, and may not have any relatives to speak for them.

A second example of where nurses might blow the whistle is where they dissent not from ongoing practices, but from organisational and institutional conditions which they believe lower standards of care. A recent example of this kind of whistle-blowing is the case of Graham Pink, a charge nurse on night duty, working in wards caring for older people in Stepping Hill Hospital in Stockport, England. After many efforts to raise the issue through the normal management procedures within the hospital, Pink eventually went public with his concerns that understaffing in the hospital caused inadequate patient care. In September 1991, he was dismissed by his employers for 'breaching confidentiality', and his case, supported by the United Kingdom Council of Nurses, received wide publicity. (Pink 1990; 1992)

Activity

a) If you were a student nurse in either of the aforementioned situations involving ongoing practices that you felt uncomfortable about, how would you express your dissent? Refuse to participate? Question the practice among the staff? Raise the matter at management level? Leave that facility?

b) If you were working in an Irish facility caring for older people, and, like Pink, were concerned about staffing levels, how might you proceed?

2. **Accusation:** Bok points out the possibility that a nurse blowing the whistle could be mistaken in the allegations made. Accusation should clearly identify those responsible and precisely what the troublesome matter is, rather than leaving the allegations in vague terms. The need for openness and clarity also tests the determination of the whistle-blower to have evidence and not simply hunches about harmful actions. Anonymous accusations are unfair to the accused. Making flippant remarks is a form of gossip and, as such, is irresponsible and a form of injustice. Making irresponsible remarks can damage a nurse's professional reputation and deny them the opportunity to defend their conduct.

A recent Irish case that underlines the accusatory feature of whistle-blowing came to light in 1998 when two midwives expressed concern about the high rate of caesarean hysterectomies being carried out by Dr Michael Neary, a consultant obstetrician at Our Lady of Lourdes Hospital, Drogheda. After an independent review, the North Eastern Health Board, which had taken over the running of the hospital from the Medical Missionaries of Mary, placed Dr Neary on leave. The consultant was subsequently struck off the medical register by the Medical Council, which found him guilty of professional misconduct over the removing of wombs of ten patients (up to one hundred women altogether claim that their wombs were removed by Dr Neary without their consent or knowledge. Many of these women are currently pursuing legal actions) (Reid 2003; Donnellan 2003).

Posing the question, 'How was Dr Neary's exceptional practice allowed continue for so long . . . without either his nursing or medical colleagues raising the alarm?', *Irish Times* medical correspondent, Dr Muiris Houston, offers the following answer:

> One of the answers lies in the hierarchical nature of medical practice. At the time of Dr Neary's professional misconduct, Our Lady of Lourdes Hospital was under the management of the Medical Missionaries of Mary. Its obstetrics unit was staffed by two to three consultant obstetricians, junior hospital doctors, midwives and other ancillary staff. The picture is one of a small unit within a larger hospital where someone with the authority of a consultant could wield enormous power. In a crisis, it was to the consultant on duty that everyone looked for a decision. Was it time to perform an emergency Caesarean section to save this baby? And if during the section the consultant announced that he had to proceed to hysterectomy, it could have been difficult for a theatre nurse or anaesthetist to question that decision.
>
> Such was the power of hierarchical medicine – and some observers would argue that this power has only slightly diminished in the last 10 years – that it would require numbers of people standing together to question a consultant's decision. (Houston 2003)

Activity

Consider the picture that Houston draws of the organisational structure and management style of the obstetrics unit in Drogheda.

a) Do you think that it is representative of many such units across Ireland?

b) If so, consider the strengths and weaknesses of this form of decision making.

c) What measures might be put in place to avoid the recurrence of a situation similar to that of the unit in Our Lady of Lourdes Hospital?

3. **Breach of Loyalty:** Deciding to inform on one's professional colleague or employer raises serious moral conflicts, including what many see as a breach of loyalty. Being part of a health-care team may seem to require that a nurse not violate team loyalty, but rather accept the values of the team. The allegation of disloyalty arises because the whistle-blower's employer (in Pink's case) or other employees (in the case involving ongoing poor practices) often do not believe that whistle-blowing is in their best interests. Unity and loyalty on a team, they might argue, may require speaking publicly with one voice or remaining silent about conflict situations for fear that the reputation of health care might suffer.

Assume that a nurse is in a situation of sufficient seriousness that they believe that they should make the events known to someone in authority. A checklist could be helpful for the nurse to reflect on what is going on here in this situation. First of all, what levels of incompetence or unethical practice are they witnessing?

Incompetence can arise out of ignorance or lack of skill, or both. There are at least five kinds of incident to which E. Haavi Morreim (1993) and Sara Fry and Megan-Jane Johnstone (2002) draw attention, which help to differentiate between different levels of accountability.

Five Levels of Accountability

1.   The first kind of incident is an accident that occurs independently of any person's decision or action. An example of this is equipment failure – often called 'mechanical error'.

2.   The second kind of incident involves a well-justified decision that unfortunately turns out badly. An example is administering an ordered blood transfusion where the patient suffers a severe reaction. This kind of incident is not evidence of a health professional's incompetence.

3.   At the third level are situations where professionals disagree. There is no consensus on what is the 'right' thing to do, and someone's decision later results in harm to the patient. For example, a nurse might decide to observe a patient longer and wait to report any troubling symptoms to the doctor if these symptoms persist. With no firm guidelines in matters such as this, the issue is left to the nurse's experience and judgement. However, a pattern or series of mishaps in this kind of situation might signal poor judgement or distracted observation powers by the nurse, and so might be indications of skill deficiencies that could harm patients over a period of time.

4.   The fourth kind of incident is when a health-care professional exercises poor, but not bad, judgement or skill. For example, a nurse might forget to inquire whether a patient is currently taking any cardiac medications. This poor judgement can be judged as incompetence if a pattern of such judgements develops.

5.   The fifth situation is where serious breaches of standards of quality care occur. An example would be if a nurse improperly restrained a confused older patient or failed to maintain adequate airways in a patient. Such breaches of the standard of care usually result in harm. (Based on Fry and Johnstone, 2002: 157–8)

In sum, setting the first two kinds of incident aside, incompetence can be understood as involving the commission of a series of errors brought about by skill deficiencies or consistently bad judgement (3 and 4), or it can involve a serious breach of standards of care (5).

Morreim also distinguishes between incompetent practice – the outcome of ignorance or lack of skill – and unethical practice. As there are levels of accountability in relation to incompetence, so too there are levels of accountability in relation to unethical practice.

1. Ethically, there are mundane misdeeds that arise out of ignorance, insensitivity or thoughtlessness – being rude, impatient or dismissive with a patient, for example.

2. There are also conscious deliberate moral wrongs, such as using one's professional power and knowledge for personal gain, or securing consent to unnecessary, dangerous, lucrative procedures. (Morreim 1993: 19–27)

Summary Learning Guide 16.1

Whistle-blowing is an act of calling to public attention abuses or dangers that jeopardise public safety.

- Three central features of whistle-blowing are: Dissent, Accusation and Breach of Loyalty.

- Incompetence involves

  § the commission of a series of errors brought about by skill deficiencies
  § or consistently bad judgement,
  § or a serious breach of standards of care.

- Unethical conduct involves

  § mundane misdeeds that arise out of ignorance, insensitivity or thoughtlessness
  § deliberate moral wrongs.

In order to apply this analysis of clinical and ethical accountability, consider the following case where a nurse friend and colleague has made a serious error. Does the situation warrant 'whistle-blowing' to a senior staff nurse? What levels of accountability in relation to competence and ethical standards do you see here?

Case 16.1: Reporting on a Colleague to Protect a Patient

Rebecca Carroll and Sarah Jansen were staff nurses on the night shift in a paediatric surgical unit. One night, as they neared the completion of their shift, Rebecca noted that a six-year-old diabetic patient recovering from minor surgery looked very pale and was perspiring. When she was unable to awaken the patient, she notified her colleague and best friend, Sarah Jansen, and together they did a blood sugar test. The results confirmed Rebecca's fears: the child was in hypoglycaemic coma. They called the doctor and the patient was immediately transferred to the intensive care unit. The child recovered and was discharged home within a week.

Later, Rebecca Carroll reviewed the incident. She stated how surprised she was to find the child in a hypoglycaemic state. At first, Sarah did not say much but finally admitted that it was all her fault. She had miscalculated the child's insulin dose and had given her too much medication. She had not gone back to check on the child and only realised her mistake when Rebecca found the child in a hypoglycaemic state.

Rebecca was shocked and asked whether her friend had completed an incident report or notified the child's doctor. Sarah said that she did not intend to report it because that would create an inquiry and trouble for her. 'I can do without that right now,' she said. She was being considered for advancement in the clinical ladder programme of the nursing division and feared that the incident would reflect unfavourably on her employment record. She looked at Rebecca and said in a pleading tone, 'And I hope that you're not going to report it, either. I told you this in confidence and as a friend, and it would be unethical for you to do anything about it.' (Variation on a case from Fry and Johnstone 2002: 158)

Sanctions as a Deterrent

While whistle-blowers are often admired and respected by their colleagues and the wider public, the consequences can sometimes be sufficiently negative that anticipating them may put off any nurse from blowing the whistle. In this case, Sarah makes clear some of the consequences for Rebecca. Such adverse consequences are, in fact, sanctions that act to discourage individuals from reporting incidents they view as problematic. They include: loss of friendships, ostracisation by fellow-workers, lowered evaluation by supervisors, demotions, punitive transfers and loss of jobs.

Rebecca's hesitation about reporting the incident seems to be based not solely on the fact of friendship but also may arise from a sense of moral unease about whether this is an appropriate situation for whistle-blowing.

Activity

a) Review the range of levels of accountability in terms of incompetent and unethical conduct discussed above, and apply them to this case. Is the incident

- simply an accident that probably needn't be reported;
- an isolated error of judgement;
- a part of a series of errors caused by Sarah's lack of skill and bad judgement;
- a serious breach of expected quality of care;
- a mundane ethical misdeed;
- a deliberate moral wrong?

b) Do the expectations of advocacy and integrity require reporting the incident?

c) Discuss the various ways in which the fact of friendship with Sarah affects Rebecca's responsibility here? Should the friendship deter Rebecca from taking further action here?

Error, Incompetence or Ethical Misconduct?

The interpretation of Sarah's actions is not straightforward. We learn from the narrative that she:

1. Miscalculated the child's insulin (error, carelessness, incompetence or all three?)
2. Gave the child too much medication (error endangering the child that follows on no. 1 above);
3. Failed to check back on the child as might have been expected (error, carelessness, incompetence or all three?)
4. Intentionally failed to complete an incident report (moral misdeed or moral wrong?)
5. Intentionally failed to notify the child's consultant (moral misdeed or moral wrong?)
6. Accuses Rebecca of betrayal if she reports the incident (moral misdeed or moral wrong?)

Looking again at the different levels of accountability in relation to competent practice described earlier, it seems a fair judgement to say that Sarah has breached the standards of due care expected of qualified nurses. However, it is unclear from the case whether her drug error was an isolated incident or a part of a series of errors indicating serious incompetence on Sarah's part. Secondly, and perhaps more significantly, if we consider the distinction we have already drawn between ordinary ethical misdeeds and deliberate moral wrongs, it seems that Sarah, in trying to hide her mistake, in refusing to notify the consultant, and in, effectively, blackmailing Rebecca, could be accused of moral misconduct.

In addition to Sarah's accountability, there is a broader issue at stake here. This relates to whether or not there are policies in place in the hospital where Sarah and Rebecca work, in relation to the reporting of drug errors. The existence or nonexistence of such policies and their scope may strongly influence Sarah's decision to report the drug error and Rebecca's decision to report Sarah. The provision of clear policies and an open culture provide concrete illustration of what has been referred to as **moral space**.

For example, were Sarah working in an institution with an open culture and policies in place which addressed the drug errors of professionals in a supportive and creative way, it is less likely that she would have difficulty in reporting the incident herself. While the Guidelines of An Bord Altranais, for example, would emphasise patient safety and require Sarah to report the drug error, they also advise health providers to support an open culture for error reporting which pays attention to the institutional context in which an error is made:

> It is of primary importance upon noting a medication error that the patient's/client's health is monitored. If a medication error has been identified medical and nursing interventions should be implemented immediately to limit potential adverse effects/reactions. Patient/client safety is of paramount importance. The nurse/midwife should be knowledgeable of the health service provider's policy for reporting such errors, including to whom errors should be reported and the necessary documentation to be completed. Nursing/midwifery management of health care settings should support an open culture for error reporting

while undertaking a comprehensive assessment of the circumstances of the error and, where appropriate, institute action plans to prevent/eradicate the contributing factors to the medication error. (An Bord Altranais 2003: 2.10)

The British Nursing and Midwifery Council (NMC)(formerly the United Kingdom Central Council for Nursing (UKCC)) is even more explicit in its commitment to the importance of a supportive and open culture in relation to drug errors by nurses and midwives:

It is important that an open culture exists in order to encourage the immediate reporting of errors or incidents in the administration of medicines. If you make an error, you must report it immediately to your line manager or employer. Registered nurses and midwives who have made an error, and who have been honest and open about it to their senior staff, appear sometimes to have been made the subject of local disciplinary action in a way that might discourage the reporting of incidents and, therefore, be potentially detrimental to patients and the maintenance of standards.

The NMC believes that all errors and incidents require a thorough and careful investigation at a local level, taking full account of the context and circumstances and the position of the practitioner involved. Such incidents require sensitive management and a comprehensive assessment of all the circumstances before a professional and managerial decision is reached on the appropriate way to proceed. If a practising midwife makes or identifies a drug error or incident, she should also inform her supervisor of midwives as soon as possible after the event. The NMC supports the use of local multi-disciplinary critical incident panels, where improvements to local practice in the administration of medicines can be discussed, identified and disseminated.

When considering allegations of misconduct arising from errors in the administration of medicines, the NMC takes great care to distinguish between those cases where the error was the result of reckless or incompetent practice or was concealed, and those that resulted from other causes, such as serious pressure of work, and where there was immediate, honest disclosure in the patient's interest. The NMC recognises the prerogative of managers to take local disciplinary action where it is considered to be necessary but urges that they also consider each incident in its particular context and similarly discriminate between the two categories described above. (Nursing and Midwifery Council 2002)

Activity

a) Take time to read each set of guidelines of An Bord Altranais and the Nursing and Midwifery Council. Do you know if there are any drug error policies in your place of work? If there are, do you think that they reflect the concerns of either the Irish or UK codes?

b) Do you think that these codes adequately address the fears that someone might have if they made a mistake in relation to patient medication? What additional provisions might be put in place to address such concerns?

Force of Friendship and Motives for Whistle-blowing

People understand the demands of friendship in very different ways. Some would argue that the close friendship between Rebecca and Sarah would make it emotionally more difficult, or indeed impossible, to report the incident to a higher superior. Consider Sarah's statements to Rebecca about confidence and the requirements of friendship. Sarah seems to be exploiting the friendship and offers a moral judgement to Rebecca: it would be moral failure, a betrayal of loyalty as a friend if she were to report. In some contexts, this would be construed as 'moral blackmail'.

If Bok's characterisation of whistle-blowing is accurate, deciding to blow the whistle requires that the nurse consider motives. Why is she taking an action that is not trivial, involves perceived disloyalty, and could threaten her own reputation and that of colleagues? As a decision that she hopes is ethical, the motive of the decision is important.

There are various motives for blowing the whistle against a work colleague.

1.   Personal gain: Make yourself appear better in the eyes of the employer or superior:
2.   Vendetta against a colleague you dislike;
3.   Concern for patient welfare and the integrity of the health-care profession;
4.   Concern about your own integrity or wellbeing as a person and professional.

Whistle-blowing to achieve personal gain or to get back at a colleague one dislikes reveals self-interested and vengeful motives. These motives lack the level of other-concern required for a moral action. These self-serving motives would most probably have the consequence of harming a colleague and compromising one's own integrity and trustworthiness. Imagine the overall consequences if a professional were rewarded for whistle-blowing in such circumstances (it does happen). The overall consequences would likely be demoralising for a level of trust required among colleagues in health-care practice.

The last two motives in the above list – concern for patient welfare and the integrity of the profession, and concern for personal and professional integrity – are decidedly different in their focus and ends to be achieved. The fact that Rebecca in the case study suffers moral unease in deliberating about informing superiors of Sarah's mistake suggests that patient welfare and the integrity of the nursing profession were central in her reasoning.

Can Loyalty be Misguided?

If we take seriously the critique of whistle-blowing as a breach of loyalty mentioned by Bok, we should recognise that we are making a significant assumption – that loyalty is always a harmless disposition or professional attitude. This may well be a false assumption. Loyalty can be understood here as commitment to a person or a set of professional standards, or adherence to policies within a health-care centre. But loyalty, in any of these examples, may be misplaced or may need to be questioned if we find that what we are committed to is no longer beneficial to others' wellbeing, or consistent with our own exercise of conscience. Before agreeing that whistle-blowing is an abuse of loyalty or breach of this 'virtue', we need to examine the very ordinary assumption that loyalty is always an admirable virtue.

A position, endorsed by authors such as Tschudin (2001) and Fry and Johnstone (2002), argues that we ought to rethink whether whistle-blowers are adequately described with such words as 'grass' or 'snitch'. Perhaps we should consider the view that whistle-blowers should be admired and respected by the public, patients and other colleagues where the motives are ones of genuine concern.

Tschudin (2001) stresses the view explained in Chapter 4 that nurse advocacy increasingly should be interpreted as an important professional and political disposition. This disposition of a nurse would show courage and conviction in standing up and opposing systems that are either unjust or are being jeopardised by the adverse actions of others. Bok argues that loyalty and confidentiality may seem unambiguous as virtues, but this may be a false generalisation. Loyalty and confidentiality may, in some situations, be dangerous – more so because of our widespread assumption that they are always worthy of praise (Bok 1978).

Appeals to loyalty or maintaining confidences might camouflage errant practices or even conceal shortcomings in patient-care practices that should be brought up for scrutiny and reassessment. Continuing in a practice or situation where conscience unease is persistent may mean that a felt loyalty to team workers is misplaced. Insistence on loyalty may mask an insecurity that insists on maintaining a united front in health care even when the professionals at front lines know that this 'united front' is an illusion and is perhaps only window-dressing for public view.

Activity

Consider the following questions as an examination of moral conscience to see whether or not you should proceed and blow the whistle where blowing the whistle involves calling public attention to a particular practice:

a) Will the benefit of 'going public' outweigh the potential harm? This question focuses us directly on consequences anticipated. If a great deal of public mistrust results in the end, is the end result more harmful than the original abuse? Personal harm can follow for the person who decides to complain and this may be substantial harm: loss of employment, loss of reputation or even physical injury.

b) What motives do we have for our action? This question encourages us to reflect on our reasons for blowing the whistle, to pause and see if there are other alternative ways of resolving a problem we notice.

As part of reflective practice in ethics, the questions remind us that the action taken is not trivial. It is an action that will have consequences – positive or negative, or both, for ourselves and others. The questions act as an examination of conscience and are not necessarily meant to be a deterrent. Consideration of them may give us pause for thoughtful deliberation and remind us of the seriousness of the action.

The nineteenth-century political philosopher, Jeremy Bentham, claimed that *publicity is the very soul of justice.* If one takes due care in thinking through the process in the ways discussed above, whistle-blowing can be assessed as an act of courage when employed as a strategy to bring about improvements in health care. The conscience conflicts and unease resulting require, as a minimum, thoughtful reflection, conversation with a trusted friend, moral courage and a keen sense of integrity to counter facile perceptions of disloyalty and 'grassing' on colleagues.

Summary Learning Guide 16.2

- Discussions on the virtue of loyalty reveal at least three claims:

    § It is an essential virtue of commitment to the profession, to others and to the practice of nursing;

    § It can too easily camouflage bad practice in the interest of presenting a united front for nursing;

    § To avoid such camouflage, responsible loyalty presupposes a requirement to question practices of the profession and colleagues where detrimental consequences would otherwise ensue.

- Whistle-blowing is a form of publicity that, when responsibly undertaken, aims at procuring the greatest good for others, oneself and the profession of nursing.

CONCLUSION

Recalling the distinctions in Chapter 15 of **micro, meso** and **macro** levels of decision making, in this chapter we considered one strategy for change that crosses over all of these levels. This essentially means that nursing accountability is expanding as professional roles are extended. Whistle-blowing is a mechanism of dissent and accusation, made with a view to bringing about improved health care but at a price. In one ethical perspective, whistle-blowing is seen as an act of advocacy and reflects the aspiration by a nurse for personal integrity. Whistle-blowing could be morally justified even if it caused considerable moral unease. The range of situations that might warrant whistle-blowing is vast and includes patterns (or even isolated incidents) of serious professional incompetence, harm-causing carelessness and abuse of power. Justification minimally requires careful deliberation on the potential consequences likely to follow in reporting the action, as well as one's motives for choosing this mechanism to improve specific situations in nursing care.

The following terms are explained in the glossary:

accountability   loyalty
advocacy   moral space
integrity   whistle-blowing

The Right to Strike?

INTRODUCTION

Strike action involves the withdrawal of labour and can take a variety of forms, from partial withdrawal to total withdrawal. The decision to engage in strike action is no easier than deciding to blow the whistle – a strategy for advocacy that we explored in Chapter 16. Strike action in nursing draws down very mixed responses from nurses and the wider public alike. These responses range from public agreement and support to moral discomfort or disdain that nurses have violated their duty to care for those who are ill. In the discussion that follows, we show how changes in the philosophy of nursing have been largely responsible for a change in this strike position.

Debates about strike action in nursing have a long and complex history. The debate has been emotive and controversial throughout the world. However, in the United Kingdom, lengthy reassessments by nurse associations have gone on since the first strike by asylum workers in 1914. The year 1995 saw a dramatic change in the official position of the Royal College of Nursing which, formerly, had not endorsed industrial action. The year 1995 also saw a change in the attitudes of professional nursing journals which, until then, had never supported industrial action (Jennings and Western 1997: 279).

The dichotomy of nurse stereotypes held sway for many years: caring, concerned, committed nurses who care too much about patients to strike, versus selfish, uncaring and militant nurses willing to put patients at risk. But why the change in policy? Karen Jennings and Glenda Western offer the following answer:

> The momentous decision by the RCN (in 1995) to discard its (non-industrial action) policy . . . reflects the pragmatism necessary to challenge what nurses, along with other health service workers, are facing in terms of the erosion of long fought-for rights. (Jennings and Western 1997: 280)

In Ireland, nurses and midwives took strike action, for the first time in the history of the Irish state, for nine days in October 1999. Involving in excess of 30,000 nurses, it was also the largest strike in the history of the state and was resolved after agreement was reached to improve working conditions and pay structures (see Clarke and O'Neill 2001).

In 1997, *Nursing Ethics* dedicated an entire issue to the question: Is it morally or ethically right to strike? (See Vol. 4, no. 4). Verena Tschudin and Geoffrey Hunt structure the articles by helpfully distinguishing three positions on the ethics of nurse strikes. In our discussion of this strategy for change, these positions are explained, and then a case study is introduced to see how the diverse perspectives might apply.

THREE VIEWPOINTS ON NURSE STRIKES

Tschudin and Hunt believe that moral reactions to nurse strikes are articulated in three different ways: **strong thesis, weak thesis** and **no-difference thesis**.

1. Strong Thesis

Nurses do not have a right to strike. A **right** is a justified claim that entitles us to demand that other people act, or desist from acting, in certain ways. In this instance, an alleged 'right' to strike would demand that Departments of Health or nurse managers provide the benefits or improvements being sought. The **strong** thesis denies that nurses have such a right.

It argues that nurses have a special kind of obligation and commitment to patients that derives from their unique vocation as nurses. Strike action and withdrawal of labour are morally incompatible with this special nurse vocation. This view is categorical and unrelenting about nurse rights to withdraw labour. As such, the strong thesis does not condone exceptions to the injunction against strike action. The strong view holds:

> A striking nurse is a contradiction in terms. A striking nurse is either not really a nurse or not really on strike.
>
> Nurses are perhaps closer in moral conception to parents; any parent capable of going on strike with their parenthood is not really a parent after all. (edited from Tschudin and Hunt 1997: 265)

According to the **strong view**, even if withdrawal of labour is purely other-concerned and focused on the good of patients, strike action is not justified. Nurses need to find ways other than withdrawal of labour to rectify inadequacies and improve their lot (Tschudin and Hunt 1997: 266).

2. Weak Thesis

Nurses do have a right to strike but it is constrained by more stringent conditions than that of other workers or employees. This position is termed 'weak' only relative to the 'strong thesis'. The weak thesis is not categorical about a unique nursing vocation. In fact, the weak thesis might see the idea of a special 'vocation' as contentious and potentially too elitist and/or prescriptive to be defensible.

Notice that the weak thesis does not **radically** distinguish nurses from other workers as the strong thesis does, but it still considers nurse activity to be sufficiently different in its responsibilities and commitments from other occupations that it can put conditions on striking. The weak thesis is more complex and requires that careful judgement be undertaken in each situation of potential dispute. Some, but not all, strike action is ethical. The morality of strike action depends on:

1. The reasons and motives for undertaking the strike, and
2. The nature and extent of anticipated consequences in terms of expected benefits relative to distress or harms caused.

The weak view further holds that, when contemplating strike action, nurses still must show a commitment to protecting patients from harm, minimising risk to patients as much as humanly possible under the circumstances. Nurses have to take special care and give due regard to how they go about this action in order to reduce potential negative consequences on patients. According to the weak view, measures that nurses might take that would protect themselves from legal and even moral liability would be: withdrawing labour in stages, cancelling all overtime, maintaining a minimal regime of work, and keeping time strictly by the letter of the law.

According to the weak thesis, moral justification will be determined by **proportionality** of a proposed specific strike action relative to the goals being sought by the action. Proportionality takes into account the special but not radically different features of nursing. Proportionality is a moral principle that has a definite role in the **weak thesis** viewpoint but has no role in the **strong thesis** since strikes are excluded without exception as an option.

Consider the following two examples that take a stand on a proportionality judgement in proposed strike action.

Proportional Justification Lacking

A large-scale sustained strike over nine months is not justified by the claim that nurses can do their jobs better if they are given a 10 per cent increase in their salaries. Using the judgement of reasonable and fair proportionality, the aim of achieving a 10 per cent salary increase does not warrant this extent of strike action. Less severe forms of action might be appropriate.

Proportional Justification Likely

Assume that there is complete closure of a large community hospital in a relatively poor area of a large city. There are no replacement plans for health centres in the area. The judgement of proportionality might argue that this situation severely compromises the level of care for a large, already struggling or deprived population. Would this serve as proportional justification for sustained and large-scale strike action?

3. No-Difference Thesis

This perspective dissents from both the strong and the weak thesis in claiming that nurses are no different from workers in other occupations. On this view, rather than strengthening nursing as a profession, the 'special vocation' thesis of the strong or weak position places nurses in an invidious and weakened negotiating position. The argument continues that employers would be delighted to be able to appeal to a special vocation of nurses to claim that nurses are violating their calling's special character by taking up industrial action.

The **no-difference** thesis, nevertheless, requires that proportionality be considered for any morally justified action. However, since it removes from nursing a special obligation to care, it would not include this feature of nursing as part of the proportionality judgement.

Strike Positions and Diverse Philosophies of Nursing

At the basis of all three positions on nurse strike action are philosophies of nursing or nursing philosophies: theories of what makes a nurse professional as distinct from a medical doctor or a missionary nun or a lawyer. What is unique to the identity of nursing? What kind of professional is a nurse? When spelling out such a philosophy, an author inevitably elaborates on the aims, goals, obligations and responsibilities of nursing. A philosophy of nursing communicates a view of nurse self-understanding that impacts on choices they make and expectations they might have of their professional and moral responsibilities. This task is complex and often leaves many assumptions about nursing unexamined (see Holt 1998: 149–157).

The first strike of Irish nurses took place on nine days in October 1999. Following the newspapers' reports on the strike, two nurse theorists recorded and analysed the language and views shown in a major newspaper, *The Irish Times*. Special notice was given to the views of nurses, understanding of what nursing is about, the notion of 'care', 'adequate care', and the gendered nature of nursing. For insight into the controversial views about the profession of nursing and philosophies of nursing, the article details a range of positions in this debate. Clarke and O'Neill argue that:

> It is regrettable that the occasion of the strike (1999) did not generate a clear debate on the nature of nursing as both expressive and technical caring . . . Individual nurses and nursing organizations need to work towards articulating the complexity of caring in order to educate the public and the media about the value of humanistic caring. Failure to do so may result in nurses being valued only as technical carers. (Clarke and O'Neill 2001: 357)

Activity

a) Reflect on how you view yourself as a nurse professional. If you were asked to prepare a discussion on a philosophy of nursing that you could endorse, what would it contain? Would it be such that it could endorse a strong, weak or no-difference view of strikes?

b) The Irish nurses' strike of 1999 did not involve a complete withdrawal of labour. Nurses, unpaid, provided emergency services and a skeleton service at night-duty staffing levels. What does this tell us about the view of nursing that underpinned the strike action? Could it be properly called a strike?

c) From your training/education in nursing, how would you characterise the philosophy of nursing that motivated the curriculum and methods of the programme?

Use the strong, weak and no-difference theses explained above and reflect on the following case.

Case 17.1: A Decision is Made to Strike: Conscience Conflicts

Claire Brady, an evening charge nurse, decided to join her nurse co-workers in a strike at their hospital. The decision to strike was reached several days ago by the majority of nurses in this rehabilitation hospital located near Dublin. The nurses were seeking higher salaries, fringe benefits including in-service study leaves, improved working conditions for all nurses employed in the hospital. Claire had personally known many frustrating evenings in the past year because of loss of nursing staff who became dissatisfied by the long hours and poor salaries. The hospital had tried to fill these vacancies by recruiting temporary agency staff. However, this affected continuity of care and the regular staff members were not satisfied with the approach.

Now that the strike was imminent, Claire wondered whether further reduction in nurse services was in the patients' immediate best interests. Any patient who might suffer because of the strike or might be harmed through care by unfamiliar nursing personnel had been moved to a special unit where non-striking and competent nurses were available. Even so, Claire anticipated that some of the patients on her unit would not do as well during the strike. They would not likely be harmed but they would not necessarily benefit either.

All of the nurses who voted to strike believed that they were doing a great service to other nurses in the country and to future patients. By striking, they were helping to making nursing practice more important, more challenging and more desirable as a profession. The striking nurses reasoned that, if staff were more contented and given responsibility for setting nursing-care standards, future patients would benefit from improved care.

By even contemplating strike action, Claire shows that she is not a proponent of the strong thesis. She seems to be closer to the weak thesis viewpoint. Considering the proportional justification required, Claire is still in doubt about whether she should proceed. The difference between immediate patient benefit and long-term benefit is crucial when making a consequential assessment and it is not an easy assessment to make. Maybe no strike action benefits patients immediately unless there is an immediate positive response to the strike action.

Activity

a) Consider the different positions on strike action discussed above. Where does Claire stand with respect to these diverse views on nursing and strike action?

b) Should nurses be willing to support a strike where safe but where the highest quality of patient care would not be provided – for the short term – to obtain a higher standard of patient care in the long term?

c) Discuss the view voiced in the case study: Striking for higher salaries, improved fringe benefits (including study leave) and better working conditions achieves benefits for patients.

Summary Learning Guide 17.1

Three positions on the ethics of strikes discussed here reflect diverse views on a philosophy of nursing:

- **Strong Thesis:** Nurses are radically different from other workers. Nursing is a unique vocation more akin to parenting than any other occupation. A striking nurse is a contradiction in terms. Nurses do not have a right to strike any more than parents have a right to withdraw care for their children.

- **Weak Thesis:** Nurses are not radically different from other workers nor is there a unique and singular vocation to nursing that explains why some become nurses. Nevertheless, nursing is sufficiently different from other occupations that it can put conditions on striking. Nurses do have a right to strike but it is constrained by stringent conditions. The weak view is more complex in requiring due care and considerable judgement about likely consequences of strike action. The principle of proportional harm to benefits must be included in deliberations here.

- **No-Difference Thesis:** Nurses are no different from other workers when it comes to their entitlements to collective bargaining, which includes a right to strike. By seeing themselves as having a special vocation, unique and different, the strong thesis puts nurses in a weakened negotiating position. There is no special obligation of care in nursing but this position still requires that proportionality be considered if any strike is to be legally and ethically warranted.

Further Considerations for Claire

Leonard Weber considers the nature of health-care organisations and supports the weak thesis, arguing that strikes by health-care workers must be viewed differently from strikes by manufacturing workers. A central feature of health care, in his view, is that it is not just like any other business that exists for money-making ends. Health care is fundamentally a service. As such, health-care organisations are best understood as community-service organisations. Because the role of health-care workers is to protect and promote a basic human need (health) of persons, the decision to take strike action requires special moral justification. On the other hand, Weber suggests that the right to bargain collectively must be preserved, and this right implies the right to strike.

> Unless unions have the ability to withhold labor as a last resort, they are in a very weak bargaining position. (Weber 2001: 114–5)

So, according to Weber, some strikes are ethically justified; some are not. It depends on the nature of the issues being addressed, the likely consequences of the strike and whether due consideration was given to other problem-resolution methods.

Graham Rumbold similarly supports the weak thesis. He argues that nurses may not have a right to strike unless very stringent conditions are observed. Some strikes are justified only if due care is taken to minimise any harm to patients. Salary increases would not justify nurse strikes.

> To strike or take any form of industrial action for the purposes of improving pay is morally unjustifiable. (Rumbold 1999: 255)

Why would Rumbold argue this? He claims that a right to strike is premised on a fundamental right to justice.

> The right to justice means that one has a right to fair terms of employment, a right to adequate working conditions and to reasonable reward. (Rumbold 1999: 255)

Why does this not justify strike action for pay where pay conditions are discouraging nurses from coming to or remaining in the profession? After all, patients suffer from increasingly reduced staffing levels.

In the final analysis, Rumbold does not believe that striking for improved pay is proportional and morally warranted. The likely harm to follow for patients – however minimal – cannot be condoned in the interest of increased pay. Other reasons for striking must be measured, reasoned and judged according to the proportionality of possible harm to patients and the type of strike action.

Rumbold cites two unambiguous justifications for strike action:

1.   If nurses were ordered by an employer or government to act in ways clearly harmful to patients, they could be justified in refusing to do so.

2.   If nurses were required to work in conditions harmful to themselves (1999: 256). Examples might include a failure in a

health-care system to provide nursing staff with correct protective clothing in radiography or hoists for lifting immobile patients.

Activity

a) Would bullying by a nurse or clinical superior over a long period of time justify strike action on the weak thesis?

b) Would Rumbold's view endorse the Irish nurses' strike action in 1999?

We conclude with the International Council of Nurses' (ICN) policy statement on strike action, which, we suggest, does allow for strikes by nurses for improved salary and other conditions of employment.

ICN Position Statement: Strike Policy

Effective industrial action is compatible with being a health professional so long as essential services are provided. Abandonment of ill patients is inconsistent with the purpose and philosophy of professional nurses and their professional organisations as reflected in the International Council of Nursing, *Code of Ethics for Nurses* (2000).

During a strike, the principles to be upheld include:

- the minimum level of disruption to the general public
- the delivery of essential nursing services
- crisis intervention by nurses for the preservation of life
- ongoing nursing care to assure the survival of those unable to care for themselves
- nursing care required for therapeutic services without which life would be jeopardized
- nursing involvement required for urgent diagnostic procedures required to obtain information on potentially life-threatening conditions.
- compliance with national or regional legislation as to procedure for implementation of strike action.
- . . . .
- . . . .

(Fry and Johnstone 2002: 156; last two bullet points added to text citation for student use)

Activity

a) This statement gives you an opportunity to see:

- If the case of Claire fulfils at least these guidelines;
- If strike action undertaken by Irish nurses in 1999 fulfilled these conditions.

b) The guidelines argue for the weak thesis and defend the need to use the proportionality model of justification. Discuss these among your colleagues and take time to construct further additions that you consider essential.

CONCLUSION

In this chapter, we have analysed three diverse positions on nurses' strike action: strong thesis, weak thesis and no-difference thesis. A principle of justification required in any judgement on strike action is that the likely harm to patients from it is fair or proportionate to the likely benefit sought by the strike action.

Each of the diverse positions on strike action reveals an underlying philosophy of nursing that motivates the strike position. Recognising this link between strike policies and philosophies of nursing allows one to realise that a philosophy of nursing is not mere rhetoric, but, by stating obligations, commitments and duties, has consequences for choices to be made by nurses. Unless one is committed to the strong thesis of nursing which argues for a special vocation position, strikes are ethically warranted after other attempts to rectify situations have been tried. Strikes are morally justified on condition that one makes a careful assessment and offers informed deliberation of proportional benefit to strike action.

The following terms are explained in the glossary:

no-difference thesis   strong thesis
proportional justification   weak thesis
strike action

Section Four:
Nursing Ethically

When we teach nursing ethics to students, we tend to leave any detailed discussion of ethical theories until the end of the module or course. We think that teaching ethical theory at the start of a course might be taken as a signal that the theory section is the most important part – that once students have a grasp of the different ethical theories, they are then equipped to apply them to cases or situations drawn from practice. We don't want to send that signal. We think that starting with theory – usually comprehensive and neat – often forces us to simplify human life so that it fits with the theory. Instead, we like to start with the messiness of life and then appeal to the languages of different theories to see if they can help us to make sense out of the mess. So, when we start our courses, we focus on practice from the outset. We ask students to consider different situations and relationships they meet with in the course of their work and draw attention to any ethical issue, question or problem to which they might give rise. Once students get the hang of seeking out and determining what might be ethically significant in their practice, we appeal to different ethical theories in order to express what might be happening from a variety of perspectives.

We have tried to keep the focus mainly on practice in this text also. Right from the outset, the challenge of working through the ethical layers of case narratives has driven the content of each chapter. In considering the ethical dimensions of each case, we have drawn on the language of a number of different ethical theories – some have focused on the need to respect commonly held values; some have emphasised the need to consider the specificity of a particular health-care situation. It is time in this final section to describe more fully the main claims of each of these ethical theories.

Chapter 18 describes and evaluates three ethical theories that have been part of the philosophical canon for many centuries: utilitarianism, deontology and virtue theory. In considering the main strengths and weaknesses of each of these frameworks, this chapter also indicates how each theory offers a response to the question of how we ought to live if we are to consider ourselves morally good.

Chapter 19 considers four ethical theories that, while indebted to the philosophical canon in different ways, nevertheless, can properly be called contemporary, because they have been informed by recent global social and cultural changes and by contemporary philosophical theories such as postmodernism and feminism. The theories considered in Chapter 19 are: principlism, narrative ethics, ethic of care and feminist ethics.

Traditional Moral Theories

Objectives

At the end of this chapter, you should be able to:

- Explain the defining features of utilitarianism;
- Identify essential elements of deontology;
- Discuss the view that virtue theory offers an agent-centred and character-focused moral theory;
- Assess the strengths and weaknesses of these three traditional theories.

INTRODUCTION

The special focus in this chapter is traditional moral theories. In particular, the lens of examining turns on three such theories: utilitarianism, deontology and virtue theory. They are termed 'traditional' because they have been in place in the canon of moral philosophy for many centuries. Moral theory is an effort to interpret our moral life and moral intuitions in a more or less formalised way. An essential connection between theory and practice is an assumption throughout this text. This connection is put well by Pojman:

> Ethical Theory and Applied Ethics are closely related: Theory without application is sterile and useless, but action without a theoretical perspective is blind. (Pojman 1990: xiv)

While giving interpretations of three theories, this chapter also has a secondary but no less important goal, which is to show the response of each theory to the question: *How ought we to live?*

UTILITARIANISM: PRODUCING THE BEST CONSEQUENCES

Utilitarianism is a moral theory that emphasises the consequences or outcomes of an act rather than the act itself. **Utilitarianism** is a **teleological theory**, a term that derives from the Greek word *telos*, meaning 'end' or 'goal'. The locus of value for utilitarians is the *outcome* or *consequences* of an act.

Good outcomes or consequences are those that yield overall benefits, pleasures and happiness for the greatest number of persons affected by an action. Good outcomes of actions also diminish overall suffering or harm. Any action that produces results of benefit, pleasure or wellbeing is a 'useful' action – useful as conducive to the greater good. Thus the term 'utility'. The choices or actions that contribute to maximal happiness or wellbeing have **instrumental value**. Instrumental values refer to something useful or important *for achieving some goal or purpose, or as a means to some end.*

The goals specified by utilitarians, of maximising pleasure, happiness, or wellbeing, are contentious. The meanings of these valued goals or human ends are not agreed. It seems clear that different people view pleasure, happiness and wellbeing with considerable disagreement. Diverse cultures might disagree even more profoundly. The utilitarians tried to specify these values or goals more fully in their social and political philosophies, but that leaves unanswered whether we can expect universal agreement on the concrete meaning of the goals.

The nineteenth-century philosopher, John Stuart Mill, in his famous essay, 'Utilitarianism', explained the meaning of goals that he believed would be universally agreed. Mill offers a 'guide to living', describing how one ought to live. Mill called utilitarianism the 'happiness theory' (Mill 1991: 134). The following quote may explain why:

> According to the Greatest Happiness Principle, the ultimate end, with reference to and for the sake of which all other things are desirable (whether our own good or that of other people) is an existence exempt as far as possible from pain, and as rich as possible in enjoyments, both in point of quantity and quality. (J. S. Mill 1991: 142)

The ultimate end sought by the utilitarian is a life described by Mill, rich in many pleasures of intellect, emotion and sensibility and spared in terms of suffering and pain. Both quantity of rich experiences and quality (range and depth) of experiences mattered in Mill's account of utilitarianism.

Does the End Justify the Means?

Utilitarians do not focus on the importance of motives for choosing when locating the moral quality of an action. Almost any motive is acceptable for a choice that delivers the positive outcome and overall best results. This point will strongly differentiate utilitarian theory from deontology. The test of the moral quality of actions is not personal motivation but objective results or outcomes: what outcomes give most pleasure, happiness, wellbeing and diminish their opposite? Saving a drowning man is always good, whatever the motivation of the rescuer. I might be doing this to get my picture in the paper and maybe get some reward from the man I save. This doesn't take away from the good result. Feeding starving people who have no subsistence is a good act and it matters not whether one's motive is primarily to get voted for the Nobel Peace Prize or whether it's from the motive of deep obligation to suffering humanity. If someone chooses to torture an innocent person with the motive of securing information that will save 150 children, utilitarians would view the beneficial outcome as the good deed. The good outcome retrospectively justifies the means taken. So, for the utilitarian, the end or outcome is what justifies any means used to get the consequences.

How Control Consequences?

Utilitarian theory is a prospective moral theory. It is forward looking, beyond the choices of the agent to outcomes of those choices. Here we look a bit more closely at the idea of how to assess outcomes. How can I know what the outcome of my actions will be? Am I responsible for whatever comes from my choices, positive and negative? Maybe the only effects or outcomes of my choices are those I foresee. Sometimes failing to foresee can be a legitimate excuse, but many times it isn't.

Utilitarians think that the consequences are the effects the agent could have *reasonably foreseen*, on the basis of information or understandings available to him or her. This aspect of the extent to which we ought to foresee consequences correctly can cause moral unease. The need to act in *anticipation of probable outcomes* requires the person to draw on many dimensions of understanding about human living, on the cultivation of moral imagination (Scott 1998). Recall the discussions of truth-telling, confidentiality, consent, abortion, sex selection and accountability. There you find illustrations of this challenging aspect of gauging consequences. What is held as a foreseeable consequence is a matter of what the agent has *sufficient grounds for believing* is likely to happen (Schick 1982: 252–3).

Stringent Demands from Utilitarian Theory

The demands of utilitarianism are stringent. In this section, two of those demands are briefly explained:

1. Sacrifice of personal projects and loved ones;
2. Requirement of negative responsibility: we are equally responsible for what we fail to do (our omissions) as what we do by positive action.

Self-Sacrifice

In the interest of effecting a maximal good of saving a city that will be bombed, the theory could expect a person to sacrifice their own family, their home or their own life if doing so would optimise an outcome. This focus on outcomes and not on the person choosing allows for the self, one's relationships and special personal projects to be subordinated to achievement of an heroic outcome. In brief, utilitarianism can endorse the situations where persons seem to violate their own integrity and character by requiring sacrifice of self, loves and life plans. From this perspective, the utilitarian demands that we act like saints without personal interests and goals (Sen and Williams 1982: 1–22). This expectation of individuals is often referred to as 'the integrity objection'.

Negative Responsibility

The distinction between positive and negative responsibility is a feature of utilitarianism that

> says something about how far we are morally accountable for our part in the way of the world. There is a distinction between positive or

negative ways of influencing events. We can act or we can fail or decline to act. We can do things, or we can forbear or neglect to do things. We can sometimes make things happen, and sometimes we allow or permit them to occur. We can set trains of events in motion or we can fail to stop them or derail them. (Harris 1985: 29)

The distinction between acts and omissions is at the root of the utilitarian distinction between positive and negative responsibility.

For example, a respirator may be off and the patient connected to it dead because someone switched it off (act or positive responsibility) or because someone did not switch it on where it was possible to do so (omission or negative responsibility). In brief, utilitarians believe we can be equally responsible for what happens because of our non-action (omissions) as what happens because of our actions. The range and scope of responsibility is thereby extended considerably, and corresponding obligations are assigned, since positive actions *and* omissions both may prove morally praiseworthy or blameworthy.

Activity

Consider the saying that is descriptive of utilitarian morality: 'The end justifies the means'. Some commentators think that this policy allows morally reprehensible acts to be committed to achieve good ends.

a) In your experience, do you think that this custom of using unjust or dishonest acts as means to achieving good ends is so unusual? What about a mother's tax evasion to save more money for a daughter's nursing studies? What about plagiarising a web essay to get first-class honours in nursing ethics or get a good position in health care? What about lying to patients to make them feel better? If these are fairly common happenings, does this mean that what is morally acceptable is changing today?

b) What does the fairly common occurrence of such events tell us? That utilitarianism is well suited to human behaviour?

Three-Step Action Formula

From what we have said, one can find in utilitarianism a three-step action formula: Taking it as a given rule or guideline spelled out by J. S. Mill in the text above, we then proceed to reflect, imagine and choose.

1. On the basis of what we know, we must project consequences of each alternative option (action or omission) open to us.
2. Calculate how much happiness, or balance of happiness over unhappiness, is likely to be produced by anticipated consequences of each action or omission.
3. Select that action which, on balance, will produce the greatest amount of happiness for the greatest number of people affected (see Yeo and Moorhouse 1996: 45).

Importance of Developing a Utilitarian Character

Developing a character or habit is important for utilitarianism as much as for the other theories we will discuss. Acting habitually for the best outcome makes it more probable that better overall outcomes will be achieved. For a utilitarian, good character is an *instrumental good*. It is useful to bring about the goal of the greatest human wellbeing. One useful way of ensuring that we are utilitarians of 'good character' is to work on self-education of natural sympathy for human beings generally. This self-education in sympathy facilitates a feeling of obligation towards achieving overall happiness and so grounds a practical utilitarian morality (Crisp 1997; Gutmann 1982).

Summary Learning Guide 18.1

Defining Features of Utilitarian Moral Theory are:

- The moral quality of our decisions (both actions and omissions) is determined entirely by the beneficial consequences following on these decisions;
- Good consequences are understood broadly to mean: outcomes such as pleasure, health, wellbeing, justice, happiness, satisfaction of preferences, and so on;
- Moral responsibility is both positive and negative – covering our actions and omissions to act.

Motives as Morally Neutral

- Motives for actions are not relevant for the moral evaluation of that action.
- Motives are simply instrumental means for achieving good ends. Ends justify means.

How Ought We to Live our Lives?

- We ought always, in our choices, to work to maximise good consequences and minimise undesirable outcomes.
- We ought to develop good habits, such as the feeling of sympathy. In doing so, we make more probable the steady pursuit of the goal of promoting human wellbeing.

Strengths and Problems in Utilitarianism

At first sight, utilitarianism seems very compelling and applicable to life. Here we review strengths and problems and encourage you to add points you think are important.

Strengths

1.   This theory specifies its goal to increase positive value and minimise evil. This goal on its own can hardly be disputed.
2.   Utilitarianism has a potential answer for most situations. There is a simple action-guiding rule or principle applicable to most occasions. We have a clear though demanding procedure for arriving at answers about what to do.

3.   Utilitarians recognise that 'the path to hell is paved with good intentions' and therefore focus moral evaluation on consequences and not on motives the agent holds.

4.   Utilitarianism is not just abstract and 'up in the clouds moralising'. It gets to the substance of morality with a material core: promote human flourishing and ameliorate suffering (Pojman 1990: 80).

5.   ??

Problems
Utilitarianism has several problems:

1.   It is a contentious issue whether we should be held equally responsible for our so-called actions and omissions. It is impractical to extend the scope of responsibility to include omissions – what we could do but fail to do.

2.   More serious is how we determine the consequences in terms of wellbeing, happiness or pleasure. Critics claim that persons simply choose their understanding of these ends to be achieved. There is no unanimous and agreed meaning to pleasures; happiness; the wellbeing of others. This seems to cast doubt on any possible objectivity to these human goods at the heart of utilitarianism (see MacIntyre 1988).

3.   Utilitarianism could sanction immoral actions as judged by the standards of common morality. If the most effective way to achieve a maximal utilitarian outcome (secure information to save fifty persons) is to perform an immoral act (torture an innocent person), then the theory seems to say not only that the torture is permissible, but that it is morally obligatory. But this requirement of the theory seems itself immoral.

4.   Utilitarianism demands too much on two fronts:
    a)   The level of skills needed is too stringent: judgement, knowledge, calculation of outcomes from actions and omissions, required imagination to envisage consequences. Given these rigorous skill requirements, utilitarianism shows itself to be an elitist moral theory.
    b)   In the interest of maximising outcomes, it requires a violation of one's character and integrity by expecting a level of heroic sacrifice of special relationships and life projects.

5.   ??

DEONTOLOGY – WHAT DUTY ASKS OF US

What makes a 'right' act right? The consequentialist answer to this question is that it is the good outcomes of an act that make it right. Moral rightness or wrongness is determined by the promotion of nonmoral values such as pleasure, wellbeing, happiness, and so on. To this extent, the end justifies the means. In many respects, deontological moral theory is diametrically the opposite of utilitarianism.

The name of the German philosopher, Immanuel Kant (1724–1804), is identified with the rigours of deontology. Kant adamantly disagreed with utilitarianism and believed it was an irresponsible theory contributing to expediency and compromises with moral evil. For deontologists, it is not consequences that determine the rightness or wrongness of an act. The emphasis is on the correctness of the action, regardless of the possible benefits or harm it might produce. There are some moral obligations that obtain absolutely, irrespective of the consequences produced.

Kant was an absolutist but he was also a rationalist. As a 'rationalist', he believed that we could always use reason to work out a consistent set of moral principles that could not be overridden. One way of describing these deontological moral principles is to say that they are 'non-negotiable'. They cannot be argued away by persuasion, rationalisations or counter-reasons.

Unlike the moral theory of consequentialism where the value of moral choices is their instrumentality, deontology finds intrinsic value in good choices. Whether they achieve good consequences is not essential to their moral quality.

> The moral worth of an action does not lie in the effect expected from it and so too does not lie in any principle of action that needs to borrow its motive from this expected effect. For, all these effects (promotion of others' happiness etc.) could have been also brought about by other causes, so that there would have been no need for this, of the will of a rational being, in which the highest and unconditional good alone can be found. (Kant 1997: 14)

The aim of the *Groundwork of the Metaphysics of Morals* (1785) is to establish a most fundamental point about morality – that there is a domain of laws applying to our conduct and that there is such a thing as non-negotiable morality. Its aim is the search for an establishment of the supreme principle of morality. That supreme principle Kant calls the categorical imperative. Categorical imperatives are commands or rules that admit of no exceptions and are binding on all rational beings.

Categorical Imperative: Four Duties
Kant's categorical imperative is not just an abstract rule. Rather, it yields four duties that must be upheld at any cost. These four duties are the rules or guidelines that answer the question we posed at the start of the chapter: How ought we to live?

1. Act in such a way as you would have others act towards you (the famous 'golden rule').
2. Treat people as ends in themselves and never solely as means to an end (people should never be simply instruments for my own ends).

3. Act so that you treat the will of every rational being as one that makes universal law (respect for autonomy of others).
4. Act in such a way that you would have all other persons act (rule of universality).

Number four states an especially challenging test for us when choosing to do something. It requires that we act not out of self-interest, but because we believe it is the right action to perform for anyone in my particular situation. So, if we are deciding to lie in order to escape a difficult task, then we must be ready to allow everyone else to lie for the same reason. If we are stealing rare lilies from our neighbour's garden to bring to a friend in hospital, we need to be ready for our neighbour to steal rare roses from our garden for her friend. Kant believed that this requirement of universality places necessary constraints on our conduct.

Here we notice clearly that Kant does not entirely ignore consequences. We take them into account in order to consider our choices. We ask: What would be the consequences of everyone acting on the principle I want to follow? So, to answer that, we need to imagine consequences for our world if everyone acted contrary to the duties spelled out above. Not every proposed reason for action can be made universal because the consequences would be defeating of all morality and yield an impossible human situation. Not every action can be squared with the requirements of acting on principle (Korskgaard 1997: x-xi). In brief, a Kantian cannot just disregard possible consequences, but the achievement of certain outcomes will *never* be the determining feature of a moral choice. Moral choices depend on choosing actions with intrinsic value and doing so with moral motives.

Intentions of a Person with Good Will

Deontological morality is grounded in human motivation, and not only in consequences. The assignment of moral worth rests totally with the person's intentional state. Even a person of niggardly disposition who has to work hard to be sympathetic with suffering people can, nevertheless, with effort, exercise their volition and do the right thing in spite of their negative inclinations. They do the right thing not because they will be praised or rewarded or otherwise gain immortal life, but simply because it is the right thing to do. Respect for the moral law is the moral motive for acting. That moral law was spelled out in the four duties given above.

We cannot discount consequences, but good outcomes will never make an immoral action moral. Our motives – whether or not we act with a good will according to the categorical imperative – determine whether we are persons of moral character or not.

Activity

Review the four duties given above that follow from Kant's understanding of the categorical imperative:
• The golden rule;

- Treating people as ends, never solely as means;
- The rule of respect for autonomy;
- The rule of universality.

a) Can you give examples where you think one or more of these four duties should not or could not be observed?

b) Do you agree with Kant that the consequences of my actions are not fully in my control and so should not count in the moral appraisal of my actions?

c) Would you add other duties to this list that would be necessary for a moral life?

The person who lives their life according to the four duties above, would, on Kant's appraisal, be judged a person of 'good will'. As they aspire to be moral, they would work to live these duties without exception. Kant's own words have no equal.

> It is impossible to think of anything at all in the world, or indeed even beyond it, that could be considered good without limitation except a good will.
>
> Power, riches, honour, even health and that complete well-being and satisfaction with one's condition called happiness, produce boldness and often arrogance unless a good will is present that corrects the influence of these on the mind, and, in so doing, also corrects the whole principle of action and brings it into conformity with universal ends.
>
> A good will constitutes the indispensable condition even of worthiness to be happy. A good will is not good because of what it effects or accomplishes, because of its fitness to attain some proposed end, but only because of its willing . . . A good will is good in itself and is to be valued incomparably higher than all else. Usefulness or fruitlessness can neither add anything to this worth nor take anything away from it. (Kant [1785] 1997: 7–8)

Do Good Inclinations Help with Being Moral?

Kant was a rigorous moralist and a religious believer. However, he too argued that religion and possible rewards of immortality could not enter into his theory intended to be universal. We could not count on certain religious beliefs to make people moral. Nor could we rely on good inclinations, feelings or sentiments in people to make them moral. We need to look to the disciplined will.

The person of good will, conscientiously working to observe the four duties spelled out above, needs to take note of the subject of natural inclinations: Natural inclinations are leanings of personality or disposition with which, for the most part we are born. Some of these inclinations are considered negative: niggardly, mean, selfish, unpleasant, discourteous, and so on. Many people judge some inclinations that we're born with to be positive: kindness, compassion, sympathy, joyfulness, and so on.

A Kantian deontologist cautions us to be wary of natural inclinations – be they negative or positive. Because we are kindly or compassionate by temperament does not give us an edge on being moral. It may make it easier to do good for other people, but that is not the yardstick Kant uses. People who have negative inclinations by temperament are considered much more praiseworthy if they succeed in doing the right thing! Moral actions done from duty are those that have true moral worth. An action one might do because one is so inclined by disposition, like telling the truth, may have no true moral worth unless it is chosen because it is one's duty and the right thing to do.

This view on inclinations offers hope to those not born with generous disposition and warns those who have such dispositions not to be complacent. Kant's deontological view on inclinations does not mean that we should not be joyous or generous if we are made that way. But no special moral value is given to positive inclinations. We did not do anything to deserve our innate inheritance of these feelings. We cannot base our morality on generous or niggardly genes and dispositions given by Nature. Morality has to be independent of natural dispositions. If we work against our niggardly disposition and succeed in acting according to duty, we are morally worthy.

Summary Learning Guide 18.2

Defining Features of Deontology:

- Actions are intrinsically right or wrong depending on whether or not right principles motivate them;
- Consequences must be considered when making a choice but can never be decisive in measuring the moral quality of an action;
- Natural inclinations (positive or negative) might make moral behaviour more or less difficult but they are not part of the moral appraisal of a person.

Motives for Acting

- The motive one has for acting is morally decisive.
- The moral motive for any action is to choose always out of respect for the moral law.

How Ought We to Live?

- We ought to work conscientiously to become persons of good will.
- A good will observes four rules or duties:
  1. Treat others as you would be treated;
  2. Treat people as ends never solely as means;
  3. Respect the autonomy of others;
  4. Observe the rule of universality.

Review the main points of Kantian deontology and see if you can add to this list of strengths and problems of the theory.

Strengths

1. Kant explains with insight how we ought to live: to be committed to a moral system of principles and rules.
2. His four duties are specific enough to give guidance where needed in many circumstances of living. The theory then is practicable.
3. The idea of universality is an undeniably helpful constraint on temptations to act solely out of self-interest. Persons cannot act morally while making themselves privileged or exempt from the duty of universality.
4. The argument that good consequences are never sufficient for the moral quality of an action offers fundamental challenges for utilitarian moral theory to respond.
5. ??

Problems

1. Kant's ethics leads to rigidly insensitive rules and so cannot take account of differences between cases.
2. Kant identifies ethical duties that are too abstract to guide action. If so, his theory is not action-guiding. Notice that a strength cited above mentioned the helpfulness of the four specific duties based on the categorical imperative. Do you think the theory is sufficiently action-guiding?
3. Some serious criticisms are directed at Kant's moral psychology. Kant says we ought to act out of the motive of duty and not out of inclination, emotion, sentiments or feeling. In fact, because these latter elements can make us confuse feeling with moral obligations, we should be wary of them. Thus Kant seems to take a negative view on the role of emotions and claims that an action we enjoy cannot be morally worthy. This problem might signal difficulties with the comprehensive nature of Kant's theory.
4. ??

Before concluding this discussion of deontology, it is important to note that there are deontologists very much alive and well today. Religious believers would often consider themselves as deontologists: accepting some actions as categorically right and others wrong. The religious believer might, additionally, have a revelation to draw on for understanding what actions are right and which to be avoided. The often uncompromising positions held by religious believers may not reflect stubbornness or close-mindedness but might demonstrate the Kantian conviction that consequences – no matter how good – cannot make evil actions good! A review of some of the positions presented in Chapter 9 on abortion and Chapter 13 on companying the chronically ill and dying illustrates the contemporary deontological perspective most clearly.

In addition, two contemporary philosophers who accept and develop a Kantian account, broadly construed, are Alan Donagan and John Rawls. Both philosophers develop their positions on the now-familiar Kantian bases of respect for persons as ends and never solely as means and the necessity to respect, and promote the autonomy of persons (see Donagan 1977; Rawls 1971).

VIRTUE THEORY:
CHALLENGING ADEQUACY OF RULE-BASED THEORIES

The third theory discussion will be more briefly developed for two reasons. Firstly, contemporary virtue theory is understood in great part as responding to the deficiencies in deontology and utilitarian theories. By focusing on virtue and moral character, it promises greater adequacy for its theory.

Secondly, Chapter 19 details several theories – narrative, care perspective and feminism – that share a number of features with virtue theory.

Virtue ethics is not altogether new. The ancient Greek philosopher, Aristotle (384–322 BC) first wrote a detailed discussion of virtue morality in the *Nichomachean Ethics*. 'Virtus' he understood as strength. Specific virtues correspondingly are seen as strengths of character. However, for many years after Aristotle, virtue theory was overshadowed by the development of utilitarianism and deontology. In the past twenty years, virtue theory has resurfaced as a major moral theory. But why is that so?

Virtue ethics has been restated and reinvigorated since 1958 by philosophers such as Philippa Foot, Alasdair MacIntrye and Elizabeth Anscombe. They and many others in the past decades became disillusioned with the promises of mainstream theories. They believe that *how we ought to live* could be much more adequately answered with virtue-based theory.

Moral Virtue: Centrality of Motives

A virtue is a trait of character that is socially valued, and a moral virtue is a trait that is morally valued. Courage might be a socially valued trait but it becomes moral courage only if the context is a moral one. Moral virtue is a disposition to act, or a habit of acting in accordance with moral ideals, principles or obligations (Pence 1991).

Aristotle distinguished between external performance and internal state. This is the difference between right action and proper motive. An action can be right without being virtuous, he said, but the action can be virtuous *only* if performed from the right state of mind of the person.

Virtue, then, is closely aligned with motives. We do care (along with Kant) how persons are motivated. We especially care about their general or habitual forms of motivation. Someone who gives donations to mental-health research and is motivated by personal concern or sympathy for suffering people meets with approval, while someone acting the same way to be able to proclaim generosity as a feature of their character would not find our endorsement. Persons who are properly motivated – not just for a single action, but by disposition or habit; persons of virtue don't simply follow rules but have a morally relevant motive and desire to act as they do. Aristotle explains the importance of learning good habits and so signalling the practical value of philosophy:

> Moral goodness . . . is the child of habit, from which it has got its very name, ethics being derived from *ethos*, 'habit' . . . The moral virtues then are produced in us neither *by* Nature nor *against* Nature. Nature, indeed, prepares in us the ground for their reception, but their complete formation is the product of habit. We are concerned . . . how we are to become good men for this alone gives philosophy its practical value – we must apply our minds to the solution of the problems of conduct. For . . . it is our actions that determine our dispositions. (Aristotle 1955, 55–7)

Virtue theorists believe that the basic instructions and emphasis on right motives and desires of virtue theory will guide us, not only about what to do but what to be (Frankena 1998: 291–6).

The person of morally good disposition is properly motivated. To be properly motivated, says Aristotle, one must experience appropriate feelings. He explains:

> We may even go so far as to state that the man [woman] who does not enjoy performing noble actions is not a good man [woman] at all. Nobody would call a person just who does not enjoy acting justly, nor generous who does not enjoy generous actions, and so on. (Aristotle 1955: 42)

Aristotelian virtue theory cautions us away from a negative view of morality that mainly requires us to do what we really don't feel like doing. Anne Thomson speaks of the critical role of emotions in developing a moral disposition of fair-mindedness. This focus on the centrality of cultivating proper feelings and emotions as ingredients of virtuous action stands in stark contrast to Kantian deontology's suspicion of feelings (see Anne Thomson 1999: 143–52).

Character More Important than Conformity to Rules

Virtue theorists believe that their views supplement deontology and utilitarianism by offering a more comprehensive moral theory for human beings, acknowledging our common intuition that motives do make a quality difference in actions and that appropriate feelings facilitate virtuous behaviour.

Writers in health-care ethics suggest that efforts to replace virtuous judgements of professionals with rules, codes or procedures will not result in better decisions and actions. For example, rather than always appealing to government regulations or international conventions to protect subjects in research, some think that the most reliable protection is a researcher with a character marked by: informed conscientiousness, responsible sensibility, and compassion. The thesis is that good habits of character are more important than conformity to rules, and such good habits are most likely to lead to behaviour consistent with rules.

The position is that virtues should be inculcated and cultivated over time, through educational interactions, role models, moral mentoring, and the like. Gregory Pence contends that the right kinds of desires, feelings and motives are best protections for client wellbeing. Almost any health professional can successfully evade a system of rules. We should create a climate in which health professionals desire by virtue of strong habit not to abuse their subjects (Pence 1991). The educational process for health-care professions is a context for modelling the virtues of good nurses and good doctors. Where adequate role models are lacking, little progress can be made by further exhortations to become a 'good (virtuous) nurse'.

This last point stresses the argument that we do not make moral decisions as isolated persons in a social vacuum. It is rather in families, schools or communities that natural affection, spontaneous sympathies, shared concerns and expectations for the virtues arise. In turn, these virtues give human nurture to these social groups.

Compatibility of Virtues and Principles
The rule-governed theories of utilitarianism and deontology are not at odds with virtue theory. They are compatible and mutually reinforcing. Persons of good moral character sometimes have difficulties discerning what is right and would recognise that they need principles, rules and ideals to help determine right or good acts.

> One often cannot act virtuously unless one makes judgements about the best ways to manifest sympathy, desire and the like. The virtues need principles and rules to regulate and supplement them. As Aristotle suggests, ethics involves judgements like those in medicine: Principles guide us to actions, but we still need to assess a situation and formulate an appropriate response. This assessment and response flows from character and training as much as from principles. (Beauchamp and Childress 1994: 67)

In order for us to progress as moral agents and justify our actions in the eyes of those affected, this need to explain and justify requires that we translate our virtuous claims into explanation of the values, duties or principles on which we base those claims. To do this, we may need to say *why* we consider it compassionate behaviour to lie, or why it is just behaviour to break confidence with patients, or loyal to keep silent when speaking out would correct wrongdoing. This requirement to justify our moral decisions reveals the intricate connection between virtue theory and rule-governed theories discussed earlier.

Activity

The concept of virtue might seem a bit of a weasel word – vague, open to multiple interpretations and unhelpful for giving practical guidance.

a) How do you understand the idea of 'virtue'? Consider someone whom you think 'virtuous'. How would you describe that person? What kinds of behaviour or attitudes of the person would you offer as moral indicators of virtue?

b) Does a 'good' nurse have certain characteristic 'virtues'? If you had to write a short essay on 'Nursing: a Life of Virtue', what would you have to say? If you believe that virtue is not relevant as a focus in nursing, try to explain why.

c) Now consider the role of feelings as expressed by Aristotle. Many times we know what we ought to do but certainly don't feel like it. Is Aristotle minimising the need for *will* to come into action when making choices? Do feelings need to accompany virtues?

Strengths

1. Virtue theory expands the moral picture by stressing the moral importance and desirability of feelings, forms of sympathy, attitudes of others and community concerns.
2. In contrast to utilitarianism which ignores the moral importance of motives, virtue theory places them at centre stage. This makes virtue theory more consistent with customary intuition that motives do make the person.
3. Virtue theory, focused on the development of good habits, provides an essential complement to the rules and duty focus of utilitarianism and deontology.
4. Virtue theory responds to social contexts of living by showing that communities both produce and find sustenance in the practice of virtuous persons.
5. ??

Problems

1. The listings of virtues are too relative to societies and cultures for us to be able to rely on them as guides to good character across cultures.
2. Virtue theory is not fully adequate to offer important moral protections where interaction between strangers is at issue. Character judgements, central to virtue theory, play a less central role than rights, duties and procedures when strangers meet.
3. Virtue theory faces difficulties in adequately justifying and explaining *why* some specific actions are right or wrong. It is not enough to say that if persons display a virtuous character, their actions are therefore morally acceptable.
4. ??

CONCLUSION

The three theories we discussed in this chapter offer different emphases in the task of assessing moral viewpoints and moral character.

Utilitarianism requires careful application of calculation skills and attention to the supreme value of promoting happiness and diminishing suffering. One's motives for acting are morally irrelevant. What counts are the consequences of one's choices. Health-care allocations are almost always determined on utilitarian grounds – a sobering realisation that calls for care in assessing this moral theory. The utilitarian view of good character takes it as a steady disposition always to attend to promoting the good of the greatest number of persons even if this means sacrifice of one's own projects and special relationships. We ought to live with a steady focus on the end value, which is happiness and the benefits we can offer to the many in promoting that happiness.

Deontology calls on its adherents to learn the particular duties of living the categorical imperative. Consequences of our actions need to be deliberated but whether they are good or adverse never affects the moral quality of our choices. Our motive for acting – in keeping with the moral law – is the sole determinant of quality of choices. Feelings and emotions are viewed with scepticism and positively discouraged as necessary elements in living the moral life.

Deontology answers the question: *how ought we to live?* by claiming that it is in the cultivation of a good will that we give example of moral character. A good will is a disposition always to act in keeping with the specific principles of the categorical imperative. The Kantian duties spelled out are illustrated in a contemporary form in principlism, discussed in Chapter 19.

Virtue theory puts less stress on duties and principles and turns the lens on states of character. With the virtue focus comes an appreciation of the role of feelings, emotions and right motives in becoming a person of virtuous character. Numerous rules and obligations can always be circumvented. These listings of duties and principles are no substitute for persons who have dispositions for courage, compassion, generosity, and so on. The inclusion of feelings, desire and emotions as valuable in moral life are positive additions of virtue theory. Virtue theory answers the question: *how ought we to live?* by insisting that cultivation of good habits makes persons better contributors to their social and professional context. Virtue theory finds contemporary expression in two theories – narrative ethics and the ethic of care, considered in Chapter 19.

In the final analysis, the three theories are seen not as adversaries but as largely complementary. Rules, duties and principles are needed to give meaning and justification to the virtues.

The following terms are explained in the glossary:

categorical imperative	teleological theory
deontological theory	utilitarianism
instrumental good	virtue theory
principlism	

Contemporary Moral Theories

Objectives

At the end of this chapter, you should be able to:

- Explain and discuss the main features of four contemporary moral theories:
  § **principlism**
  § **narrative ethics**
  § **ethic of care**
  § **feminist ethics**;

- Consider the way in which each of these moral theories highlights different features of moral life;
- Assess the different ways in which each of these theories might enhance the moral decision making of nurses.

INTRODUCTION

The discussion in Chapter 18 of three 'traditional' theories offered moral perspectives that are supported by the authority and durability of years. They were called 'traditional' simply because they have been in place in the canon of moral philosophy for centuries. Duration is not enough to make them adequate to the tasks required of moral theories. Moral theories need to interpret human efforts to live a moral life. Utilitarianism, deontology, and virtue theory have not remained fixed and static as theories. Volumes are written that assess elements of these theories, sharpening them for greater clarity, and attuning them more to the fullness of human living. The conclusion of Chapter 18 stated that it is counterproductive to understand these traditional theories as competing for the best theory marks! Rather, the theories can largely be seen as complementary – each interpreting our moral lives in ways that offer different emphases but also challenge us to look again at our own understanding of moral living.

However, insights into moral living come in fresh forms, breathing new life into the traditional moral canon. This chapter offers four contemporary ethical theories. In these, we find new insights that attempt a number of tasks:

1. To offer developments (and improvements) on essential features in traditional theories;
2. To fill in the dimensions of human living that were often omitted or understated in traditional theorising;

3.   To acknowledge that the challenges of moral development require that we move from a realm of moral abstractions to concrete situations. This allows us to see whether or how much the resources of moral theory help to guide our decision making.

PRINCIPLISM

What is known as the principlist approach to ethical decision making has dominated western bioethics for the past twenty years. It emerged with the publication of several well-known texts in the 1970s and 1980s. One of these was the *Belmont Report* which identified basic principles that would underlie and guide the regulation of research involving human subjects (National Commission for the Protection of Human Subjects of Biomedical and Behavioral Research 1979). Three books, also published at that time, outlined and defended a principlist ethical framework – those of Tom Beauchamp and James Childress (1979), Robert Veatch (1981) and H. Tristram Engelhardt (1986).

Of these three, the account developed by Beauchamp and Childress in their book, *The Principles of Biomedical Ethics*, is the most well known. What is particularly attractive about this principlist model (hereafter called the PBE model) is that, since its first appearance in 1979, the authors have continuously refined and honed its central elements in response to numerous objections that have been made to it over the years. This reworking of their position has, we think, made it more resistant to the problems endemic to principlism generally, and more inclusive of other features of the moral world that it had, initially, ignored.

The PBE model is an ethical decision-making process which negotiates between fundamental principles, on the one hand, and the unique nature of specific moral situations on the other. These principles oblige the health professional to behave in certain ways in relation to patients.

1.   The principle of autonomy obliges nurses to respect the views, choices and actions of individuals in their care.
2.   The principle of nonmaleficence obliges nurses not to harm patients.
3.   The principle of beneficence obliges nurses to act for the benefit of, or in the interests of, patients.
4.   The principle of justice obliges nurses to treat people in their care equally and to ensure that resources are distributed fairly.

A good deal of the *Principles of Biomedical Ethics* text is taken up with an analysis and discussion of each of the four principles in terms of its nature and scope. In particular, the specific rules that are supported by these principles and that permit, prohibit or require particular kinds of action are delineated. These include rules governing truth telling, confidentiality and informed consent (Beauchamp and Childress 2001: 57–112).

What is special about the four principles, according to Beauchamp and Childress, is their universal or objective nature. Beyond tradition, individual vagaries and culture, the authors claim that these principles have been drawn from a 'common morality', the set of norms that 'all morally serious persons share' (2001: 3). According to Beauchamp and Childress: 'The common morality contains moral norms that bind all persons in all places; no norms are more basic in the moral life' and they refer to the notion of international human rights as an example of such universal norms (2001: 3). Having grounded their four principles, they justify their particular choice by pointing out that these four have been presupposed by traditional ethical theories and medical codes throughout history.

The most immediate way to decide on the merits of a proposed course of action, on the PBE model, is to determine whether or not that course of action obeys the moral rules that are derived from the four principles. For example, in this view, a nurse might consider that it is, generally, morally required to provide a patient with information about their illness because this action obeys the moral rule 'Tell the truth' which is, in turn, derived from the principle, 'Respect patient autonomy'.

In morally difficult situations, however, where there is a conflict between principles, or between principles and particular judgements, the PBE model stipulates that none of the principles is *a priori* privileged. In any given situation, each principle must be specified and weighed relative to the particular context in which it is applied, and informed by generally accepted background theories of human nature and moral life. Following John Rawls, this weighing and balancing is described as a process of **reflective equilibrium** and the principles are described as **prima facie** rather than absolute (Beauchamp and Childress 2001: 398). This is to express the idea that any one principle is, on first impression, morally obligatory but that it may be modified or overridden in certain situations. In the case of Sean, the patient with Alzheimer's in Case 2.1, Chapter 2, for example, a nurse might initially believe that keeping Sean in the hospital might be the morally correct thing to do. However, on consideration of all of the circumstances surrounding the patient, she might reconsider. In this case, it could be argued that it is her particular judgement in the concrete situation which prompts her to reconsider whether the principle of beneficence, or some other rule, such as autonomy, should apply here.

The process of reflective equilibrium involves the specification, reciprocal weighing, testing, revising and balancing of principles, rules, background theories and particular judgements. For Beauchamp and Childress, the objective here is to reduce any conflict among our beliefs by fitting them into a coherent whole:

> So-called wide reflective equilibrium occurs when we evaluate the strengths and weaknesses of all plausible moral judgments, principles, and relevant background theories. Here we incorporate as wide a variety of kinds and levels of legitimate beliefs as possible, including hard test cases in experience [. . .] No matter how wide the pool of beliefs, we have no reason to anticipate that the process of pruning, adjusting, and rendering coherent will either come to an end or be

perfected. A moral framework is more a process than a finished product; and moral problems [. . .] should be considered projects in need of continual adjustment by reflective equilibrium. (Beauchamp and Childress 2001: 399)

On this understanding, the processes of moral deliberation are akin to scientific processes: plausible beliefs and possible decisions are considered and accepted, rejected and modified on the basis of reflection and experience. Also, analogous to the scientific goal of achieving theoretical consistency and unity, the aim of reflective equilibrium is to unify all one's moral beliefs and background commitments.

Positively, the PBE model provides a method of supporting ethical decisions that has a strong justificatory force. Put simply, according to this view, the force of the imperative, 'Respect autonomy', derives from its grounding in universally accepted norms, not, for example, in the subjective viewpoint or intuition of the nurse.

Moreover, even in situations of doubt and uncertainty, such as in the case of Sean in Chapter 2, the deliberative process which comes into play appeals to reasoning strategies and goals that are also considered objective, not intuitive. In addition, the course of action that would be considered the most successful, in this view, would be one that manages to meet as many of the relevant principles as possible. The challenge in Sean's case is both to respect his autonomy, and, at the same time, to act in his best interests.

Finally, principlism has received the critical attention of theorists working in nursing ethics. Steven Edwards, for example, proposes that nurses should adapt and adopt the PBE model developed by Beauchamp and Childress, and he defends principlism on several grounds including the following: that it provides a clear and coherent framework for ethical decision making; that it is easily applicable to very many problems that nurses face; that it requires that nurses consider moral problems in the light of the different perspectives, such as the perspectives of autonomy and justice, for example; and that it is consistent with the norms of international nursing codes (Edwards 1996: 1, 48–9).

Summary Learning Guide 19.1

Principlism claims that:

- Basic commonly shared principles – autonomy, nonmaleficence, beneficence and justice – and the specific action-guiding rules that are derived from them are central to the ethical decision-making process in health-care situations;
- In any given health-care situation, any decision or course of action is morally justified if it is consistent with relevant principles, rules, background theories and judgements in particular situations;
- The success of any chosen course of action, on the part of the nurse, can be measured by the degree to which it achieves an overall cohesion of all of the elements of the decision-making process.

NARRATIVE ETHICS

While different shades of principlism have dominated the health-care landscape in the past twenty years, an increasing number of theorists have begun to turn their attention to alternative approaches to describing and understanding the various elements of moral life. One such approach deploys, as tools of moral understanding and assessment, narrative concepts and methodologies drawn from literary criticism and philosophy. In common with contemporary thinkers in other disciplines (anthropology, philosophy, cognitive psychology and history, for example) who have turned their attention to narratives, narrativists in the health-care arena argue that the first-person narrative, or personal story, is a rich medium for qualitative data about the unique lives of individual people. Further, for some of these theorists, the narrative is not only an important form of communication, it is also a means of making human life, and specifically the moral life, intelligible. While they deploy narrative tools in different ways, we suggest that all of these thinkers are engaged in 'narrative ethics'.

Martha Nussbaum (1992), for example, views literature as a vast resource of moral knowledge and a means of sensitising people to the responsibilities, obligations and challenges of a full moral life. Alternatively, the narrative approaches of Albert Jonsen and Stephen Toulmin (1988) and John Arras (1991) take a **casuistic** turn and resolve ethical dilemmas by comparing each new situation with others and with paradigm cases. These authors argue that local, contingent moral rules and maxims to guide action can be derived from paying attention to the morally relevant similarities and differences between cases.

More recently, Rita Charon (1994) has suggested that our understanding of health-care situations will be greatly enhanced if we pay attention to their narrative elements – for example, the function of the narrator; who tells the story; the development of plot; how the story unfolds; the relationship with the audience; who hears and interprets the story. In addition to supporting Charon's view, Tod Chambers (1999) has sparked a lively debate in the bioethics community, arguing that the task of reporting cases is itself not a neutral enterprise. He argues that the process of describing any set of events involves decisions about including or excluding certain pieces of information and making choices about the way different facts are presented. Consider, for example, the way in which we treated Bill Murphy's story in Chapter 5 (Case 5.1) and then again in Chapter 6 (Case 6.2).

Finally, narrativists such as Howard Brody (1987), Arthur Frank (1995), Kathryn Montgomery Hunter (1992, 1995), Alasdair MacIntyre (2000) and Paul Ricoeur (1988) argue that not only does the narrative approach to morally difficult situations enhance existing models of decision making, such as principlism, but that the approach itself is theoretically robust. At the very least, it radically challenges the theoretical adequacy of models such as principlism. At best, it provides an alternative means of justifying ethical decisions which focus on the relational and communicative dimensions of moral situations.

Because narrative ethics is in its early stages of development, there is, as yet, no ready-to-hand canonical position that best expresses its central tenets. Indeed, as we have indicated, 'narrative ethics' comprises a very diverse range of thinkers, from those who view narratives as a rich resource for existing ethical theories to those who see the concepts and methodologies associated with the study of narratives as the foundation of a health-care ethics theory that can serve as an alternative to traditional models. Even so, in what follows, we will roughly sketch what we see as the most plausible and defensible account of narrative ethics. It is also one that highlights the tensions between narrative ethics and principlism and exposes the congruities and incongruities between these, supposed, competing positions.

For narrativists, understanding an individual's life as a narrative, and deploying narrative methodologies to read and interpret it, broadens and enriches our understanding of that life and deepens our insight into the relationship between the unravelling of human life and moral agency. Anne Scott (1999), for example, argues that in addition to skills of moral reasoning, what is required for an adequate moral engagement in many health-care situations is **moral imagination**. She defines moral imagination as:

> the human faculty that allows 'gut reaction' to be used and moderated into the perceptual schema, enabling a moral agent to build up multidimensional understandings of a situation. (Scott 1999: 149)

Like Nussbaum, mentioned above, Scott argues that literature, especially poetry and short stories, can provide a rich critical resource for the development of the moral imagination of nursing and medical students.

According to the narrative view also, when ethically challenging situations arise, it is the whole journey of an individual's life as they conceive it themselves that is privileged. Howard Brody, for example, sees the practice of health care, in part, 'as a storytelling enterprise':

> The concept of 'story' suggests appreciation of a narrative mode – that certain sorts of events can be fully understood only as portions of certain ongoing narrative and not as disconnected events occurring in isolation. In contrast, much of modern medical ethics is 'rule' and 'decision'-oriented, suggesting that precisely such an ahistorical, nonnarrative form of ethical analysis is optimal. (Brody 1987: xiii)

For Brody, actions are made meaningful in the context of an individual life story. As such, it is difficult to isolate any given decision or choice, uncouple it from the whole person who acts, and evaluate it in terms of abstract and general rules. In health-care settings, this means that, where it is possible to hear it, the patient's own account – of their illness, their preferences, their needs – is considered profoundly important. However, not any tall tale will do, and personal stories are tested against various criteria such as the stories of others and the medical chart. Why? Firstly because, as we all know, we are wont to be naïve, mistaken and delusional about our beliefs and self-understandings. Secondly, as Nelson argues

(2001: 93–5), our self-conceptions rely on the conceptions of others to make them genuinely identity-constituting – for example, a nurse might find it difficult to take a patient's blood pressure if the patient did not believe that they were a nurse. Thirdly, our self-conceptions are contextual – they get constructed within culturally available narratives which both enable and limit the kinds of people we can imagine ourselves to be.

According to this narrative account, the more credible stories are those that capture what it is about our lives that matters most to us. They are intelligible, consistent with biographical events and consistent with what we actually do. They also explain best why we take responsibility for our actions, why some things matter to us more than others, why we love what we love, why we are happy or hurt (Nelson 2001: 92–105).

We liken this idea of testing personal narratives against various criteria to the way in which the principlist model tests its principles through the application of the process of reflective equilibrium. In the case of the PBE model, the four principles are prima facie privileged, and may be modified subsequently. In the narrative view, it is first-person narratives that are prima facie privileged; however, like principles, they can be challenged and modified in the process of what we call, a 'narrative reflective equilibrium'. The final story, or account of a life that emerges from such evaluation, Ricoeur describes, recalling the Socratic ideal, as 'the fruit of an examined life' (1988: 246–7).

In recent years, a narrative approach of this kind has contributed to discussion and debate in relation to surrogate decision making in end-of-life situations. For example, it informs one of the recent recommendations of the US Council on Ethical and Judicial Affairs which suggests that, when it comes to making decisions for incompetent patients, one of the tasks of a surrogate decision maker is to consider 'how the patient constructed his or her identity or life story' in order to reach a decision about a proposed course of treatment that continues the story 'in a manner that is meaningful and consistent with the patient's self-conception' (Council on Ethical and Judicial Affairs 2001). In addition, the Council argues that it is precisely the fact that a number of different options might be consistent with a person's life story that makes the narrative approach so attractive because it avoids having to predict only a single course of action as compatible and, therefore, morally acceptable.

Finally, the task of moral justification for narrative ethics is not, primarily, a unifying one. Rather, its focus is on acknowledging and embracing the multiplicity of, often contested, meanings that are available in any given situation. What is key for this narrativist account is the idea that many different voices and readings of moral situations and individual lives are possible. And, generally, narrativists focus less on trying to reduce competing perspectives to a commonly shared view, and more on involving as many people as possible in the dialogue. Anne Hudson Jones summarises this view as:

> In ideal form, narrative ethics recognizes the primacy of the patient's story but encourages multiple voices to be heard and multiple stories

to be brought forth by all those whose lives will be involved in the resolution of a case. Patient, physician, family, health professional, friend, and social worker, for example, may all share their stories in a dialogical chorus that can offer the best chance of respecting all the persons involved in a case. (Hudson Jones 1988: 222)

What is refreshing about the account of narrative ethics outlined above is that it introduces the idea that the aim of ethics is not necessarily to reduce discord, disunity and disagreement. Where principlism is lauded because of its justificatory force – its supposed objective rules distinguishing between good and bad actions – and its theoretical consistency, narrative ethics, as we have seen, slides towards relativism and diversity, with seeming wild abandon. Some might see this slide as good reason to be cautious in relation to narrative ethics and to favour the more stable and theoretically satisfying priniciplist position. However, what if one were to view the relativism of narrative ethics not as a failure of comprehensiveness or probity or insight, but rather as pointing the way toward a reframing of what we understand the task of ethics to be?

Activity

a) Does the narrative model demand too much of nurses? Are the demands on nurses' time realistic?

b) An important communication process is presupposed here. Nurses need to come to understand their patients, work colleagues, and so on. Does nurse scheduling allow for this?

c) Does education in nursing equip nurses for the communication, listening and responding skills needed to implement the richness of this ethical framework?

Summary Learning Guide 19.2

Narrative ethics claims that:

- Every moral situation is unique and unrepeatable and its meaning cannot be fully captured by appealing to law-like universal principles;
- In any given health-care situation, any decision or course of action is justified in terms of its fit with the individual life story or stories of the patient. The credibility of these, in turn, is determined on the basis of narrative reflective equilibrium.
- The objective of narrative reflective equilibrium is not necessarily to unify moral beliefs and commitments, but to open up dialogue, challenge received views and explore tensions between individual and shared meanings.

ETHIC OF CARE

In similar ways to narrative ethics, the ethic of care puts particularity, relationship, interdependence and emotion at the heart of the moral life. It rejects the idea that moral decision making is best done by rational agents applying general ethical rules impartially, as deontological, utilitarian and principlist approaches would have us do. Instead, it proposes a contextualist approach that pays attention to the particularity of each moral situation, to the relationships involved and to the task of maintaining those relationships throughout the decision-making process.

Carol Gilligan (1982, 1987), Annette Baier (1994) and Nel Noddings (1984) were key contributors to the early development of modern care-based ethical approaches. Gilligan's work, in particular, radically challenged classical theories of moral development, and set the parameters of a debate about the nature of morality, and the different ways in which women and men engage with it – a debate which has been raging since. In brief, Gilligan challenged the widely accepted paradigm of moral development, propounded by her mentor, Lawrence Kohlberg (1981a, 1981b). Assuming that humans move through different developmental stages in moral understanding, from childhood to adulthood, Kohlberg's theory associated moral immaturity with what he saw as the self-centredness of children – who do not see beyond the satisfaction of their own needs. He identified a second stage with the conventional behaviour of the adolescent, who conforms to social norms and expectations. Moral maturity, in his view, was the ability to think beyond personal need and convention, in order to apply universal rules of justice impartially. These he associated with the Kantian deontological principle of respect for others, arguing that an individual's progress through the different stages of moral development could be measured by determining the degree to which they had acquired, could understand and use this conception of justice in their moral deliberations. Although his initial empirical research measured the moral development of males, Kohlberg argued that his understanding of moral maturity and his account of the different stages of moral development could be applied to both sexes.

On the basis of her own empirical research with females and males, Gilligan (1982) argued that not only was Kohlberg's model of moral development limited because it was generated from the findings of empirical studies with only male samples, but it was also deeply problematic at its core. According to Gilligan, Kohlberg relied on one significant assumption: that there was only one model of moral reasoning, one way of describing what was involved in the exercise of moral agency. Instead of equating moral deliberation with the ability to take a justice stance, Gilligan proposed that the justice stance ought to be viewed as only one way of seeing moral problems, the care stance being another (different voice). From her research, Gilligan suggests that women predominantly adopt the care perspective to guide their moral judgements and actions.

If the justice perspective involves 'judging the conflicting claims of self and others against a standard of equality or equal respect', the care perspective involves viewing the self in the context of relationship: 'the self as a moral agent perceives and responds to the perception of need' and the moral question changes from 'What is just?' to 'How to respond?' (Gilligan 1987: 23). From the care stance, priority is given not to the perspective of the detached stranger, but to that of the involved intimate. In addition, importance is attributed not to the intellectual capacity to detach, but to interpersonal experiences where values are formed by dependent relations with others, paradigmatically, the mother–child relationship. Feminine virtues usually associated with that relationship are, in turn, validated, such as compassion, empathy, kindness and nurturance.

Tong summarises this perspective in the following terms:

> An ethics of care is directly concerned neither with doing duty for duty's sake nor with maximizing the good of the aggregate; rather, it is focused on attending to the specific needs of particular individuals and on weaving thick webs of human relationships and responsibilities. (Tong 1999: 33)

In sum, the justice perspective and the care perspective can be cast as two different ways of seeing and understanding moral problems. Concerns about justice focus on some aspects of a moral situation; concerns about care focus on other aspects. Crudely applying these perspectives to the cases on confidentiality in Chapters 5 and 6 of this text, for example, the justice stance would focus on balancing the rights and interests of Bill and his wife, Mary, and on identifying whose rights ought to be respected (Case 5.1), whereas the care stance would focus on maintaining the relationships among all involved and on enabling Bill's responsiveness to his own and his family's situation (Case 6.2).

Nursing Ethics and the Ethic of Care

From a nursing ethics perspective, the ethic of care such as that propounded by Gilligan, has stimulated great interest and debate. Positively, it is seen as an approach to ethical situations that validates virtues long associated with nursing. This validation of the caring and nurturing dimensions of nursing practice have been greatly welcomed by many nurse theorists such as Watson (1988), Gadow (1985, 1990) and Fry and Johnstone (2002: 28–30). Fry and Johnstone, drawing on the work of both Watson and Gadow, for example, privilege care as a central concept in nursing ethics:

> [A] theory of nursing ethics should emphasise caring as a moral obligation . . . the value of caring supports a nursing ethic that will protect and enhance the human dignity of patients receiving health care. [C]aring is demonstrated in the nursing actions of truth-telling and touch . . . Caring implies a commitment on the part of the nurse to protect human dignity and preserve humanity. (Fry and Johnstone 2002: 30)

Feminist theorists too, such as Alisa Carse and Hilde Lindemann Nelson (1999) and Rosemarie Tong (1992, 1999), argue that the ethic of care can make a significant contribution to the broad field of health-care ethics. One reason for this, according to Tong, is that the care ethic provides a language within which to talk about the relationships of dependency in a way that other ethical frameworks cannot.

> [T]he bulk of our human relationships . . . after all, are mostly between unequals. [. . .] When we relate to aging parents, young children, ailing siblings, and distraught friends, for example, we do not relate as if we were perfectly rational adults negotiating business deals. (Tong 1982: 45)

Agreeing with Tong, we would argue that central notions developed by adherents of the ethic of care can provide nursing ethics with a rich language for capturing and articulating the patient–nurse relationship. The ethic of care:

- Highlights features of human life that other frameworks ignore, such as our interdependency and vulnerability;
- Pays attention to the needs of concrete particular individuals in their specific situations;
- Takes the experiences of women seriously;
- Validates traditionally feminine virtues, such as nurturance and empathy;
- Affirms the importance of being actively concerned with the welfare of others;
- Recognises the role of emotion in moral life.

However, granted its strengths, we would advise caution in adopting the ethic of care. Even as theorists such as Carse and Nelson extol its positive features, they also express concerns in relation to the uncritical deployment of the language of care (1999: 17–31). The ethic of care has also received strong criticism from within and without nursing ethics (Edwards 1996: 133–40; Holm 1997: 16–17; Brown et al. 2004: 134–5).

One of the most comprehensive theoretical challenges to the idea that nursing ethics should privilege the care ethic is articulated by Helga Kuhse (1997). Kuhse takes issue with the ethic of care because, she argues, it is not sufficiently comprehensive to ground the moral decision making of nurses. She advances a number of different reasons for this and we will briefly outline two that we see as key.

The Arbitrariness of Care

First of all, she asks, how can we be sure that all caring is intrinsically good? We may care about dubious objectives and our 'caring' relationships may perpetuate patterns of domination and exploitation. She states:

> [W]ithout a substantive notion of the good, and universal principles to guide us towards that good, relational care is not only blind – unable to tell us what we should be caring about – but also unable to provide non-arbitrary reasons for our actions. (Kuhse 1997: 154)

Taking the example of Liz, the Ward of Court case (Case 13.1), discussed in Chapter 13, it could be argued that the ethic of care cannot settle the question of what is the morally right thing to do in that situation. Clearly both Liz's family who argued in favour of treatment withdrawal and at least some of the nurses caring for Liz, who argued in favour of continuing treatment, cared deeply and profoundly for Liz. There was care involved in both letting Liz die and keeping her alive: further reasons were needed to arrive at a final decision.

The Sexist Nature of Care

Kuhse is also concerned that the ethic of care deploys a language that is part of a tradition which celebrates maternal values. That tradition, on Kuhse's view, is not an innocent celebration but a means of perpetuating the cultural assumption that women and nurses have a natural aptitude for caring and that they willingly undertake the caring role. Such an assumption means that they can easily be accused of failing to care when they, for example, focus on their own careers, hand over the main parenting role after a divorce, and as we have seen in Chapter 17, go on strike for better conditions. For Kuhse, along with the notion of nurses as good women and natural carers comes the notion of them as naturally inferior and subservient to men. Ultimately, she fears that the language of care perpetuates traditional notions of the limited role of nurses and women in social and political life. She warns:

> If nurses eschew all universal principles and norms, they will not be able to participate in ethical discourse. They will not be able to speak on behalf of the patients for whom they care, nor will they be able to defend their own legitimate claims – and the motto of the first Canadian school of nursing, 'I see and I am silent,' will have continuing relevance for nurses. (Kuhse 1997: 166)

Activity

The care model seems indisputable in encouraging nurses to incorporate emotions, empathy and nurturance more fully in their moral lives. However, Kuhse raises a challenge to care models by asking: does the exhortation to 'care' provide guidance in disagreement situations. For example, consider:

a) What happens when nurses disagree about what 'care' requires? What happens when family considers 'care' for their loved one to mean using all the medical systems available to prolong life and the health-care staff know this to be futile? Perhaps health-care workers believe that what is needed is comfort care and companying with the dying or chronically ill.

b) How do you go about the task of adjudicating these different understandings of what 'care' requires?

Summary Learning Guide 19.3

The ethic of care:

• Claims that human interdependency and vulnerability are fundamental features of human life that moral theory must highlight;

- Focuses on concrete particular individuals in their specific situations;
- Takes the experiences of women seriously;
- Validates traditionally feminine virtues such as nurturance and empathy;
- Affirms the importance of being actively concerned with the welfare of others;
- Recognises the role of emotion in moral life.

FEMINIST ETHICS

If the ethic of care focuses attention on relationships, on women and on feminine virtues, **feminist ethics** considers the impact of gender roles and gendered understandings on the moral lives of individual human beings and draws attention to the power and power differentials inherent in moral relationships at individual, societal and organisational levels. Feminist ethics, in short, is the application of feminist theory to understanding the ethical realm: it critiques traditional ethical frameworks from a feminist perspective such as those we have already discussed: deontology, utilitarianism, principlism and, as Kuhse's objections illustrate, the ethic of care itself. The diversity of theoretical starting points when tackling the subject of ethics makes it difficult to identify or talk about a single 'feminist perspective' in ethics. However, as we indicated, what all of these approaches share is a common concern with the marginalisation and disempowerment of women in sexist societies and a transformative concern to change those societies for the better (Murphy 2004). In addition, as Sharon Murphy points out:

> Given their sensitivity to the oppression of women, feminist perspectives also often share a sensitivity to the oppression and marginalisation of other social groupings based on age, race, class, sexual orientation, etc. With this sensitivity comes an interest in feminist ethics in analysing how moral authority and the status and power that goes with it, has traditionally been constructed, aligned and divvied out, moral authority and moral agency having traditionally been inequitably distributed among different social groups, with women in particular being deemed less morally capable than men. (Murphy 2004)

In general, feminist ethics has widened the scope of health-care ethics to include consideration of the social, cultural and political dimensions of moral decision making in health-care settings. Susan Sherwin makes this point in the following way.

> [M]edical and other health-care practices should be reviewed not just with regard to their effects on the patients who are directly involved but also with respect to the patterns of discrimination, exploitation, and dominance that surround them. (Sherwin 1992: 4–5)

This broadening of the scope of health-care ethics that feminist theory has enabled is evidenced throughout this nursing text. For example, our discussion, in Chapter 11, of the moral warrant for sex selection pays close attention to the impact of sex selection on the lives of girls and women. While the chapter acknowledges the force of the libertarian argument of

John Robertson in favour of parents' rights to select the sex of their children, our key objection to his position is prompted by a feminist concern that sex selection might ultimately perpetuate sexist practices and thus restrict or harm the lives of both sexes, but especially the lives of girls and women.

In a similar way, in Chapter 6 on the Confidentiality Process, we took a feminist (and narrativist) approach to the case of the Somali woman with HIV. There, we widened the lens of our exploration of Chi Chi's narrative (Case 6.1) beyond a narrow concern with confidentiality in order to consider the context within which Chi Chi and the midwife involved were trying to engage as moral agents. We paid attention, for example, to the power imbalance between Chi Chi and the health professionals caring for her. We also considered economic and cultural obstacles that might prevent Chi Chi from getting the health-care support she and her family needed.

Feminist theory has also been recruited by other contemporary writers who see it as a rich resource for the development of nursing ethics theory. Elizabeth Peter and Joan Liaschenko, for example, take a feminist approach to nursing ethics when they make the claim that:

> [S]tandard bioethical theory fails to reflect nurses' moral concerns; [. . .] we believe that it is part of the process through which nurses' moral concerns actually 'get disappeared'. (Peter and Liaschenko 2003: 259)

Peter and Liaschenko argue that having knowledge of ethical theories does not mean that nurses can participate fully in the process of ethical decision making. In their view, the very naming of what is or is not morally relevant is not neutral – different theories highlight different concerns and ignore or 'disappear' others. Moreover, even after a particular feature of a moral situation is highlighted, the processes of reflection and analysis that are invoked play a role in the eventual outcome of the deliberations. Their particular concern is that adherence to moral frameworks, such as principlism, leads nurses to doubt their own moral reading of situations, and they fear that they will become 'morally paralysed in their attempt to embrace theoretical ideas far removed from their world' (Peter and Liaschenko 2003: 261). They propose the work of feminist philosopher, Margaret Urban Walker, as an antidote to the empty generalising and silencing entailed in more traditional ethical approaches.

Briefly, Walker (1997, 1998) rejects the possibility of there being any objective or near objective moral system of decision making, and tries, instead, to offer an account of morality that is contextual but not relativist. Walker critiques moral frameworks such as principlism described above, which, in her view, represent morality as a compact code of impersonal propositions guiding the actions of moral agents. She replaces it with a moral framework that represents morality as a process, rather than a set of prescriptions or outcomes. For Walker, morality and politics cannot be separated. Individuals are not the bounded integrated decision makers that traditional moral approaches seem to presuppose. Rather, who we are and how we decide upon a course of action at any given time must be understood contextually. Morality, for Walker, is a socially embedded process which determines what is morally significant, who is assigned responsibility for decision making and who is permitted and enabled to participate (Walker 1998: 7–9; Peter and Liaschenko 2004).

Peter and Liaschenko, pointing to the contested role of nurses in decision making in health-care situations, argue that Walker's work can be usefully deployed to help nurses to navigate their way in the moral and social spaces where they work, and to support them in identifying, articulating and defending their moral concerns (Peter and Liaschenko 2003: 262; 2004).

Taking an example from this text, recall the case, in Chapter 3, involving the deception of a young woman. There a decision was made by the husband of a patient, Sarah, not to inform her that she had a terminal illness. The doctor in the case agreed to the husband's request and the nurses caring for the patient were asked to collude in the deception. A feminist approach to this case might be concerned with truth telling as we have been, but it would highlight the power balance inherent in the relationships among the individuals involved. It would attach significance to the role of the husband who makes a decision without consulting his wife and the role of the doctor, who makes a decision without consulting the nurses. In each of these cases, the decision maker is a man who is in a position of power over those who must live with the consequences – the patient Sarah and the people who nurse her. Any adequate moral engagement with this case, from a feminist perspective, would have to address the power imbalances that provide the context in which the decision to deceive is made. Further, it would have to recognise the limits which the hierarchical arrangements in the unit place on the nurse's decision-making capacity: she believes that telling Sarah the truth about her condition is the right thing to do, but what moral space is available to her to exercise her agency?

Activity

Feminist theory highlights the significance of power structures and hierarchies in moral situations. These elements of power seem intractable and yet they are found in educational settings, in health-care contexts and indeed in families. In the context of health care, hierarchies of authority seem resistant to change. But are they?

a) Consider a situation where some moral disagreement occurs in a health-care setting where power imbalances are at play. These power factors greatly diminish your opportunities to speak, to offer suggestions for resolution of a moral disagreement. What do you do? What would you suggest be done if asked by a nurse colleague or friend of yours?

b) It seems that power structures and health-care hierarchies are culturally relative. Does nursing in some countries suffer more from power imbalances than nursing in others? If so, how do you explain these cultural differences?

Summary Learning Guide 19.4

Feminist ethics:

- Is the application of feminist theory to understanding the ethical realm;
- Considers the impact of gender roles and gendered understandings on the moral lives of individual human beings, especially, the moral lives of women;
- Is sensitive to and examines the power/power differentials and politics inherent in moral relationships;
- Highlights the contextual socially embedded nature of moral decision making;
- Is argued to be a moral framework that has particular relevance for nursing ethics.

CONCLUSION

Søren Holm (1997) summarises two common complaints directed at health-care ethics theory: that it is too simple-minded and that it does not sufficiently engage with reality. He adds a third, even more damning, objection that

> the actions prescribed by bioethicists must be carried out by actual human beings with an independent mind and independent moral reasoning; and that these human beings (also known as health care professionals) work within elaborate organisational structures which constrain their actions in various ways. (Holm 1997: 3)

It is evident from our brief survey of some contemporary moral theories – principlism, narrative ethics, ethic of care and feminist ethics – that the theorists who are currently engaged in forging and refining these perspectives are attempting to address the objections identified by Holm. In different ways, and to different degrees, they are all concerned with the concrete realities of human life and the huge challenges that living that life in a critically engaged and emotionally alive way can present. In turn, each aims to provide conceptual resources – tools of thought – to enable nurses and other health professionals to negotiate better the moral challenges that human illness, death and loss inevitably present.

What is of particular interest to the development of nursing ethics is the fact that contemporary ethical theories such as narrative and feminist ethics directly address many of the key problems that have exercised nurses ethically, but also personally and professionally. That ethical theories take increasing account of the way in which gender bias, oppressive hierarchies, discriminatory practices and structural injustices limit the moral agency of individuals indicates a shift in ethical thinking that we especially welcome. It also challenges nurses and other health professionals no longer to see and be silent, but to engage more ethically, with greater accountability and deeper humanity.

The following terms are explained in the glossary:

care

casuistry

ethic of care

feminist ethics

narrative model of ethics

prima facie

reflective equilibrium

Glossary

Accountability: the requirement to give reasons for one's actions. One can be called on to give reasons for both actions and omissions.

Acts and Omissions Doctrine: the view that there is a significant moral difference between actions we do and actions we omit or fail to do. The doctrine is controversial among ethicists.

Advance Directive: a document in which a person gives their preferences for what medical decisions they wish taken in the event that they become incapacitated and unable to express their wishes. These directives have no legal status in Ireland at present. However, they may play a valuable role in the assessment of patients' best interests and provide a statement of patients' wishes in regard to future health decisions.

Advocacy: assuming the role of speaking for another. Nurses act as advocates in representing the views of patients to others – often others on the health-care team. Advocacy also refers to the work of connecting patients and services for the purposes of facilitating patient outcomes.

An Bord Altranais: The Nursing Board of Ireland, responsible for the official registration of nurses and the accreditation of nurse courses.

ANH: This acronym refers to 'artificial nutrition and hydration' which provides feed to patients who are unable to take food through the conventional oral route. ANH covers both the naso-gastric tube and the gastrostomy tube inserted in the abdomen when patients cannot tolerate a naso-gastric tube. ANH is ethically controversial in terms of one's moral obligations to sustain life, especially in circumstances of terminal illness.

Applied Ethics or **Practical Ethics:** the application of moral theories to particular behaviours, professions or policies.

***Attorney General* v. *X*:** The Irish Supreme Court Judgement (1992) on the restricted permissibility of abortion in the Republic of Ireland.

Autonomy: the capacity of self-determination; the ability to make choices about one's own life. The principle of autonomy states that those choices should be respected (contrast paternalism). The principle of autonomy obliges health-care professionals to refrain from interfering or constraining the autonomy of patients, except where the exercise of this autonomy might seriously limit or harm others.

Beneficence: that feature of actions whereby the wellbeing of others and promotion of their interests is paramount.

Best-Interest Standard: A mechanism for surrogate decision making for currently non-autonomous patients. The goal is to protect another's wellbeing by assessing risks and benefits of various treatments and alternatives to treatment. The surrogate decision maker must determine the highest net benefit among available options. This standard is a quality-of-life criterion of decision making.

Biological v. Biographical Life: A distinction that differentiates between two levels of human existence: the biological includes all physical functions minus mental functioning such as cognitive awareness and consciousness; biographical life refers to the capacity to be aware of one's own meaning in life, one's plans and aspirations.

Care: a concept that some authors privilege in nursing ethics in order to validate and positively to reinforce the nurturing and relational dimensions of nursing practice. Care ethics argues that this privileging of care protects and enhances the human dignity of patients receiving health care.

Casuistry: a model of decision making that was very popular in medieval and early modern philosophy. It has again found favour in contemporary health-care ethics. Casuists claim that moral knowledge and understanding are wrought from concrete situations and particular cases and circumstances. They claim that the task of moral reasoning begins not with the application of principles or general rules to specific cases, but with determining the similarities and differences between cases and identifying some cases to serve as paradigms against which others can be compared.

Categorical Imperative: from Kantian ethics, this is reason at work commanding actions that are necessary of themselves, for their own sakes, without reference to other ends. Categorical commands or principles are those that cannot be negotiated or qualified, no matter what the circumstances.

Competence: the core meaning of 'competence' is the ability to perform a task. The criteria of particular competencies vary from context to context because the criteria are relative to specific tasks. The competence to decide is relative to the particular decision to be made. Competence also may vary over time and be intermittent.

Confidential Information: usually understood to be private information that a person confides in another who promises not to disclose the information to a third party without the permission of the confider. Where a patient *authorises* a professional to disclose information, their right to confidentiality has not been violated even though there is loss of both confidentiality and privacy.

Conscience: refers to a person's professed beliefs about what is right and wrong. It is usually formed by education, upbringing, religion, and personal reflection.

Consent: Agreement to an action based on knowledge of what the action involves and its likely consequences.

Consequentialism: a label attached to theories holding that actions are right or wrong according to the balance of their good and bad consequences. The most noted consequence-based theory is utilitarianism.

Contested Concepts: concepts where the meaning or applications are disputed.

Contractual Model: refers to one model for promoting autonomy within the patient–nurse relationship. In the contractual model, this relationship is viewed as nurse-provider and patient-consumer, or expert and non-expert. On this model, the challenge for the nurse is to ensure that the patient is fully informed of the nature of their illness, risks and benefits of any proposed treatment and alternative procedures available. The patient is then encouraged to be the decision maker.

Corrective Justice also called **Remedial Justice:** one of Aristotle's two species of justice, the other being distributive justice.

CPR: acronym referring to cardio-pulmonary resuscitation, a medical method of restarting a heart that has arrested. Guidelines for the application of CPR are often presented to doctors and nurses. Central questions in ethics about CPR are who authorises CPR and whether conscious patients give consent to having a CPR on their record.

Crisis Pregnancy: a pregnancy that a woman does not wish for or voluntarily choose. Such pregnancies may bring the woman to a nurse or doctor for advice or to a family planning clinic or Well-Woman centre for counselling and assistance.

Deontological Theory: (from Greek *deon*, what is due) describes moral systems which judge actions according to their intrinsic (non-instrumental) merit or demerit and which emphasise duties and the rights to which they give rise. Deontological theories determine the rightness or wrongness of an act by something other than the consequences – by God's commands or intuition, for example. Deontology differs from teleological ethical theories such as utilitarianism that hold that the rightness or wrongness of an act is determined by its consequences.

Dialogical Model: an approach to promoting autonomy, which involves viewing the patient as an interdependent decision maker. Information is seen as shared communication, and the nurse practitioner recognises the vulnerability of the patient as decision maker.

Dichotomous Thinking: a form of thinking that tends to simplify ways of approaching issues by restricting alternatives to two: either this or that. This form of thinking unduly limits the potential of moral imagination to consider other than two alternatives.

Distributive Justice: the problem or theory of how to allocate or distribute goods and services in a society. Should there be an equal distribution, or should some people be allowed to have more goods and services than others?

DNR: acronym referring to 'Do Not Resuscitate' orders. They can be included in a patient's notes, indicating that, should the patient have a cardiac arrest, they should not be resuscitated.

Donor Insemination (DI): the use of sperm donated for the purposes of achieving a pregnancy. Donor insemination normally refers to the sperm of someone who is not known by the woman who is attempting to conceive a child.

Dualist: a person holding the position that human beings are made up of two distinct substances: a body and a non-material soul or spirit.

Durable Power of Attorney (DPOA): the power vested in an agent who is legally designated by a competent individual to act on behalf of them in specified matters of health care if and when they become incompetent.

Embedded: located in a context of meaning such as one's culture, history, tradition, relationships with others, language, social and political arrangements.

Embryo: the developing human organism between conception and eight weeks, after which it is often referred to as a foetus up to the time of birth.

Embryo Research: studies and/or experiments conducted on human embryos.

Ethic of Care: an ethical theory that argues that particularity, relationship, interdependence and emotion are at the heart of moral life. It is a contextualist approach that pays attention to the particularity of each moral situation, to the relationships involved and to the task of maintaining those relationships throughout the ethical decision-making process.

Ethics: seeks to explain and understand the moral life.

Ethnic Monitor: an individual or group given the task of ensuring that a health-care system or other state body does not adversely discriminate against any particular ethnic group.

Evidence-Based Ethics: phrase borrowed by analogy with 'evidence-based medicine'. Evidence-based ethics refers to the awareness of relevant empirical matters for ethical judgements made. Evidence-based ethics calls for a recognition that empirical accuracy about a patient's diagnosis, prognosis, mental state, etc., can make the difference between good moral decisions and careless decisions.

Express Consent: consent expressed orally or in writing (except where patients cannot write or speak, when other forms of communication may be sufficient).

Extraordinary Treatments: those treatments that are considered morally non-obligatory. This judgement is usually based on the clinical evidence and/or patient's decision that they would be of no benefit to the patient.

Feminist Ethics: theory approach to ethics which considers the impact of gender roles and gendered understandings on the moral lives of individuals. It draws attention to the power differentials inherent in moral relationships at societal, organisation and individual levels.

Free Will: a capacity that human beings are widely supposed to have and use in deciding the course of their lives; a feature of human beings that enables them to be held responsible for decisions they make and the actions they take.

Gender: a culturally shaped group of attributes and behaviours given to the female or the male. Many contemporary feminist theorists distinguish between sex and gender, taking the view that sex is biological while gender is socially constructed.

Gillick Competence: refers to a principle that informs the relationships between nurses, doctors, minors and parents. The Gillick principle of competence recognises the evolving maturity of children. The Gillick court judgement of 1985 provided five criteria to be used in assessing the maturity that individual minors have reached. This means that, in practice, health professionals can decide in each case whether the child in front of them can give valid consent for a particular intervention requested.

Good Will: a term from Immanuel Kant's moral theory. According to Kant, the only thing that is good without qualification is a good will. A person acquires a good will by acting out of respect for the moral law.

Gradualist Position on Moral Status of the Human Embryo: sees the human embryo as a potential human life. The seriousness and moral gravity of abortion increases as the embryo develops from fertilisation to birth.

Holism: a complex concept in nursing theory and research. 'Holism' is not a single, unitary concept but has a meaning that has evolved and continues to evolve in nursing theory. Many authors claim that we should refer to a number of 'holisms' rather than think of it in the singular.

Identifiable Data: data from which a patient can be identified. Name, address and full postcode will identify patients. Combinations of data may also do so, even where name and address are not included.

Impartiality: that capacity of individuals to decide the best course of action independently of their own personal preferences or inclinations.

Informed Consent: the principle or rule widely used by ethical and legal theorists, as well as practitioners, to communicate the idea that a person should be informed about and should freely consent to any health-care treatment that they receive or any research in which they participate.

Instrumental Good: something that is useful or important for achieving some goal or purpose, or as a means to some end. This type of 'good' is in contrast with an 'intrinsic good'.

Integrity: in the context of ethical theory, means soundness, reliability, and integration of moral character. In a more restricted sense, moral integrity means fidelity in adherence to one's moral norms or convictions and standing up in the defence of such norms.

Intrinsic Good: something is intrinsically good if it is good considered in and of itself, apart from any consequences. Intrinsic good is contrasted with 'instrumental good'.

In Vitro Fertilisation (IVF): literally, the achievement of fertilisation of a human egg and sperm in a laboratory test-tube.

Justice Ethics: Refers to a framework or set of core principles designed to best achieve a fair or just system of health-care provision.

Justification: the process of explaining and giving reasons for a position or argument.

Loyalty: often considered a strength of character or virtue. Loyalty implies commitment to colleagues and the recognised practice of one's own profession. Loyalty can camouflage bad practice, but to avoid this, responsible loyalty recommends questioning practices that have discernible detrimental consequences.

Metaethics: the analysis of concepts (such as right and justice) and modes of reasoning in ethics, and the evaluation of ethics as, for example, subjective or objective, universal or relative.

Moral Distress: a complex concept in nursing theory and practice. It is a type of concern or anxiety that can occur when a nurse, having chosen what she or he sees as the right course of action, is unable to act because of varying kinds of constraints. These constraints may arise because of personal, situational or institutional limitations.

Moral Space: refers to a complex set of provisions within any institution that, when put in place, can facilitate ethical decision making and respect for individual moral conscience.

Narrative Ethics: an approach to moral situations that sees them as unique and unrepeatable. Any decision or course of action in health care would be defended in terms of its fit with the individual life story or stories of the patient in focus. This fit is termed 'narrative reflective equilibrium'.

No-Difference Thesis: a position that rejects the view that nurses have a 'special vocation' and argues rather that nurses should see themselves as no different from workers in other occupations. The no-difference thesis puts nurses in precisely the same negotiating position as any other worker in situations of considered strike action.

Nonmaleficence: the principle of ethics that exhorts us to 'do no harm'. This principle is one of four rules or guidelines comprising 'principlism'.

Normative Ethics: concerned with the identification and justification of the moral norms or rules that might be used to guide and evaluate human conduct. In other words, normative ethics attempts to determine what we *ought* to do.

Opportunity Cost: the loss of other opportunities that were sacrificed when one alternative is chosen in preference to another.

Ordinary Means of Treatment: a distinction from as far back as fifteenth-century medical ethics. 'Ordinary means of treatment' are those treatment forms that are morally obligatory. They refer to medicine, treatments and operations that can be given without excessive pain, expense or other inconvenience. Most importantly the medical therapies considered to be 'ordinary means' of treatment (and obligatory) must offer a reasonable hope of benefit and that benefit must be more than the burden or distress experienced by the particular patient receiving these medical treatments.

Paradigm Case: an ethical case or legal precedent that yields new moral insight that changes future practices.

Partner Notification: The activity of partner notification and contact tracing is identical and so the terms may be used interchangeably. Partner notification is the spectrum of public health activities in which the sexual partners of an individual with a Sexually Transmitted Infection (STI) are notified, counselled and offered services (World Health Organisation (WHO) 1986). It contributes to the control of STIs by identifying and treating previously undiagnosed infection. Because of lack of policy, custom and practice have to a great extent guided partner notification methods. There are three approaches to partner notification:

1) *Patient referral*: individuals diagnosed with an STI are encouraged to notify their partners of their possible exposure to the infection, without the direct involvement of the health adviser.

2) *Provider referral*: Infected individuals give partner information to the health adviser who then notifies the partners directly – always being aware of the importance of confidentiality for all parties concerned.

3) *Conditional referral*: A combination of both of these methods. (Woodman 2004)

Paternalism: the overriding of someone's autonomy for what is considered to be their own good.

Paternalism with Permission: agreement or generalised consent on the part of a patient that a health-care professional (or team) can take decisions about their treatment and care without further conversations about consent. This trust is based on the patient's belief that the health professional will act only in their view of the patient's best interest

Person: a contested concept. This means that there is basic disagreement among philosophers about precisely what features are necessary for someone to be considered a 'person' and so treated as a person. One definition given by John Locke defines a person as an individual who possesses a range of biological and psychological capacities. These include the ability to think, communicate and reason, and the ability to consider oneself as the same person at different times and places.

Personal Information: information about people that health professionals learn in a professional capacity and from which individuals can be identified.

Pluralistic Society: a society whose members may have many different and, often, competing world-views and values.

Pre-implantation Genetic Diagnosis (PGD): the use of genetic testing on a live embryo to determine the presence or absence of a particular gene or chromosome prior to implantation of the embryo in the uterus.

Prenatal Diagnosis: also known as antenatal screening, prenatal diagnosis refers to a group of tests offered to pregnant women to screen the unborn human embryo for genetic disorders and malformations. Several of the more common types of developed genetic testing are: amniocentesis, CVS (chorionic villus sampling), maternal serum screening, fetal ultrasound scanning. Newer techniques of prenatal screening are under development.

Prima Facie: literally meaning 'at first sight' or on the first impression. Principles that are *prima facie* binding, are not absolute principles, but are considered sufficiently defensible that they should be given first consideration in a situation requiring a decision. Departure from prima facie principles in favour of some other rules in any given situation requires reasons or justification.

Principle: a fundamental rule or basic norm that is considered so general that it can be applied to a wide range of circumstances or situations. For example, the rule, 'Respect autonomy', applies to all autonomous persons and actions, and so, is considered a basic rule or principle. On the other hand, the rule, 'Do not lie to children', applies to a more particular action and a particular group of people. Finally, a particular judgement refers to the judgement one makes in a specific concrete situation – for example, 'I will not lie to Mary about her diagnosis.'

Principle of Equality of Consideration: a principle for equality of treatment of other persons. This principle requires that we act justly when we treat similar cases. It follows that we can treat persons unequally or differently only if there are some morally relevant differences between them.

Principle of Proportionality: a principle or guide used in decision making about prolongation of life. The health-care professional and patient (if competent) determine whether the means of treatment offered are proportional to the prospects for patient improvement. The principle of proportionality is often abbreviated to state that the risks of distress or further suffering for a particular patient from a treatment given must have a clear and proportionate benefit for the patient.

Principle of Truth Telling: a guideline stating that a doctor or nurse should tell the patient the truth about their diagnosis – in a measured manner, and in language the patient can understand. This would not be required *if* there were good reasons to believe that a degree of harm more serious than a temporary emotional depression would follow as a result of telling the diagnosis.

Principlism: involves the application of one or more basic principles to moral issues and situations, in order to determine a justifiable or morally correct course of action with regard to them.

Privacy: a right or claim to privacy is a right to control access to one's personal domain. That domain may involve informational privacy (e.g. of personal medical records); physical privacy (e.g. of the person or personal space); decisional privacy (e.g. of personal choices); or proprietary privacy (e.g. of personal property).

What is kept private does not have to be secret, and what is kept secret does not have to be private. For example, a private house or a private life is not always a secret house or a secret life. In turn, a secret ballot for government elections is not a private concern, nor is a secret plan to assassinate a president.

Professional Standard: also called 'standard medical practice'. This is one of the competing standards for determining informed consent. The professional standard holds that a health professional is not wrong in withholding information from a patient *if* other health professionals with the same expertise generally think she or he is doing the right thing.

Pro-natalism: within the context of abortion positions, this view argues for a special primacy of commitment to the protection of the unborn foetus. Usually pro-natalism rejects the view that women should have a right to control their reproduction by access to abortion if they choose.

Proportional Justification: a moral principle particularly applicable to considerations of strike action by nurses. The principle affirms the view that a proposed strike has to find justification (if at all) by looking at the goals sought by strike action and weighing those against the negative consequences (on patients and public trust) of the strike.

Public Interest: the interests of the community as a whole.

PVS: an acronym that means 'persistent vegetative state'. This condition causes an individual to suffer the loss of higher cortex activity and yet, because the brain stem is usually intact, the patient is able to breathe spontaneously (without ventilator assistance). Ethical issues are considerable, including questions about whether a patient who is in a persistent vegetative state ought to be kept alive indefinitely with all support systems available.

Rational: that feature of individuals whereby they are able to decide a course of action on the basis of careful reflection and in the absence of coercion from authority or custom.

Reasonable Person Standard: one of the competing standards for determining how to approach informed consent. Under this standard, the focus shifts to the patient and asks: what would a reasonable person expect to know about this patient's condition and choices for treatment? The challenge of this standard is in the question of who is the 'reasonable person'. Can we assign universal, definite features for 'reasonable persons'? This question becomes especially acute in view of cultural diversity and difference of value perspectives now recognised as part of many countries.

Reflective Equilibrium: a term introduced by John Rawls to refer to attempts to justify general principles on the grounds that they accord with our intuitive judgements concerning particular cases. In this process of reflective equilibrium, we weigh, test, revise and balance our principles against background theories and particular judgements.

Respect for Persons: a principle that sets out the ways in which it is appropriate to treat those who are considered to have an important moral status. That persons have a high moral value and significance is an assumption that is practically universally held. There may be disagreement in relation to defining personhood and in determining when a person begins or ceases to exist, but it is generally agreed that persons have an ultimate moral value.

Right: an entitlement that prohibits or obliges the actions of others. It is a justified claim that individuals or groups can make on other individuals or society generally. If a person is considered to have a right – to freedom or bodily integrity, for example – they may be considered to be inviolable in some sense. On the other hand, a right may entitle a person to make certain claims on others for support or service – to a minimum standard of education or health care, for example.

Rule: a principle or guideline used as a general norm to follow in circumstances of moral decision making. Examples would be the rule of truth telling, the rule of confidentiality, the rule of consent. As with all rules, there are possible exceptions but if the rule stands as defensible, the exception must be morally justified.

Sex: refers to a person's physical make-up – biological, anatomical, and hormonal. The sex of an individual is usually determined by the genital properties of the person: female or male (some ambiguous cases arise). In gender theory, this physical element of the self (sex) is often distinguished from the 'gender' of an individual, where gender refers to 'man' or 'woman', masculinity or femininity that develops from within socio-cultural contexts.

Sexism: a form of prejudice that applies to one's skewed perceptions or judgements about women *or* men. They are biased judgements because they are not based on the character qualities of individuals but are founded on negative assumptions about the individuals precisely as female or male.

Slippery-Slope Argument: in general, a form of argument that includes an assumption that, when we make a choice, A, that we believe is desirable, we have to recognise that making choice A may make it very difficult to draw a line and avoid choosing B which is not correspondingly good or desirable. For instance, if one allows some sick people to be killed, one must allow all sick people to be killed – one will slide down a slope of killing. If one allows competent individuals to choose the timing of their own dying, then, before we're aware of it, we will go down the 'slippery slope' of actively causing the involuntary dying of older patients, or of infirm or severely disabled patients. This argument is often criticised for its emotive appeal which prevents some measures from being taken which are not harmful in the way suggested in these examples.

Stem Cells: long-living cells that have varying capacities to differentiate into specialised tissues and parts of the body, such as organs, blood, nerves, skin or bone. Some stem cells are present in early human (embryonic) development while others can also be derived from children and adults.

Stem-Cell Research: research studies on *stem cells*. These seem to offer varying degrees of 'promise' in the therapeutic application of stem cells. There are extensive ethical, social and legal debates, particularly about the promise of stem-cell research where cells are derived from human embryos that are not implanted after IVF.

Strike Action: a decision to withhold labour in varying degrees for a range of reasons, such as, for example, to draw attention to poor conditions for patients and staff or to strengthen one's bargaining position for certain improvements in staffing ratios or salaries.

Strong Paternalism: action or intervention in decision making and choices of an autonomous patient where the intervention is carried with the motive of doing good for the patients. What distinguishes strong paternalism from weak paternalism is that strong paternalism intervenes with patients who are definitely autonomous.

Strong Thesis: a position in one philosophy of nursing which claims that nurses, by virtue of their special vocation and commitments to care, are radically different from other workers. This strong thesis has consequences on the question of whether strike action is permissible for nurses.

Subjective Standard: one of the standards that applies to the process of making decisions about providing information to patients in order to achieve informed consent. The subjective standard focuses on the individual patient and specific values that a patient holds that they prefer not to risk in any treatment or care plan.

Substantial Autonomy: a degree of autonomy that is sufficient for an individual's decision making. The substantially autonomous person is neither coerced nor ignorant and is reasonably aware of the consequences of their decision.

Substituted Judgement: a surrogate decision standard used when a patient is not competent to decide for himself or herself. The substituted judgement standard requires the decision maker 'to don the mantle of the incompetent' and try to make a decision as the incompetent would have made it if competent.

Surrogate Decision Standards: guidelines and procedures to guide decision making where a patient is not competent to speak their preferences regarding treatment or refusal. Several such decision mechanisms for those not competent are: advance directives, substituted judgement and the best-interest judgement.

Teleological Theory: a theory that determines moral rightness or wrongness by looking at consequences of actions. The standard teleological theory in ethics is utilitarianism. Teleological theories are usually contrasted with deontological theories that don't look at consequences in determining moral rightness or wrongness.

Therapeutic Privilege: that right of health-care professionals to withhold information from a patient if they think that providing the information would run the risk of seriously harming them. This privilege does *not* allow a health professional to remain silent simply because divulging information might prompt a patient to forgo therapy the professional feels the patient really needs.

Tolerance: that character feature of a person that recognises both that he or she is fallible in moral matters, and that respect for differences of moral perspective is a necessary means to living in society with some measure of peace. Many writers in ethics and politics assume that tolerance is a virtue that should assume a privileged place in any list of political virtues.

Two-Tier Health System: an organisation of health care that provides for a basic, universal minimum of health care for all citizens (or residents) of a state but, in addition, also allows for individuals to use their income to buy more services and avail of them more quickly than the basic minimum in health care. The two-tier system is sometimes criticised on the grounds that it is unjust in giving special opportunities of health care for individuals simply because they can afford to pay for those extra services.

Utilitarian: a proponent of utilitarianism.

Utilitarianism: a consequentialist moral theory which judges actions according to their outcome or consequences and states that the morally best outcomes are those that maximise the happiness or interests of all concerned with the action.

Veracity: the disposition of being truthful.

Virtue Theory or **Virtue Ethics:** tells us what traits of character dispose a person towards choosing the good (virtues) and what traits make a person disposed to wrongdoing (vices). Different writers pick out different traits of character as virtues. The Greeks emphasised courage; the Christians stressed theological virtues such as faith, hope and charity; modern moral philosophers think that justice and benevolence are most important.

Vitalism: a position that holds that the presence of biological life is an intrinsic good. It should be valued until all life has ceased, with the implication that quality-of-life judgements are morally wrong.

Waiver: literally, a removal of something. In health-care ethics, a waiver refers to a decision by a competent patient or legitimate proxy not to seek information leading to consent. The waiver of a patient effectively is 'paternalism with permission'.

Ward of Court: refers to a legal process whereby an individual is placed under the jurisdiction of the courts for certain decision-making processes.

Weak Paternalism: refers to a form of intervention that limits the freedom of substantially non-autonomous individuals.

Weak Thesis: a philosophy of nursing that believes that nurses are not radically different from other workers and do not have a unique, singular vocation to nursing. However, on the weak thesis, nursing is believed to be sufficiently different from other occupations that nurses must have strong and justified conditions for any decision to engage in strike action.

Weakness of Will: failure of someone, through insufficient motivation or strength of character, to do something that they believe is the right thing to do.

Whistle-blowing: an attempt by an employee, a former employee or patient to bring a wrongful practice to the attention of those who one believes have power to remedy the situation – for example, it can involve calling to public attention abuses or dangers that jeopardise public safety and that would not otherwise be publicised.

Appendix 1

Gillick Competence

Victoria Gillick took the Department of Health and Social Services in Great Britain to the Courts because they had sent out a circular to GPs saying that they were entitled to prescribe contraceptives to minors if certain conditions were fulfilled in the character of the young person coming to see them. Mrs Gillick took the case all the way to the House of Lords and lost – but not by much.

In the Gillick case (1984–86), the idea of chronological age was challenged. It was found not to be a sufficient indicator of 'maturity' to give consent. Listed below are criteria for judging whether a minor is competent to give consent. These criteria are often referred to as a definition of 'Gillick competence'.

Lord Scarman in the Gillick case said:

> If the law should impose upon the process of growing up fixed limits where nature knew only a continuous process, the price would be artificiality and a lack of realism in an area where the law must be sensitive to human development and social change.

A doctor would be justified in proceeding with contraceptive advice without parents' consent or even knowledge provided that the doctor was satisfied that:

a) The girl would, although under 16, understand his advice.

b) He could not persuade her to inform her parents or to allow him to inform the parents that she was seeking contraceptive advice [so effort should be made to involve parents in discussion with young person].

c) She was very likely to have sexual intercourse with or without contraceptive treatment [she showed determination and clarity about her future plans].

d) Unless she received contraceptive advice or treatment, her physical or mental health or both were likely to suffer [you judge that it is in the young girl's overall best interest to be assisted].

e) Her best interests required the doctor to give her contraceptive advice, treatment, or both, without parental consent.

Some or all of the Gillick criteria can be applied to:

- minors refusing blood (Jehovah's Witnesses), or
- minors wishing to consent to certain treatments or decline others.

Many pressures increasingly seem to encourage the young to seek a status of miniature adults and a readiness for sexual activity as part of that perceived identity. In 2003, medical evidence in the UK and Ireland recorded a significant increase in sexually transmitted diseases, a point that is noticed as well in the experience of public health and general practice nurses.

While general practitioners in Ireland might be aware of the Gillick judgement, and may have to make difficult judgements about contraceptive advice to minors, the law deriving from the case does not, strictly speaking, apply in the Republic of Ireland. The Irish Constitution states clearly that the family has primacy in making decisions on the comprehensive welfare of children. Health-care professionals within the Irish Republic would need to be aware that the Constitution gives considerable rights to 'the Family'.

Appendix 2
The History of Abortion in Ireland: 1861 to present

I LEGAL SITUATION
a) British Law:

Offences Against the Person Act 1861
Strict prohibition against abortion with prison penalties.

Infant Life Preservation Act 1929
Reiterated 1861 Act but said that abortion should not be an offence 'when such act is done in good faith with the intention of saving the mother's life'.

R. v. Bourne 1939
Gynaecologist Alex Bourne performs abortion on a young victim of rape.

Abortion Act of 1967
Abortion is no legal offence when two registered medical practitioners certify in good faith that continuance of pregnancy would constitute a risk to the life or health of the pregnant woman or to the health of her existing children greater than if the pregnancy were terminated. Termination may also be carried out if there is a risk that the child, if born, would suffer serious physical or mental handicap. The Act became effective in 1968. Immediate effect was a large increase in notified abortions and a significant decrease in post-abortion mortality.

b) Irish Law:

Abortion Statistics regarding Irish Women
     1975 – 1,562 reported with Irish addresses
     1980 – 3,480
     1988 – estimated 4,400 annually
     1994 – estimated 5,600 annually
     2004 – estimated 12,000 annually

Since 1967, Irish women choosing abortion have most often gone to England or Wales. Ireland has operated with the 1861 Act and continues to do so with the addition of the following:

II EIGHTH AMENDMENT OF THE CONSTITUTION (passed 1983)
Article 40 of the Constitution (*context* for 1983 amendment)

40.3.1   The State guarantees in its laws to respect and, as far as practicable, by its law to defend and vindicate the personal rights of the citizen. [In the original constitution, 1937]

40.3.2   The State shall, in particular, by its laws protect as best it may from unjust attack and, in the case of injustice done, vindicate the life, person, good name and property rights of every citizen. [In the original constitution, 1937]

40.3.3   The State acknowledges the right to life of the unborn and, with due regard to the equal right to life of the mother, guarantees in its laws to respect and, as far as practicable, by its laws to defend and vindicate that right. [Passed in 1983]

III   *ATTORNEY GENERAL v. X AND OTHERS*

In March 1992: The Supreme Court gave a judgement of 4–1 that abortion is not always unlawful in Ireland. By a 4–1 decision, the Supreme Court argued that abortion is legal in limited cases. The substantial risk of suicide allowed this appeal to be taken by a 14-year-old girl.

In this decision, the Supreme Curt decided:

' . . . if it is established as a matter of probability that there is a real and substantial risk to the life as distinct from the health of the mother, which can only be avoided by the termination of her pregnancy, that such termination is permissible, having regard to the true interpretation of Article 40.3.3 of the Constitution'. (Read: *The Irish Times,* 6 March 1992, 4–13.)

In October 1992: Another referendum was held *following* the Supreme Court judgement in Attorney *General* v. *X and Others.*

The Proposed Constitutional Amendments were to amend article 40.3.3 (see above). The amending subsections were proposed as follows:

Travel Issue: 'Subsection 3 of this section shall not limit freedom to travel between the State and another State.'

[Passed]

Information: 'Subsection 3 of this section shall not limit freedom to obtain or make available, in the State, *subject to such conditions as may be laid down by the law*, information relating to services lawfully available in another state'.

[Passed]

'It shall be unlawful to terminate the life of an unborn unless such termination is necessary to save the life, as distinct from the health of the mother where there is an illness or disorder of the mother giving rise to a real and substantial risk to her life, not being a risk of self-destruction . . .'

[This amendment known as the 'substantive issue' was *not passed*]

The Passing of the *Information* amendment meant that the Government had to introduce legislation to allow for the control of information distribution in keeping with the Constitution.

Note: Subsequently, an Abortion Information Bill was proposed, called Regulation of Information (Services Outside the State for Termination of Pregnancies) Bill 1995. This Bill would give GPs and others the right of providing information on where abortions could be obtained. However, GPs could not make appointments for women to have a termination.

Objectors argued that even this provision of information was contrary to the Constitution's commitment to protect unborn life. Others objected that the information provisions, by forbidding her doctor from making an abortion appointment, did not go far enough in protecting the woman's right to protect her health and life.

President Mary Robinson referred this Bill to the courts for a decision on whether it was consistent with the provisions in the Constitution.

In May 1995: The decision of the Supreme Court on this Information Bill was: 'that the Regulation of Information Bill, 1995, is not repugnant to the Constitution or to any provision thereof'.

Appendix 3

a. Standard Form of a General Advance Directive

In recognition of the dignity and privacy which patients have a right to expect, the Legislature hereby declares that the laws of the State of _____ shall recognise the right of an adult person to make a written directive instructing his physician to withhold or withdraw life-sustaining procedures in the event of a terminal condition.

Directive made this _____ day of _____

I, _____, being of sound mind, wilfully and voluntarily make known my desire that my life shall not be artificially prolonged under the circumstances set forth below. I do hereby declare:

1. If at any time I should have an incurable injury, disease, or illness certified by two physicians to be a terminal condition, and where the application of life-sustaining procedures would serve only to prolong artificially the moment of my death and where my physician determines that my death is imminent whether or not life-sustaining procedures are utilised, I direct that such procedure be withheld or withdrawn, and that I be permitted to die naturally.

2. In the absence of my ability to give directions regarding the use of such life-sustaining procedures, it is my intention that this directive shall be honoured by my family and physician(s) as the final expression of my legal right to refuse medical or surgical treatment and accept the consequences from such refusal.

3. If I have been diagnosed as pregnant and that diagnosis is known to my physician, this directive shall have no force or effect during the course of my pregnancy.

4. I have been diagnosed at least 14 days ago as having a terminal condition by _____, M.D., whose address is _____ and whose telephone number is _____. I understand that if I have not filled in the physician's name and address, it shall be presumed that I did not have a terminal condition when I made out this directive.

5. This directive shall have no force or effect five years from the date filled in above.

6. I understand the full import of this directive and I am emotionally and mentally competent to make this directive.

Signature of Declarant _____

The declarant has been personally known to me and I believe him or her to be of sound mind.

Signature of Witness _____

b. Health-Care Advance Directive
for Jehovah's Witnesses

(1) I, _____

Print your full name

Born the _____ th day of _____, 19 _____, am of sound mind and I voluntarily make this Health-Care Advance Directive. This document revokes any prior Health-Care Advance Directive and shall take effect upon my incapacity. It will remain in force unless and until specifically revoked in writing by me.

(2) I am one of Jehovah's Witnesses. On the basis of my firmly held religious convictions (see Acts 15:28, 29) and on the basis of my desire to avoid the numerous hazards and complications of blood transfusions, **I absolutely, unequivocally and resolutely REFUSE allogenic blood** (another person's blood); stored **autologous blood** (my own stored blood); under any and all circumstances, no matter what my medical condition. This means **no whole blood, no red cells, no white cells, no platelets and no blood plasma; no matter what the consequences.** Even if health-care providers believe that only blood transfusion therapy will preserve my life or health, I refuse it. Family relatives or friends may disagree with my religious beliefs and with my wishes as expressed herein. However, their disagreement is legally and ethically irrelevant because it is my subjective choice which is determinate. Any such disagreement should in no way be construed as creating ambiguity or doubt about the strength or substance of my wishes.

(3) With respect to minor blood fractions* or products containing minor blood fractions, according to my conscience I ACCEPT: [Initial <u>one</u> of the three choices below.]

_____ (a)   **NONE**

_____ (b)   **ALL**

_____ (c)   **SOME** That is, **I ACCEPT**: [initial choice(s) below]

_____   Products that may have been processed with, or contain small amounts of albumin (e.g. streptokinase, and some recombinant products [such as erythropoietin (EPO, epoetin-α) and synthesised clotting factors], and some radionuclide scan preparations may contain albumin).

_____   Immunoglobulins (e.g. Rhesus immune globulin [anti-D], gammaglobulin, horse serum, snake bite anti-venoms).

_____   Clotting factors (e.g. fibrinogen, Factors VII, VIII, IX, XII). Warming: use of blood-derived clotting factors has been associated with transmission of infections/complications (e.g. HIV, hepatitis and clotting disorders) which could be avoided by using recombinant products, if available.

*Warning: Consult your doctor regarding potential health risks.

_____   Other: _____

(4)   **I accept and request alternative non-blood medical or surgical management** to stop, avoid or minimise blood loss; to replace lost circulatory volume; and/or to build up or conserve my own blood. For example, volume expanders such as dextran, saline or Ringer's solution, modified fluid gelatine, hetastarch and perflurochemicals; and oral or parenteral iron would be acceptable to me.

(5)   With respect to **non-stored autologous blood** (my own non-stored blood), according to my conscience **I ACCEPT**: [Initial choice(s) below]

———————— (b)   HAEMODILUTION

———————— (a)   HAEMODIALYSIS AND HEART-LUNG MACHINERY
(diversion of my own blood within an extracorporeal circuit *that does not involve storage* or more than a brief interruption of blood flow and that is constantly linked to my circulatory system, provided any equipment used is not primed with stored blood).

———————— (b)   HAEMODILUTION
(dilution of my blood within an extracorporeal circuit *that does not involve storage* or more than a brief interruption of blood flow and that is constantly linked to my circulatory system, provided any equipment used is not primed with stored blood).

———————— (c)   INTRAOPERATIVE OR POSTOPERATIVE BLOOD SALVAGE
(contemporaneous recovery and reinfusion of blood lost during or after surgery *that does not involve storage* or more than a brief interruption of blood flow, provided any equipment used is not primed with stored blood).

(6)   With respect to **end-of-life decisions, I CHOOSE**: [Initial <u>one</u> of the three choices below]

———————— (a)   NOT TO PROLONG LIFE, *if to a reasonable degree of medical certainty my condition is hopeless.* (For example, if to a reasonable degree of medical certainty I have an incurable and irreversible condition that will result in my death within a relatively short time, or if I am unconscious and to a reasonable degree of medical certainty will not regain consciousness, or if I have brain damage or a brain disease that makes me unable to recognise people or communicate and to a reasonable degree of medical certainty my condition will not improve.) If to a reasonable degree of medical certainty my condition is hopeless, I refuse mechanical respiration (ventilation), cardiopulmonary resuscitation (CPR), tube feeding (artificial nutrition or hydration), etc., but I accept basic palliative care — treatment for comfort.

———————— (b)   TO PROLONG LIFE, as long as possible within the limits of generally accepted health-care standards but subject to my absolute refusal of blood and those blood components described herein, although I realise this means that I might be kept alive on machines for years in a hopeless condition.

———————— (c)   OTHER, [If you do not completely agree with either (a) or (b) above, initial and write your own end-of-life instructions in the space provided.]

—————————————————————————————

—————————————————————————————

(7)   Other instructions: [Write any other health-care instructions here.]

_____

_____

_____

_____

(8)   I am primarily concerned that my refusal of blood and choice of alternative non-blood management be respected, regardless of my medical condition. My rights under the Constitution of Ireland, 1937, statute and common law require health-care providers to respect and comply with my treatment decisions. My rights are not dependant on, and do not vary with my medical condition. In *In the Matter of Ward of Court* [1955] 2 ILRM 401 at 426, the Supreme Court (per Hamilton CJ) stated that a competent adult patient has the right 'to forego [medical] treatment or at any time, to direct that it be withdrawn, even though such withdrawal would result in . . . death', and at p. 427, 'a competent adult, if terminally ill has the right to forego or discontinue life-saving treatment'. Denham J. stated at p. 454 that 'medical treatment may be refused for other than medical reasons. Such reasons may not be viewed as good medical reasons, or reasons most citizens would regard as rational, but the person of full age and capacity may make the decision for their own reasons'.

(9)   MY DECISION to refuse blood and choose non-blood management MUST BE RESPECTED EVEN IF MY LIFE OR HEALTH IS THREATENED by my refusal. Any attempt to administer blood contrary to my instructions will be a violation of my constitutional rights of bodily self-determination and personal autonomy, and accordingly will constitute an actionable trespass to my person.

(10)   If my health-care providers will not or cannot undertake a surgical operation or administer any other form of medical treatment, without the use of blood or those blood products specifically prohibited by myself in this document, I direct my health-care providers to cooperate fully with the appointed representative(s) of the local Hospital Liaison Committee for Jehovah's Witnesses and to assist in transferring me promptly to another health-care provider that will respect my health-care instructions herein. In such circumstances, I direct that all my medical records, including a copy of this document, be transferred promptly to the other health-care provider.

(11)   A copy of this document shall be as valid as the original. I ask that a copy of this document be made part of my permanent medical record. I have provided a copy of this document to my registered general practitioner.

(12)   The provisions of this entire document are separable, so that the invalidity of one or more provisions shall not affect any others.

(13)   I understand and believe the full import of this document and verily aver that it accurately reflects my personal informed choice and that it expresses a firm and settled decision (after careful consideration of the options) of my wishes.

(14)   SIGNED: _____

          Your signature   Date

          _____

          _____

          Address

(15)   STATEMENT OF WITNESSES: The person who signed this document whose health-care wishes are reflected herein (the principal) is known to me and

voluntarily signed or voluntarily directed another to sign this document in my presence, and the presence of the other witnesses. The principal appears to be of sound mind and free from duress, fraud or undue influence. I am aged 18 years and upwards and am not related to the principal by blood, marriage or adoption.

_____   _____
Signature of Witness 1   Signature of Witness 2

_____   _____
Print Name   Print Name

_____   _____
Occupation or Profession   Occupation or Profession

_____   _____
_____   _____
_____   _____
Home Address   Home Address

_____   _____
Home Telephone   Home Telephone

_____   _____
Work Telephone   Work Telephone

Appendix 4

Statements following Supreme Court Decision in 'Ward of Court' case (1995)

a. Medical Council Statement of 4 August 1995
On 4 August 1995, the Medical Council considered the recent Supreme Court decision in the matter of a Ward of Court.

The Council wishes to draw attention to its publication *A Guide to Ethical Conduct and Behaviour and to Fitness to Practise* and emphasise the following paragraphs:

13.01	Doctors must do their best to preserve life and promote the health of the sick person....
12.05	'Medical Care must not be used as a tool of the State to be granted or withheld or altered in character under political pressure. Regardless of the type of their practice, the responsibility of all doctors is to help the sick and injured. Doctors must practise without consideration of religion, nationality, race, politics or social standing. Doctors should not allow their professional actions to be influenced by any personal interest'.
43.01	'Where death is imminent, it is the doctor's responsibility to take care that a patient dies with dignity and with as little suffering as possible. Euthanasia, which involves deliberately causing the death of a patient, is professional misconduct and is illegal in Ireland.'

Appendix J (Principles of Medical Ethics in Europe)

Article 2	'In the course of his professional practice a doctor undertakes to give priority to the medical interest of the patient. The doctor may use his professional knowledge only to improve or maintain the health of those who place their trust in him; in no circumstances may he act to their detriment'.
Article 4:	... The doctor must not substitute his own definition of the quality of life for that of his patient....

It is the view of the Council that access to nutrition and hydration is one of the basic needs of human beings. This remains so even when, from time to time, this need can only be fulfilled by means of long established methods such as nasogastric and gastrostomy tube feeding.

The Council sees no need to alter its Ethical Guide.

b. An Bord Altranais Statement of 18 August 1995
Guidance issued by An Bord Altranais to the nursing profession following An Bord's consideration of the Supreme Court decision in the matter of A Ward of Court, delivered on 27th July 1995.

1.   Section 51(2) of the Nurses' Act, 1955 provides that:
                'It shall be a function of the Board to give guidance to the nursing profession generally on all matters relating to ethical conduct and behaviour.'

2.   'The aim of the nursing profession is to give the highest standard of care possible to patients. An Bord is satisfied that The Code of Professional Conduct for each Nurse and Midwife affirms and protects this aim and sees no reason to change the code following consideration of this judgement. The code provides that specific issues will be considered when they arise and the Board considers the decision of the Supreme Court to be one such issue.

3.   The decision of the Supreme Court refers to a specific case where the wishes of the family and the best interest of the patient have been considered by the Supreme Court. In this specific case the Supreme Court has consented to the withdrawal of and termination of nutrition and hydration by tube from the patient and to the withdrawal of other treatments save as palliative treatment and declared such action to be lawful and consistent with the patient's Constitutional rights and to be in her best interest.

4.   The Board reaffirms the principle laid out in the Code that:

                The Nurse must at all times maintain the principle that every effort should be made to preserve human life both born and unborn. When death is imminent care should be taken to ensure that the patient dies with dignity.

This ethical principle requires that so long as there remains a means of nutrition and hydration of this patient it is the duty of the nurse to act in accordance with the Code and to provide nutrition and hydration. In this specific case, a nurse may not participate in the withdrawal and termination of the means of nutrition and hydration by tube. In the event of the withdrawal and termination of the means of nutrition and hydration by tube the nurse's role will be to provide all nursing care.

Interpretative Statement 1   18 August 1995

References and Further Reading

Introduction

Fowler, Marsha, *Ethics in Nursing, 1893–1984: The Ideal of Service, the Reality of History*, Los Angeles: University of Southern California 1984.

Fowler, Marsha, 'Nursing Ethics' in A. Davis, M. Arosakar, J. Liaschenko, and T. Drought, *Ethical Dilemmas and Nursing Practice* (4th edition), Stamford, CT: Appleton & Lange 1997, 17–34.

Fry, Sara T., 'Toward a Theory of Nursing Ethics', *ANS* 11/4 (1989), 9–22.

Fry, Sara T., 'Nursing Ethics' in Warren Thomas Reich, ed., *Encyclopedia of Bioethics*, New York: Simon and Schuster Macmillan 1995.

Fry, Sara T. 'Defining Nurses' Ethical Practices in the 21st Century', International Council of Nurses, *International Nursing Review*, 49 (2002), 1–3.

Fry, Sara T. and Megan-Jane Johnstone, *Ethics in Nursing Practice* (2nd edition), Oxford: Blackwell 2002.

Holm, Søren, *Ethical Problems in Clinical Practice*, Manchester: Manchester University Press 1997.

Nelson, Siobhan, 'The Search for the Good in Nursing? The Burden of Ethical Expertise', *Nursing Philosophy* 5/1 (2004), 12–22.

Rodney, Patricia, Bernadette Pauly and Michael Burgess 'Our Theoretical Landscape: Complementary Approaches to Health Care Ethics' in Janet L. Storch, Patricia Rodney and Rosalie Starzomski. eds, *Toward a Moral Horizon*, Toronto: Pearson Education Canada 2004, 77–97.

Storch, Janet L., 'Nursing Ethics: A Developing Moral Terrain' in Janet L. Storch, Patricia Rodney and Rosalie Starzomski, eds, *Toward a Moral Horizon*, Toronto: Pearson Education Canada 2004, 1–14.

1: Respecting Patient Autonomy

Beauchamp, Tom and James Childress, *Principles of Biomedical Ethics* (5th edition), Oxford: Oxford University Press 2001, 57–112.

Berlin, Isaiah 'Two Concepts of Liberty' in Isaiah Berlin, *Four Essays on Liberty*, Oxford: Oxford University Press 1992 [1969], 11–25.

Burckhardt, Margaret A. and Alvita K. Nataniel, *Ethics and Issues in Contemporary Nursing*. Albany NY; London: Delmar 2001.

Dworkin, Ronald, *Life's Dominion*, London: Harper Collins 1993.

Edwards, Steven D., *Nursing Ethics, A Principle-Based Approach*, Basingstoke: Macmillan 1996.

Fry, Sara T. and Megan-Jane Johnstone, *Ethics in Nursing Practice* (2nd edition), Oxford: Blackwell 2002.

Hill, Thomas E., *Autonomy and Self-Respect*, Cambridge: Cambridge University Press 1991.

Kant, Immanuel, *Groundwork of the Metaphysics of Morals*, Mary Gregor, ed., Cambridge: Cambridge University Press 1997 [1785].

Kukathas, C. and P. Petit, *Rawls: A Theory of Justice and its Critics*, Cambridge: Polity 1990.

Mill, John Stuart, *On Liberty*, Harmondsworth: Penguin 1981 [1859].

Rawls, John, *A Theory of Justice*, Oxford: Oxford University Press 1971.

2: Autonomy and Vulnerability

American Nurses Association, *Code for Nurses with Interpretive Statements*, Kansas City, MO: American Nurses Association 1985.

An Bord Altranais, *The Code of Professional Conduct for Each Nurse and Midwife*, Dublin: An Bord Altranais 2000(a). *www.nursingboard.ie* Accessed 1 May 2004.

An Bord Altranais, *Scope of Nursing and Midwifery Practice Framework*, Dublin: An Bord Altranais 2000(b).

Beauchamp, Tom and James Childress, *Principles of Biomedical Ethics* (5th edition), Oxford: Oxford University Press 2001, 57–112.

Berlin, Isaiah 'Two Concepts of Liberty' in Isaiah Berlin, *Four Essays on Liberty*, Oxford: Oxford University Press 1992 [1969], 11–25.

Brody, Howard, *Stories of Sickness*, New Haven and London: Yale University Press 1987.

Dickenson, Donna, 'Three Different Models in European Medical Law and Ethics' in Michael Parker and Donna Dickenson, eds, *The Cambridge Medical Ethics Workbook*, Cambridge: Cambridge University Press 2001, 284–9.

Donnelly, Mary, *Consent: Bridging the Gap Between Doctor and Patient*, Cork: Cork University Press 2002.

Frank, Arthur W., 'How Can They Act Like That, Clinicians and Patients as Characters in Each Other's Stories', *Hastings Center Report*, (November–December 2002), 14–22.

Fry, Sara T. and Megan-Jane Johnstone, *Ethics in Nursing Practice* (2nd edition), Oxford: Blackwell 2002.

Goldman, Alan, 'The Refutation of Medical Paternalism' in Bonnie Steinbock, John D. Arras and Alex John London, eds, *Ethical Issues in Modern Medicine* (6th edition), Boston: McGraw Hill 2003, 56–64.

Hill, Thomas E., *Autonomy and Self-Respect*, Cambridge: Cambridge University Press 1991.

Kitwood, Tom, *Dementia Reconsidered*, Maidenhead UK: Open University Press 1997.

MacKenzie, Catriona and Natalie Stoljar, *Relational Autonomy*, Oxford: Oxford University Press 2000.

McCarthy, Joan, 'Principlism or Narrative Ethics: must we choose between them?', *Journal of Medical Humanities* 29/4 (2003), 65–71.

Oberlie, Kathleen and Sandra Tenove, 'Ethical Issues in Public Health Nursing', *Nursing Ethics* 7/5 (2000), 425–39.

Scott, P. A., 'Autonomy, Power and Control in Palliative Care', *Cambridge Ethics Quarterly* 8/2 (1999): 139–47.

Mendus, Susan, 'Out of the Doll's House' in Michael Parker and Donna Dickenson, eds, *The Cambridge Medical Ethics Workbook*, Cambridge: Cambridge University Press 2001, 290–94.

Parker, Michael, 'A Deliberative Approach to Bioethics' in Michael Parker and Donna Dickenson, eds, *The Cambridge Medical Ethics Workbook*, Cambridge: Cambridge University Press 2001, 304–10.

Schwartz, Robert L., 'Autonomy, Futility, and the Limits of Medicine' in Helga Kuhse and Peter Singer, eds, *Bioethics*, London: Blackwell 1999.

3: Truthful Conversations

Beauchamp, Tom and James Childress, *Principles of Biomedical Ethics* (3rd edition), New York: Oxford University Press 1989.

Bok, Sissela, *Lying: Moral Choice in Public and Private Life*, Sussex: Harvester Press 1978.

Cassell, Eric J., 'The Nature of Suffering and the Goals of Medicine', *New England Journal of Medicine* 306 (1982), 639–45.

Chadwick, Ruth and Win Tadd, *Ethics & Nursing Practice*, London: Macmillan 2000.

Frith, Lucy, ed., *Ethics and Midwifery*, Oxford: Butterworth 1996.

Higgs, Roger, 'On Telling Patients the Truth' in Helga Kuhse and Peter Singer, eds, *Bioethics: An Anthology*, Oxford: Blackwell Publishers 1999, 507–12.

Hill, Thomas E., *Autonomy and Self-Respect*, Cambridge: Cambridge University Press 1991.

Kant, Immanuel, *The Metaphysical Principles of Virtue*, trans. J. Ellington and W. Wick, Indianapolis, Indiana: Bobbs-Merrill Co. 1968.

Katz, Jay, *The Silent World of Doctor and Patient*, Baltimore: Johns Hopkins University Press 2002.

Mill, John Stuart, *On Liberty*, Indianapolis, Indiana: Hackett Publishing Co. 1978.

Rumbold, Graham, *Ethics in Nursing Practice*, Edinburgh: Baillière Tindall 1999.

Seedhouse, David, *Ethics: The Heart of Health Care*, Chichester: John Wiley & Sons 1988.

Tadd, Win, *Ethical Issues in Nursing and Midwifery Practice*, London, Macmillan Press 1998.

Tschudin, Verena, *Deciding Ethically*, London: Baillière Tindall 1994.

Yeo, Michael and Anne Moorhouse, *Concepts and Cases in Nursing Ethics*, Ontario: Broadview Press 1996.

4: Advocacy and Integrity

An Bord Altranais, *The Code of Professional Conduct for Each Nurse and Midwife*, Dublin: An Bord Altranais, 2000.

Bandman, Elsie and Bertram, *Nursing Ethics through the Life Span*, New Jersey: Prentice Hall 2002.

Bartter, Karen, 'The Midwife Advocate' in Lucy Frith, ed., *Ethics and Midwifery*, Oxford: Butterworth 1996, 221–36.

Beauchamp, Tom and James Childress, *Principles of Biomedical Ethics* (5th edition), New York: Oxford University Press 2001.

Chadwick, Ruth, Mairi Levitt and Darren Shickle, eds, *The Right to Know and the Right Not to Know*, Aldershot: Avebury 1997.

Gadow, S. A., 'Clinical Subjectivity: Advocacy with Silent Patients', *Nursing Clinics of North America* 24/2 (1989), 535–41.

Hudak, Carolyn, Barbara Gallo and Patricia Gonce Morton, *Critical Care Nursing: A Holistic Approach*, Philadelphia: Lippincott Williams and Wilkins 1998.

Kasenene, Peter, 'African Ethical Theory and the Four Principles' in Robert M. Veatch, *Cross-Cultural Perspectives in Medical Ethics* (2nd edition), Sudbury, Massachusetts: Jones and Bartlett 2000, 347–57.

Kuhse, Helga, *Caring: Nurses, Women and Ethics*, Oxford: Blackwell 1997.

Liaschenko, Joan 'The Shift from the Closed to the Open Body: Ramifications for Nursing Testimony', in Steven Edwards, ed., *Philosophical Issues in Nursing*, London: Macmillan 1998, 11–30.

Mallik, M., 'Advocacy in Nursing – A Review of the Literature', *Journal of Advanced Nursing* 25/1 (1997), 130–38.

Moazam, Farhat, 'Families, Patients, and Physicians in Medical Decision-making: A Pakistani Perspective', *Hastings Center Report* 30/6 (2000), 28–37.

Rumbold, Graham, *Ethics in Nursing Practice*, Edinburgh: Baillière Tindall 1999.

Tschudin, Verena, *Nurses Matter: Reclaiming our Professional Identity*, London: Palgrave 1999.

United Kingdom Central Council for Nursing, Midwifery and Health Visiting, *Exercising Accountability*, London: UKCC 1989.

Willard, C., 'The Nurse's Role as Patient Advocate: Obligation or Imposition?', *Journal of Advanced Nursing* 24/1 (1996), 60–66.

Yarling, R. R. and B. J. McElmurry, 'The Moral Foundations of Nursing', *Advances in Nursing Science* 8/2 (1986), 63–73.

Yeo, Michael and Anne Moorhouse, *Concepts and Cases in Nursing Ethics* (2nd edition), Ontario, Canada: Broadview Press 1996.

5: Respecting Patient Confidentiality

An Bord Altranais, *The Code of Professional Conduct for Each Nurse and Midwife*, Dublin: An Bord Altranais, 2000.

An Bord Altranais, *Scope of Nursing and Midwifery Practice Framework*, Dublin: An Bord Altranais 2000.

Ainslie, D. C., 'Questioning Bioethics, Aids, Sexual Ethics and the Duty to Warn, *Hastings Center Report* 29/5 (1999), 26–35.

Beauchamp, Tom and James Childress, *Principles of Biomedical Ethics*, (5th edition), Oxford: Oxford University Press 2001.

Bok Sissela, *Secrets*, New York: Vintage Books 1989.

Council of Europe, *Data Protection Directive 95/46/EC*. Strasbourg: Council of Europe 1995. *http://europa.eu.int/ISPO/legal/en/dataprot/directiv/directiv.html* Accessed 1 May 2004.

Council of Europe, *European Convention on Human Rights*. Strasbourg: Council of Europe 1950. *http://conventions.coe.int/treaty/en/Treaties/Html/005.htm* Accessed: May 2004.

Department of Health, *A Charter of Rights for Hospital Patients*, Dublin: Department of Health 1990.

Department of Health and Children, *Confidentiality – Ethical Considerations in HIV Transmission: Guidelines for Professionals*, prepared by Anne Marie Jones 2001.

Edelstein, Ludwig, *The Hippocratic Oath, Translation and Interpretation*, Baltimore: Johns Hopkins Press 1943. See also *http://hsc.virginia.edu/hslibrary/historical/antiqua/texto.htm* Accessed 1 May 2004.

General Medical Council (UK), *Confidentiality: Protecting and Providing Information*, London: GMC 2004. *http://www.gmc-uk.org/standards/default.htm* Accessed 1 May 2004

Government of Ireland, *Data Protection Act*, Dublin: Government Stationery Office 1988. *http://www.irishstatutebook.ie/ZZA25Y1988S8.html* Accessed 1 May 2004.

Government of Ireland, *Data Protection (Amendment) Act*, Dublin: Government Stationery Office 2003. *http://www.justice.ie/802569B20047F907/vWeb/wpMJDE5NKDM9* Accessed 1 May 2004

Irish Medical Council, *A Guide to Ethical Conduct and Behaviour*, (6th edition), Dublin: IMC 2004. *http://www.medicalcouncil.ie/professional/ethics.asp* Accessed 1 May 2004.

Kennedy & Arnold v. *Ireland* [1987] IR1 per Hamilton P.

Kuhse, Helga, 'Confidentiality and the AMA's New Code of Ethics: An Imprudent Formulation?' in Helga Kuhse and Peter Singer, eds, *Bioethics, An Anthology*, London: Blackwell 1999, 493–6.

Madden, Deirdre, *Medicine, Ethics & the Law*, Dublin: Butterworths 2002.

Mason, T., 'Tarasoff Liability: Its Impact for Working with Patients who Threaten Others, *International Journal of Nursing Studies* 35 (1998), 109–14.

Mills, Simon, *Clinical Practice and the Law*, Dublin: Butterworths 2002.

Nightingale, Florence, *Notes on Nursing: What it is, and what it is not*, Philadelphia: J. B. Lippincott 1859. *http://www.nursingcenter.com/library/JournalArticle.asp?Article_ID=270233#13* Accessed 1 May 2004.

Nightingale, Florence, *Notes on Nursing: What it is, and what it is not*, commemorative edition, Philadelphia: J. B. Lippincott 1992.

Society of Sexual Health Advisers (UK), *Code of Professional Conduct*, UK: SSHA 2004. *http://www.ssha.info/member/code.htm* Accessed 1 May 2004.

Tarasoff v. *the Regents of the University of California, et al.*, 551 P.2d 334, 131 Cal. Rptr. 14 (1976). [Tarasoff II]

Woodman, Margaret Antoinette, 'Partner Notification for Sexually Transmitted Infections in the Republic of Ireland', M.Comm thesis, University College Cork, 2003.

Woodman, Antoinette, Personal communication, 2004.

6: The Confidentiality Process

Cain P., 'The Limits of Confidentiality', *Nursing Ethics* 5/2 (1998).

Fry, Sara T. and Robert M. Veatch, *Case Studies in Nursing Ethics* (2nd edition), Sudbury, Massachusetts: Jones and Bartlett 2000.

Society of Sexual Health Advisers (UK), *Code of Professional Conduct*, UK: SSHA 2004. *http://www.ssha.info/member/code.htm* Accessed 1 May 2004.

Woodman, Margaret Antoinette, 'Partner Notification for Sexually Transmitted Infections in the Republic of Ireland', M.Comm thesis, University College Cork, 2003.

7: Informed Consent to Nursing and Medical Procedures

An Bord Altranais, *The Code of Professional Conduct for Each Nurse and Midwife*, Dublin: An Bord Altranais, 2000. *www.nursingboard.ie* Accessed 1 May 2004.

American Nurses' Association, *Code of Ethics with Interpretive Statements*, Washington, DC: American Nurses Publishing 2001. *http://www.nursingworld.org/ethics/code/ethicscode150.htm#* Accessed 1 May 2004.

Aveyard, Helen, 'Implied Consent Prior to Nursing Care Procedures', *Journal of Advanced Nursing* 39/2 (2002), 201–7.

Beauchamp, Tom and James Childress, *Principles of Biomedical Ethics* (5th edition), Oxford: Oxford University Press 2001.

Bolam v. *Friern Hospital Management Committee* (1957) 1 WLR 582.

Canterbury v. *Spence* [1972] 464 F 2d 772.

Donnelly, Mary, *Consent: Bridging the Gap Between Doctor and Patient*, Cork: Cork University Press 2002.

Draper, Heather, 'Consent in Childbirth' in Lucy Frith, ed., *Ethics and Midwifery*, Oxford: Butterworth-Heinemann 1996, 17–35.

Faden, Ruth R. and Tom L. Beauchamp, *A History and Theory of Informed Consent*, Oxford: Oxford University Press 1986, Ch. 8.

Frith, Lucy, ed., *Ethics and Midwifery*, Oxford, Butterworth-Heinemann 1996.

Fry, Sara T. and Robert M. Veatch, *Case Studies in Nursing Ethics* (2nd edition), Sudbury Massachusetts: Jones and Bartlett 2000.

Geoghegan v. *Harris* (2000) 3 IR 536. *http://www.bailii.org/ie/cases/IEHC/2000/129.html* Accessed 1 May 2004.

Gillick v. *West Norfolk and Wisbech AHA* (1986) AC 112, (1985) 3 ALL ER 402.

Harris, John, 'Consent and End of Life Decisions', *Journal of Medcial Ethics* 29/1, (2003): 10–15.

Lewison, Helen, 'Choices in Childbirth: Areas of Conflict' in Lucy Frith, ed., *Ethics and Midwifery*, Oxford, Butterworth-Heinemann 1996, 36–49.

O'Neill, Onora, 'Some Limits of Informed Consent', *Journal of Medical Ethics* 29/1 (2003): 4–7.

Madden, Deirdre, *Medicine, Ethics & the Law*, Dublin: Butterworths 2002.

McParland, J. and P. A. Scott, 'Consent and Nursing Interventions', *British Journal of Nursing* 9/10 (2000), 660–65.

Non-Fatal Offences against the Person Act 1997 Section 23 (1). *http://www.irlgov.ie/bills28/acts/1997/a2697.pdf* Accessed 1 May 2004.

Nursing and Midwifery Code of Professional Conduct, 2002, from the UK *http://www.nmcuk.org/nmc/main/publications/codeOfProfessionalConduct.pdf* Accessed 1 May 2004.

Parker, Michael, and Donna Dickenson, eds, *The Cambridge Medical Ethics Workbook*, Cambridge: Cambridge University Press 2001.

Re a Ward of Court (1995) 2 ILRM 401, 431.

Re C (adult: refusal of treatment) (1994) 1 All ER 819.

Rothman, D., *Strangers at the Bedside: A History of How Law and Ethics Transformed Medical Decision-making*, New York: Basic Books 1991.

Schloendoff v. *Society of New York Hospital* (1914) 211 NY 125.

Tadd, Win, ed., *Ethical Issues in Nursing and Midwifery Practice*, London: Macmillan 1998.

Tuma v. *Board of Nursing*, 100 Idaho 74, 593 P.2d 711 (Idaho Apr 17, 1979)
Walsh v. *Family Planning Services Ltd.* (1992)1 IR 496.

8: Informed Consent in Research

An Bord Altranais, *The Code of Professional Conduct for Each Nurse and Midwife*, Dublin: An Bord Altranais 2000.

Boomgaarden, Jürgen, Pekka Louhiala and Urban Wiesing, *Issues in Medical Research Ethics*, Oxford: Berghahn Books 2003.

Brandt, Allan M., 'Racism and Research: The Case of the Tuskegee Syphilis Study', *Hastings Center Report*, December 1978, 21–9.

Canadian Nurses' Association, *Ethical Guidelines for Nurses in Research Involving Human Subjects*, Ottowa: CNA 2002.

Coney, Sandra, *The Unfortunate Experiment*, Auckland, New Zealand: Penguin 1988.

Control of Clinical Trials Act, Annotated by Robert A. Pearce, London: Sweet and Maxwell 1987. Reprinted from *Irish Current Law Statutes Annotated*.

Council of Europe, *European Convention for Protection of Human Rights and Dignity of the Human Being with Regard to the Application of Biology and Biomedicine: European Convention on Human Rights and Biomedicine*, Strasbourg: Texts of the Council of Europe 1996.

Council of Europe, Clinical Trials Directive 2001/20/EC. *Official Journal of the European Communities.* L121 (2001), 34–44. *http://www.europa .eu.int/eur-lex/en/search/search_lif.html* Accessed 1 May 2004.

Department of Health, *Report on Three Trials Involving Babies and Children in Institutional Settings 1960/61, 1970 and 1973*, 2000. This Report has since been referred to the Commission to inquire into child abuse 2000. Web address: *http://www.irishstatutebook.ie/ZZA7Y2000.html* Accessed 1 May 2004.

Donnelly, Mary, *Consent: Bridging the Gap Between Doctor and Patient*, Cork: Cork University Press 2002.

Doyal, Len and Jeffrey S. Tobias, eds, *Informed Consent in Medical Research*, London: BMJ Books 2001.

Heller, Jean, 'Syphilis Victims in US Study Went Untreated for 40 years: Syphilis victims got no therapy', *New York Times*, 26 July 1972, 1–2.

International Council of Nurses, *Code of Ethics for Nurses*, Geneva: ICN 2000.

International Council of Nurses, *Ethical Guidelines for Nursing Research*, Geneva: ICN 2003. *http://www.icn.ch/icncode.pdf* Accessed 1 May 2004.

Irish Council for Bioethics, *Operational Procedures for Research Ethics Committees: Guidance 2004*, 2004. Website: *http://www.bioethics.ie*

Jones, James H., *Bad Blood: The Tuskegee Syphilis Experiment*, New York: Free Press 1993.

Madden, Deirdre, *Medicine, Ethics & the Law*, Dublin: Butterworths 2002.

Montgomery, Jonathan, 'Informed Consent and Clinical Research with Children' in Len Doyal and Jeffrey S. Tobias, eds, *Informed Consent in Medical Research*, London: BMJ Books 2001.

National Commission for the Protection of Human Subjects of Biomedical and Behavioral Research, *Belmont Report*, Washington DC: Government Printing Office 1979. *www.http://ohsr.od.nih.gov/mpa/belmont.php3* Accessed 1 May 2004.

National Disability Authority, *Guidelines for Including People with Disabilities in Research*, Dublin: NDA 2002. *http://www.nda.ie/CntMgmt.nsf/0/ 2B766F9C159E070680256C7B00640CFF/$File/Inclusion.pdf* Accessed 1 May 2004.

Nuremberg Code, *Trials of War Criminals before the Nuremberg Military Tribunals under Control Council Law*, 10/2, 181–2. Washington, DC: US Government Printing Office 1949. *http://ohsr.od.nih.gov/nuremberg.php3* Accessed 1 May 2004.

Pellegrino, Edmund, 'The Nazi Doctors and Nuremberg, Some Moral Lessons Revisited', *Annals of Internal Medicine* 127/4 (1997), 307–8.

Rivers, Eunice, Stanley Schuman, Lloyd Simpson and Sidney Olansky, 'Twenty Years of Followup Experience in a Long-Range Medical Study', *Public Health Reports* 68/4 (1953), 391–5. *http://www.dc.peachnet.edu/~shale/humanities/ composition/assignments/experiment/rivers.html* Accessed 1 May 2004.

Royal College of Paediatrics, Child Health Ethics Advisory Committee, *Archives of Disease in Childhood* 82 (February 2000), 177–82.

Savage, Eileen, Personal Communication, 2003 (a).

Savage, Eileen, 'Children's and Parents' Perspectives of Food and Eating in the Management of Cystic Fibrosis', PhD thesis, Manchester University, 2003 (b).

Smith, Susan L., 'Neither Victim nor Villain: Nurse Eunice Rivers, The Tuskegee Syphilis Experiment, and Public Health Work', *Journal of Women's History* 8/1 (1996): 95–105.

Tuskegee Syphilis Study Legacy Committee, *Final Report*, 20 May 1996. *http://hsc.virginia.edu/hs-library/historical/apology/report.html* Accessed 1 May 2004.

World Medical Association Helsinki Declaration, *Declaration of Helsinki* (Document 17.C), 1964. This is an official policy document of the World Medical Association, the global representative body for physicians. It was first adopted in 1964 (Helsinki, Finland) and revised in 1975 (Tokyo, Japan), 1983 (Venice, Italy), 1989 (Hong Kong), 1996 (Somerset-West, South Africa) and 2000. *http://www.wma.net/e/policy/b3.htm* Accessed 1 October 2003.

9: Abortion and Moral Space

Beauchamp, Tom L. and James F. Childress, *Principles of Biomedical Ethics* (3rd edition), Oxford: Oxford University Press 1989.

Beauchamp, Tom L. and James F. Childress, *Principles of Biomedical Ethics* (5th edition), Oxford: Oxford University Press 2001.

Bok, Sissela, 'Ethical Problems of Abortion', *Hastings Center Studies* 2/1 (1974), 33–52.

Clarke, Liam, 'The Person in Abortion', *Nursing Ethics* 6/1 (1999), 1–37.

Dooley, Dolores, 'Abortion and the Law in Ireland' in Desmond Clarke, ed., *Morality and the Law*, Cork: Mercier Press 1982.

Dooley, Dolores, 'Conscientious Refusal to Assist with Abortion', *British Medical Journal* 309/6955 (1994), 622–3.

Fry, Sara T. and Robert M. Veatch, *Case Studies in Nursing Ethics* (2nd Edition), Sudbury Massachusetts: Jones and Bartlett 2000.

Grisez, Germain and Joseph Boyle, *Life and Death with Liberty and Justice*, Notre Dame, Indiana: University of Notre Dame Press 1979.

Rumbold, Graham, *Ethics in Nursing Practice* (3rd edition), Edinburgh: Baillière Tindall 1999.

10: Personal Conscience and Public Policy

Attorney General v. *X and Others* [1992] IESC 1; [1992] 1 IR 1 (5 March 1992)

Bok, Sissela, 'Ethical Problems of Abortion', *Hastings Center Studies* 2/1 (1974), 33–52.

Clarke, Desmond, *Morality and the Law*, Cork: Mercier Press 1982.

Clarke, Liam, 'The Person in Abortion', *Nursing Ethics* 6/1 (1999), 1–37.

Dooley, Dolores, 'Abortion and the Law in Ireland' in Desmond Clarke, ed., *Morality and the Law*, Cork: Mercier Press 1982.

Dooley, Dolores, 'Conscientious Refusal to Assist with Abortion', *British Medical Journal* 309/6955 (1994), 622–3.

Dworkin, Ronald, *Life's Dominion*, London: Harper Collins 1993.

Edmondson, Ricca, 'Moral Debate and Social Change', *Doctrine and Life* 42/5 (1992), 233–43.

Fletcher, Ruth, 'The Significance of Irish Women's Silence About their Experiences of Abortion', MA thesis in Women's Studies, National University of Ireland at Cork, Ireland, 1993.

Grisez, Germain and Joseph Boyle, *Life and Death with Liberty and Justice*, Notre Dame, Indiana: University of Notre Dame Press 1979.

Haring, Bernard, *Free and Faithful in Christ*, Vol. 3, St Paul, Minnesota: Slough Publishers 1978.

Hunt, Geoffrey, 'Abortion: Why Bioethics Can Have No Answer: A Personal Perspective', *Nursing Ethics* 6/1 (1999).

Irish Council for Civil Liberties, 'The Need for Abortion Law Reform in Ireland: Position Paper', 2002. *http://www.iccl.ie/women/abortion/abortion_paper*2002.html Accessed 1 May 2004.

Irish Family Planning Association, *The Irish Journey: Women's Stories of Abortion*, Dublin: IFPA 2000.

Mahon, Evelyn, Catherine Conlon and Lucy Dillon, *Women and Crisis Pregnancy: A Report Presented to the Department of Health and Children*, Dublin: Stationery Office 1998.

Petchesky, Rosalind Pollack, *Abortion and Woman's Choice*, London: Verso Press 1986.

Rumbold, Graham, *Ethics in Nursing Practice*, 3rd ed., Edinburgh: Baillière Tindall 1999.

Smyth, Ailbhe, ed., *The Abortion Papers Ireland*, Dublin: Attic Press 1992.

Treacy, Bernard, ed., 'Abortion, Law and Conscience', collection of articles in *Doctrine and Life*, Kildare, Ireland: Dominican Publications, 42/5 (1992) 31–47.

11: Selecting for Sex

Berkowitz, J. M., 'Sexism and Racism in Preconceptive Trait Selection', *Fertility and Sterility* 71/3 (1999), 415–7.

Buchanan, Allen, Dan W. Brock, Norman Daniels and Daniel Wikler, *From Chance to Choice*, Cambridge: Cambridge University Press 2000.

Colapinto, J., *As Nature Made Him: The Boy who was Raised as a Girl*, New York: Harper Collins 1999.

Commission on Assisted Human Reproduction, *Conference Transcript*, Dublin: CAHR, 31/35 Bow Street, Dublin 7, 6 February 2003.

Council of Europe, European Convention on Human Rights. Strasbourg: Texts of the Council of Europe 1950. *http://conventions.coe.int/treaty/en/Treaties/Html/005.htm* Accessed 1 May 2004.

Council of Europe, *European Convention for Protection of Human Rights and Dignity of the Human Being with Regard to the Application of Biology and Biomedicine: European Convention on Human Rights and Biomedicine*, Strasbourg: Texts of the Council of Europe 1997. *http://conventions. coe.int/treaty/en/treaties/html/164.htm* Accessed 1 May 2004.

Daniels, Norman, 'It isn't just the sex' *American Journal of Bioethics* 1/1 (2001), 10–11.

De Beauvoir, Simone, *The Second Sex*, London: Vintage 1997.

Dickens, Bernard M., 'Can Sex Selection Be Ethically Tolerated?' *Journal of Medical Ethics* 8/6 (2002), 335–6.

Dooley, Dolores, Joan McCarthy, Tina Garanis-Papadatos and Panagiota Dalla-Vorgia, *The Ethics of New Reproductive Technologies*, Oxford: Berghahn Books 2003, 55–73.

Fugger, E. F., S. H. Black, K. Keyvanfar and J. D. Schulman, 'Births of Normal Daughters after Microsort Sperm Separation and Intrauterine Insemination, In-vitro Fertilization, or Intracytoplasmic Sperm Injection', *Human Reproduction* 13 (1998), 2367.

Guttentag, M. and P. Secord, *Too Many Women? The Sex Ratio Question*, Beverley Hills, CA: Sage Publications 1983.

Hanmer, Jalna, 'Sex Predetermination and Male Dominance' in Helen Roberts, ed., *Women, Health and Reproduction*, London: Routledge and Kegan Paul 1981, 163–90.

Human Fertilisation and Embryology Authority (HFEA), *Sex Selection: Options for Regulation*, London: HFEA 2003. *http://www.hfea.gov.uk/AboutHFEA/Consultations/Final%20sex%20selection%20main%20report.pdf* Accessed 1 May 2004.

Irish Medical Council, *A Guide to Ethical Conduct and Behaviour*, 6th ed., Dublin: IMC 2004. *http://www.medicalcouncil.ie/professional/ethics.asp* Accessed 1 May 2004.

Kant, Immanuel, *The Moral Law: Groundwork of the Metaphysics of Morals*, trans. H. J. Paton, London: Routledge 1991 [1785].

Madden, Deirdre, *Medicine, Ethics & the Law*, Dublin: Butterworths 2002.

Mill, John Stuart, *On Liberty*, New York: Penguin 1981 [1859].

President's Council on Bioethics, *Report on Human Cloning and Human Dignity: An Ethical Inquiry*, Washington: President's Council on Bioethics 2002. *http://www.bioethics.gov/reports/cloningreport/index.html* Accessed 1 May 2004.

Robertson, John A., *Children of Choice*, Princeton: Princeton University Press 1994.

Robertson, John A., 'Preconception Gender Selection', *American Journal of Bioethics* 1 (2001), 2–9.

Robertson, John A., 'Sex Selection for Gender Variety by Preimplantation Genetic Diagnosis', *Fertility and Sterility* 78 (2002), 463.

Taylor, Charles, *Sources of the Self*, Cambridge: Cambridge University Press 1989.

United Nations, *Universal Declaration of Human Rights*, Geneva: Office of the High Commissioner for Human Rights 1948. *http://www.unhchr.ch/udhr/miscinfo/carta.htm* Accessed 1 May 2004.

United Nations, *International Covenant on Civil and Political Rights*, Geneva: Office of the High Commissioner for Human Rights 1976. *http://www.unhchr.ch/html/menu3/b/a_ccpr.htm* Accessed 1 May 2004.

Warren, Mary Anne, 'Sex Selection: Individual Choice or Cultural Coercion?' in Helga Kuhse and Peter Singer, eds, *Bioethics*, Oxford: Blackwell 1999, 137–42.

12: Surrogate Pregnancy

Anderson, Elizabeth, *Value in Ethics and Economics*, Cambridge Massachusetts: Harvard University Press 1993.

Barret, Robert L. and Bryan E. Robinson, 'Gay Dads' in Adele E. Gottfried and Allen W. Gottfried, eds, *Redefining Families: Implications for Children's Development*, New York: Plenum Press 1994, 157–70.

Bigner, J. J., and F. W. Bozett, 'Parenting by Gay Fathers', *Marriage and Family Review* 14(3/4) (1990), 155–75.

Brazier Committee Review, *Surrogacy: Review for Health Ministers of Current Arrangements for Payments and Regulation* (Cm. 4068), London: Department of Health 1998.

Clarke, Victoria, 'What About the Children? Arguments Against Lesbian and Gay Parenting', *Women's Studies International Forum* 24/5 (2001) (a), 555–70.

Clarke, Victoria, 'The Normalisation of Lesbian and Gay Parenting' in Adrian Coyle and Celia Kitzinger, eds, *Lesbian and Gay Psychology, New Perspective*, Oxford: Blackwells British Psychological Society Books 2001 (b).

Cramer, D., 'Gay Parents and Their Children: A Review of Research and Practical Implications', *Journal of Counseling and Development* 64 (1986), 504–7.

Childlessness Overcome Through Surrogacy (COTS), *Information for Surrogates*, London: COTS 1997.

Dooley, Dolores, Joan McCarthy, Tina Garanis-Papadatos and Panagiota Dalla-Vorgia, *The Ethics of New Reproductive Technologies*, Oxford: Berghahn Books 2003, 55–73.

Gottman, Julie Schwartz, 'Children of Gay and Lesbian Parents,' *Marriage and Family Review* 14(3/4) (1990): 177–96.

Green, G. Dorsey and Frederick W. Bozett, 'Lesbian Mothers and Gay Fathers' in J. C. Gonsiorek and J. D. Weinrich, eds, *Homosexuality: Research Implications for Public Policy*, Newbury Park, CA: Sage 1991, 197–214.

Human Fertilisation and Embryology Act (1990), Section 13, 5. *http://www.hmso.gov.uk/acts/acts1990/Ukpga_19900037_en_1.htm* Accessed 1 May 2004.

Human Fertilisation and Embryology Act (1990), Section 27, 1.

Jerusalem Bible, Genesis, Chapter 16, London: Darton, Longman & Todd 1985.

Johnson and Calvert (1993) 851 P.2d 776 Cal.

Knight, Robert H. and Daniel S. Garcia, 'Homosexual Parenting: Bad for Children, Bad for Society, *Insight*, 25 July 1994, Washington: Family Research Council, 1–13.

MacCallum, Fiona and Deirdre Madden, 'Contract Pregnancy' in Dolores Dooley , Joan McCarthy, Tina Garanis-Papadatos and Panagiota Dalla-Vorgia, *The Ethics of New Reproductive Technologies*, Oxford: Berghahn Books 2003, 55–73.

Madden, Deirdre, *Medicine, Ethics & the Law*, Dublin: Butterworths 2002, 293–340.

Patterson, C., 'Children of Lesbian and Gay Parents', *Child Development*, 63 (1992), 1025–42.

Philpott, Ger, 'In the Name of the Fathers', *The Irish Times*, 20 August 2001.

Purdy, Laura M., 'Children of Choice: Whose Children?' *Washington Lee Law Review* 52/1 (1995), 197–224.

Purdy, Laura, 'Surrogate Mothering: Exploitation or Empowerment?' in Helga Kuhse and Peter Singer, eds, *Bioethics*, Oxford: Blackwell 2000, 103–12.

Robertson, John A., *Children of Choice*, Princeton: Princeton University Press 1994.

13: Companying the Chronically Ill and Dying

Andrews, Keith, 'Managing the Persistent Vegetative State', *British Medical Journal* 305 (1992), 486–7.

Andrews, Keith, et al., 'Misdiagnosis of the Vegetative State: Retrospective Study in a Rehabilitation Unit', *British Medical Journal* 313 (1996), 13–16.

Courts Service, *Office of Wards of Court: An Information Booklet*, Dublin: Courts Service Information Office 2003.

Donnelly, Mary, *Consent: Bridging the Gap between Doctor and Patient*, Cork: Cork University Press 2002.

Dooley, Dolores, 'The Primacy of Spirit in Decisions at the End of Life', paper presented at Second International Conference on PVS in Bonn, Germany 1995.

Grubb, Andrew, Pat Walsh, Neil Lambe, Trevor Murrells and Sarah Robinson, 'Doctors' Views on the Management of Patients in Persistent Vegetative State: report of a small survey in Ireland' collaborative project between Dolores Dooley, National University of Ireland at Cork and the Centre for Medical Law & Ethics, King's College, London 1997. Report unpublished but available from Dolores Dooley.

Hanafin, Patrick, *Last Rights: Death, Dying & the Law in Ireland*, Cork: Cork University Press 1997.

Iglesias, Teresa, 'Ethics, Brain-Death, and the Medical Concept of the Human Being', *Medico-Legal Journal of Ireland* 1/2 (1995), 51–7.

Jennett, Bryan, *The Vegetative State*, Cambridge: Cambridge University Press 2002.

Kendrick, Kevin David, 'Ethical Issues in Critical Care Nursing' in Win Tadd, ed., *Ethical Issues in Nursing and Midwifery Practice*, London: Macmillan 1998, 216–32.

Keown, John, ed., *Euthanasia Examined: Ethical, Legal and Clinical Perspectives*, Cambridge: Cambridge University Press 1995.

Kübler-Ross, Elisabeth, *Death: The Final Stage of Growth*, Englewood Cliffs, New Jersey: Prentice-Hall 1975.

Kuczewski, M. G., 'Commentary, Narrative Views of Personal Identity and Substituted Judgement in Surrogate Decision Making', *Journal of Law, Medicine and Ethics* 27/1 (1999), 32–6.

Mappes, Thomas, 'Persistent Vegetative State, Prospective Thinking, and Advance Directives', *Kennedy Institute of Ethics Journal* 13/2 (2003), 119–39.

McCarthy, Hannah Teresa, 'Narrative Theories of the Self', Ph.D. thesis, Department of Philosophy, National University of Ireland, Cork, 2001.

Rachels, James, *The End of Life*, Oxford: Oxford University Press 1986.

Ramsey, Paul, *The Patient as Person*, New Haven: Yale University Press 1970.

Scott, P. A., 'Moral Judgement, Emotion and Nursing Practice' in *Nursing Philosophy* 1/2 (2000), 123–31.

Supreme Court of Ireland, *In the Matter of a Ward of Court*, 2 ILRM, 401 (1995). *www.irlii.org* Accessed 1 May 2004.

Tomkin, David and Adam McAuley, 'Re a Ward of Court: Legal Analysis', *Medico-Legal Journal of Ireland* 1/2 (1995), 45–50.

Tschudin, Verena, 'Nursing Ethics at the End of Life' in Win Tadd, ed., *Ethical Issues in Nursing and Midwifery Practice*, London: Macmillan 1998, 233–55.

14: Falling Down the Slippery Slope

Ashley, Benedict, and Kevin O'Rourke, *Health Care Ethics: A Theological Analysis* (4th edition), Washington DC: Georgetown University Press 1997.

British Journal of Nursing editorial, 'What do nurses feel about end of life decisions? An Ethical Debate', *British Journal of Nursing* 6/14 (1997).

Congregation for the Doctrine of the Faith, 'Declaration on Euthanasia' (5 May 1980).

Cusack, Denis, 'Re a Ward of Court: Medical Law and Medical Ethics', *Medical Legal Journal of Ireland*, 60 (1995), 43–4.

Derr, Patrick, 'Why Food and Fluids Can Never Be Denied', *Hastings Center Report* 16/1 (1986), 28–30.

Dooley, Dolores, 'The Primacy of Spirit in Decisions at the End of Life', unpublished paper presented at Second International Conference on PVS in Bonn, Germany 1995.

Grubb, Andrew, Pat Walsh, Neil Lambe, Trevor Murrells and Sarah Robinson, 'Doctors' Views on the Management of Patients in Persistent Vegetative State: report of a small survey in Ireland' collaborative project between Dolores Dooley, National University of Ireland at Cork and the Centre for Medical Law & Ethics, King's College, London 1997. Report unpublished but available from Dolores Dooley.

Hanafin, Patrick, *Last Rights: Death, Dying & the Law in Ireland*, Cork: Cork University Press 1997.

Iglesias, Teresa, 'Ethics, Brain-Death, and the Medical Concept of the Human Being', *Medico-Legal Journal of Ireland* 1/2 (1995), 51–7.

JM v. *Board of Management of St Vincent's Hospital* [2003] 1IR 321.

John Paul II, *Evangelium Vitae*, known as *The Gospel of Life*, 1995.

Kearney, Michael, *Mortally Wounded: Stories of Soul Pain, Death and Healing*, New York: Scribner 1996.

Keown, John, ed., *Euthanasia Examined: Ethical, Legal and Clinical Perspectives*, Cambridge: Cambridge University Press 1995.

Kübler-Ross, Elisabeth, *On Death and Dying*, London: Macmillan 1969.

Lamb, David, *Down the Slippery Slope: Arguing in Applied Ethics*, London: Croom Helm 1988.

Lynn, Joanne, ed., *By No Extraordinary Means*, Bloomington, Indiana: Indiana University Press 1989.

McCormick, Richard A., *The Critical Calling*, Washington DC: Georgetown University Press 1989.

Meilaender, Gilbert, 'On Removing Food and Water: Against the Stream', *The Hastings Center Report*, December 1984.

O'Brien, Tony, 'Supreme Court Decision in Respect of a Ward of Court', *Irish Medical Journal* 6 (1995), 183–4.

O'Rourke, Kevin D., 'On Prolonging Life', *Doctrine and Life* 39/7 (1989), 352–66.

O'Rourke, Kevin D. and Patrick Norris, O.P., 'Care of PVS Patients: Catholic Opinion in the United States', *The Linacre Quarterly* 68/3 (2001), 201–17.

Panicola, Michael, 'Catholic Teaching on Prolonging Life', *Hastings Center Report* 31/6 (2001), 14–25.

Paris, John J., 'When Burdens of Feeding Outweigh Benefits', *Hastings Center Report* 16/1 (1986), 30–32.

Pius XII, Allocution 'Le Dr. Bruno Haid', 24 November, *Acta Apostolicae Sedis*, 49 (1957), 1031–2.

President's Commission for the Study of Ethical Problems in Medicine and Biomedical and Behavioral Research, March (1983), *Deciding to Forego Life-Sustaining Treatment*, Washington, DC: US Government Printing Office 1983.

Råholm, Maj-Britt and Lisbet Lindholm, 'Being in the World of the Suffering Patient: A Challenge to Nursing Ethics', *Nursing Ethics* 6/6 (1999), 528–39.

Randall, Fiona and R. S. Downie, *Palliative Care Ethics: A Good Companion*, Oxford: Oxford University Press 1998.

Rumbold, Graham, *Ethics in Nursing Practice* (3rd edition), Edinburgh: Ballière Tindall 1999.

Sabatino, Charles, 'Reflections on the Meaning of Care', *Nursing Ethics* 6/5 (1999), 374–82.

Sacred Congregation for the Doctrine of Faith, *Declaration on Euthanasia* 1980.

Scott, P. A., 'Autonomy, Power and Control in Palliative Care' in *Cambridge Ethics Quarterly* 8/2 (1999): 139–47.

Sheikh, Asim A. 'The Status of the "Do Not Resuscitate" Orders in Irish Law and Medicine', *Do Not Resuscitate! Who Decides?*, Dublin: St Paul Ireland 2001, 5–8.

Tilden, Virginia, Susan Tolle, Christine Nelson and Jonathan Fields, 'Family Decision-Making to Withdraw Life-Sustaining Treatments from Hospitalized Patients', *Nursing Research* 50/2 (2001), 105.

Weber, L. J., 'Who Shall Live?' in J. Walter and T. Shannon, eds, *Quality of Life: The New Medical Dilemma*, New York: Paulist Press 1990, 111–18.

15: Allocating Scarce Health Resources

Campbell, Alastair, Grant Gillett and Gareth Jones, *Medical Ethics* (2nd edition), Oxford: Oxford University Press 1997.

Daniels, Norman, *Just Health Care: Studies in Philosophy and Health Policy*, Cambridge: Cambridge University Press 1985.

Daniels, Norman, 'Is There a Right to Health Care, and, if so, what does it encompass?' in Helga Kuhse and Peter Singer, *A Companion to Bioethics*, Oxford: Blackwell Publishers 2001, 316–25.

Dickenson, Donna, 'Nurse Time as a Scarce Health Care Resource' in Geoffrey Hunt, ed., *Ethical Issues in Nursing*, London: Routledge, 207–17.

Dooley, Dolores, *Equality in Community*, Cork: Cork University Press 1996.

Fletcher, Nina, Janet Holt, Margaret Brazier and John Harris, *Ethics, Law and Nursing*, Manchester: Manchester University Press 1995.

Fry, Sara T. and Robert M. Veatch, *Case Studies in Nursing Ethics*, (2nd Edition), Sudbury Massachusetts: Jones and Bartlett 2000.

Gillon, Raanan, *Philosophical Medical Ethics*, Chichester: Wiley 1985.

Hendrick, Judith, *Law and Ethics in Nursing and Health Care*, Cheltenham: Stanley Thornes 2000.

Holland, Kitty, 'Plea for Ethnic Monitor in Health Services' *The Irish Times*, 30 June 2004, 5.

Hope, Tony, Julian Savulescu and Judith Hendrick, *Medical Ethics and Law*, Edinburgh: Churchill Livingstone 2003.

Hussey, Trevor, 'Efficiency and Health', *Nursing Ethics* 4/3 (1997), 181–90.

Kuhse, Helga and Peter Singer, eds, *A Companion to Bioethics*, Blackwell: Oxford 2001.

McIntosh, Peggy, 'White Privilege: Unpacking the Invisible Knapsack', excerpt from *Working Paper 189*, Wellesley College Center for Research on Women, Wellesley, Massachusetts 1988, 02181.

Newdick, Christopher, *Who Should We Treat?*, Oxford: Clarendon Press 1995.

Nozick, Robert, *Anarchy, State and Utopia*, Oxford: Blackwell 1974.

O'Keeffe, Cormac and Michael O'Farrell, 'Shocking State of Mental Homes Under Fire', *Irish Examiner*, 9 September 2004, 1.

Parker, Michael and Donna Dickenson, *The Cambridge Medical Ethics Workbook*, Cambridge: Cambridge University Press 2001.

Rawls, John, *A Theory of Justice*, Oxford: Clarendon Press 1972.

Rumbold, Graham, *Ethics in Nursing Practice* (3rd edition), Edinburgh: Baillière Tindall 1999.

Schwartz, Lisa, Paul Preece and Rob Hendry, *Medical Ethics: A Case Based Approach*, Saunders: Edinburgh 2002.

Scott, P. Anne, 'Allocation of Resources: Some Issues for Nurses' in Win Tadd, ed., *Ethics in Nursing Education, Research and Management: Perspectives from Europe*, London: Palgrave 2003, 145–62.

Shickle, Darren, 'Resource Allocation' in *Encyclopedia of Applied Ethics*, Vol. 3, London: Academic Press 1998, 861–73.

Tschudin, Verena, *Deciding Ethically*, London: Baillière Tindall 1994.

Wilkinson, Richard, *Unhealthy Societies: The Afflictions of Inequality*, London: Routledge 1996.

Wilmot, Stephen, *Ethics, Power and Policy: The Future of Nursing in the NHS*, London: Palgrave 2003.

Wren, Maev-Ann, *Unhealthy State: Anatomy of a Sick Society*, Dublin: New Island 2003.

Yeo, Michael and Ann Moorhouse, eds, *Concepts and Cases in Nursing Ethics* (2nd edition), Ontario, Canada: Broadview Press 1996.

16: Accountability and Whistle-blowing

An Bord Altranais, *Guidance for Nurses and Midwives on Medication Management*, 2003. Web address: *www.nursingboard.ie* Accessed 1 May 2004.

Bok, Sissela, *Lying: Moral Choice in Public and Private Life*, Sussex: Harvester Press 1978.

Chadwick, Ruth and Win Tadd, *Ethics and Nursing Practice*, London: Macmillan 1992.

Donnellan, Eithne, 'Patient Group Says up to 100 Women Could Sue', *The Irish Times*, 29 October 2003.

Fletcher, Nina, Janet Holt, Margaret Brazier and John Harris, *Ethics, Law and Nursing*, Manchester: Manchester University Press 1995.

Fry, Sara T. and Megan-Jane Johnstone, *Ethics in Nursing Practice* (2nd edition), Oxford: Blackwell 2002.

Houston, Muiris, 'Power in the Wrong Hands?' *The Irish Times*, 2 August 2003.

Nursing and Midwifery Council (NMC), *Management of Errors or Incidents in the Administration of Medicines*, 2002. Web address: *www.cybernurse. org.uk/nmc_drug_policy.html* Accessed 1 May 2004.

Morreim, E. Haavi, 'Am I My Brother's Warden? Responding to the Unethical or Incompetent Colleague', *Hastings Center Report* 23/3 (1993): 19–27.

Pink, Graham, Correspondence, *Guardian*, 11 April 1990. Web address: *http://society.guardian.co.uk/societyguardian/story/0,7843,1304327,00.html* Accessed 1 May 2004.

Pink, Graham, *Truth from the bedside*, London: Charter 88 1992. Web address: *www.charter88.com/pubs/violations/pink.html* Accessed 1 May 2004.

Reid, Liam, 'Pressure for Inquiry into Doctor Guilty of Misconduct', *The Irish Times*, 30 September 2003.

Thompson, Ian, Kath Melia and Kenneth Boyd, *Nursing Ethics* (4th edition), Edinburgh: Churchill Livingstone 2000.

Tschudin, Verena, *Deciding Ethically*, London: Baillière Tindall 1994.

Tschudin, Verena and Geoffrey Hunt, 'Editorial', *Nursing Ethics* 4/4 (1997), 265–7.

Tschudin, Verena, 'Special Issues Facing Nurses' in Helga Kuhse and Peter Singer, eds, *A Companion to Bioethics*, Blackwell: Oxford 2001.

Weber, Leonard, *Business Ethics in Health Care: Beyond Compliance*, Bloomington, Indiana: Indiana University Press 2001.

Wilmot, Stephen, *Ethics, Power and Policy: The Future of Nursing in the NHS*, Basingstoke: Palgrave Macmillan 2003.

World of Irish Nursing, 'No Place for Bullying', 12/8 (September 2004), on Irish Nursing Organisation web page, 1–5.

Yeo, Michael and Ann Moorhouse, *Concepts and Cases in Nursing Ethics* (2nd edition), Ontario, Canada: Broadview Press 1996.

17: The Right to Strike?

Clarke, Jean and Catherine O'Neill, 'An Analysis of How the *Irish Times* Portrayed Irish Nursing During the 1999 Strike', *Nursing Ethics* 8/4 (2001), 350–59.

Fry, Sara T. and Megan-Jane Johnstone, *Ethics in Nursing Practice* (2nd edition), Oxford: Blackwell 2002.

Goold, Susan Dorr, 'Trust: and the Ethics of Health Care Institutions', *Hastings Center Report*, November–December 2001, 26–33.

Hendrick, Judith, *Law and Ethics in Nursing and Health Care*, Cheltenham: Stanley Thornes 2000.

Holt, Janet, 'The Unexamined Life is Not Worth Living' in Steven Edwards, ed., *Philosophical Issues in Nursing*, London: Macmillan 1998, 149–57.

Jennings, Karen and Glenda Western, 'A Right to Strike', *Nursing Ethics* 4/4 (1997), 277–81.

Kuhse, Helga and Peter Singer, eds, *A Companion to Bioethics*, Blackwell: Oxford 2001.

Martin, Ann, 'Industrial Action Could Return by End of Year', *World of Irish Nursing* 12/6 (June 2004), 1–3.

Nursing Ethics: 'Ethics of Strike Action' 4/4 (1997). This entire issue is devoted to articles on the topic of strike action.

Rumbold, Graham, *Ethics in Nursing Practice* (3rd edition), Edinburgh: Baillière Tindall 1999.

Thompson, Ian, Kath Melia and Kenneth Boyd, *Nursing Ethics* (4th edition), Edinburgh: Churchill Livingstone 2000.

Tschudin, Verena, *Deciding Ethically*, London: Baillière Tindall 1994.

Tschudin, Verena and Geoffrey Hunt, 'Editorial', *Nursing Ethics* 4/4 (1997), 265–7.

Tschudin, Verena (2001), 'Special Issues Facing Nurses' in Helga Kuhse and Peter Singer, eds, *A Companion to Bioethics*, Blackwell: Oxford 2001.

Weber, Leonard, *Business Ethics in Health Care: Beyond Compliance*, Bloomington, Indiana: Indiana University Press 2001.

Wilmot, Stephen, *Ethics, Power and Policy: The Future of Nursing in the NHS*, Basingstoke: Palgrave Macmillan 2003.

Yeo, Michael and Ann Moorhouse, *Concepts and Cases in Nursing Ethics* (2nd edition), Ontario, Canada: Broadview Press 1996.

18: Traditional Moral Theories

Aristotle, *The Nicomachean Ethics*, trans. J. A. K. Thomson, Middlesex: Penguin 1955.

Baron, Marcia, Philip Pettit and Michael Slote, *Three Methods of Ethics*, Oxford: Blackwell 1997.

Beauchamp, Tom and James Childress, *Principles of Biomedical Ethics* (5th edition), New York: Oxford University Press 2001.

Beauchamp, Tom and James Childress, *Principles of Biomedical Ethics* (4th edition), Oxford: Oxford University Press 1994.

Crisp, Roger, Mill. *On Utilitarianism*, London: Routledge 1997.

Donagan, Alan, *The Theory of Morality*, Chicago: University of Chicago Press 1977.

Downie, R. S. and K.C. Calman, *Healthy Respect: Ethics in Health Care* (2nd edition), New York: Oxford University Press 1995.

Edwards, Steven D., ed., *Philosophical Issues in Nursing*, London: Macmillan 1998.

Frankena, William, 'A Critique of Viritue Based Ethical Systems' in James Sterba, ed., *Ethics: the Big Questions*, Oxford: Blackwell 1998, 291–6.

Gutmann, Amy, 'What's the Use of Going to School?' in Amartya Sen and Bernard Williams, eds, *Utilitarianism and Beyond*, Cambridge: Cambridge University Press 1982, 261–77.

Harris, John, *The Value of Life: An Introduction to Medical Ethics*, London: Routledge 1985.

Kant, Immanuel, *Groundwork of the Metaphysics of Morals*, edited by Mary Gregor, Cambridge: Cambridge University Press 1997 [1785].

Kekes, John, *Moral Wisdom and Good Lives*, Ithaca: Cornell University Press 1995.

Korsgaard, Christine, 'Introduction to the Groundwork of the Metaphysics of Morals' in Mary Gregor edition of *Groundwork*, Cambridge: Cambridge University Press 1997, vii–xxxvi.

Kuhse, Helga, *Caring: Nurses, Women and Ethics*, Oxford: Blackwell, 1997.

MacIntyre, Alasdair, *Whose Justice? Which Rationality?* London: Duckworth 1988.

MacIntyre, Alasdair, *After Virtue* (2nd edition), London: Duckworth 1999.

McCarthy, Joan, 'Principlism or Narrative Ethics: Must We Choose Between Them?', *Medical Humanities* 29/2 (2003), 65–71.

Mill, John Stuart, *On Liberty and Other Essays*, edited by John Gray, Oxford: Oxford University Press 1991.

Pence, Greg, 'Virtue Theory' in Peter Singer, ed., *A Companion to Ethics*, Oxford: Basil Blackwell 1991, 249–58.

Pojman, Louis P., *Ethics: Discovering Right and Wrong*, Belmont, California: Wadsworth 1990.

Rawls, John, *A Theory of Justice*, Cambridge, Massachusetts: Harvard University Press 1971.

Rumbold, Graham, *Ethics in Nursing Practice* (3rd edition), Edinburgh: Baillière Tindall 1999.

Schick, Frederic, 'Under Which Description?' in Amartya Sen and Bernard Williams, eds, *Utilitarianism and Beyond,* Cambridge: Cambridge University Press 1982, 251–60.

Schwartz, Lisa, Paul Preece and Robert A. Hendry, *Medical Ethics: A Case-Based Approach*, Edinburgh: Saunders 2002.

Scott, P. Anne, 'Nursing Narrative, and the Moral Imagination', in Trish Greenhalgh and Brian Hurwitz, eds, *Narrative Based Medicine*, London: BMJ Books 1998, 149–58.

Sen, Amartya and Bernard Williams, eds, *Utilitarianism and Beyond*, Cambridge: Cambridge University Press 1982.

Statman, Daniel, *Virtue Ethics: A Critical Reader*, Edinburgh: Edinburgh University Press 1997.

Sterba, James P., ed., *Ethics: The Big Questions*, Oxford: Blackwell, 1998.

Tad, Win, ed., *Ethical Issues in Nursing and Midwifery Practice*, London: Macmillan 1998.

Thomson, Anne, *Critical Reasoning in Ethics: A Practical Introduction*, London: Routledge 1999.

Yeo, Michael and Anne Moorhouse, *Concepts and Cases in Nursing Ethics*, Ontario, Canada: Broadview Press 1996.

19: Contemporary Ethical Theories

Arras, John, 'Getting Down to Cases: The Revival of Casuistry in Bioethics', *The Journal of Medicine and Philosophy* 16 (1991), 29–51.

Baier, Annette, *Moral Prejudices: Essays on Ethics*, Cambridge, Massachusetts: Harvard University Press 1994.

Beauchamp, Tom and James Childress, *Principles of Biomedical Ethics*, New York: Oxford University Press 1979.

Beauchamp, Tom and James Childress, *Principles of Biomedical Ethics* (5th edition), Oxford: Oxford University Press 2001.

Benner, Patricia, 'The Role of Experience, Narrative and Community in Skilled Ethical Comportment', *Advances in Nursing Science* 14/2 (1991), 1–21.

Bishop, A. H. and J. Scudder, *The Practical, Moral and Personal Sense of Nursing: A Phenomenological Philosophy of Practice*, Albany, New York: State University of New York Press 1990.

Bishop, A. H. and J. Scudder, *Nursing, the Practice of Caring*, New York: NLM Press 1991.

Brody, Howard, *Stories of Sickness*, New Haven and London: Yale University Press 1987.

Brown, Helen, Patricia Rodney, Bernadette Pauly, Colleen Varcoe and Vicki Smye, 'Working within the Landscape: Nursing Ethics', in Janet L. Storch, Patricia Rodney and Rosalie Starzomski, eds, *Toward a Moral Horizon*, Toronto: Pearson Education Canada 2004, 126–53.

Carse, Alisa L. and Hilde Lindemann Nelson, 'Rehabilitating Care' in Anne Donchin and Laura M Purdy, eds, *Embodying Bioethics*, Lanham, Maryland: Rowman & Littlefield 1999.

Charon, Rita, 'Narrative Contributions to Medical Ethics: Recognition, Formulation, Interpretation, and Validation in the Practice of the Ethicist' in E. R. DuBose, R. P. Hamel and L. J. O'Connell, eds, *A Matter of Principles?*, Valley Forge, Pennsylvania: Trinity Press International 1994, 260–83.

Chambers, Tod, *The Fiction of Bioethics: Cases as Literary Texts*. New York: Routledge 1999. See also *American Journal of Bioethics*. 2001; 1(1) for a range of open peer commentaries drawn from philosophy, sociology, literature and medicine, on Chambers' book.

Cooper, M. C., 'Principle-Oriented Ethics and the Ethic of Care: A Creative Tension', *Advances in Nursing Science* 14/2 (1991), 22–31.

Clouser, K. D., 'Philosophy, Literature, and Ethics: Let the Engagement Begin', *The Journal of Medicine and Philosophy* 21 (1996): 321–40.

Clouser, K. D. and B. Gert, 'A Critique of Principlism', *The Journal of Medicine and Philosophy* 15 (1990), 219–36.

Council on Ethical and Judicial Affairs, *Surrogate Decision Making*. No. 119, (June 2001).

DuBose, E. R., R. P. Hamel and L. J. O'Connell, eds, *A Matter of Principles? Ferment in US Bioethics*, Valley Forge, Pennsylvania: Trinity Press International 1994.

Edwards, Steven D., *Nursing Ethics, A Principle-Based Approach*, Basingstoke: Macmillan 1996.

Edwards, Steven D., *Philosophy of Nursing*. Basingstoke: Palgrave 2001.

Doane, Gweneth, Bernadette Pauly, Helen Brown and Gladys McPherson, 'Exploring the Heart of Ethical Nursing Practice: Implications for Ethics Education', *Nursing Ethics* 11/3 (2004): 240–53.

Engelhardt, H. Tristram, *The Foundations of Bioethics*, New York: Oxford University Press 1986.

Frank, Arthur, *The Wounded Storyteller: Body, Illness and Ethics*, Chicago: Chicago University Press 1995.

Fry, Sara T. and Megan-Jane Johnstone, *Ethics in Nursing Practice* (2nd edition), Oxford: Blackwell 2002.

Gadow, Sally, 'ANS Open Forum: The Most Pressing Ethical Problem Faced by Nurses', *Advances in Nursing Science* 1/3 (1979): 92–5.

Gadow, Sally, 'Nurse and Patient: The Caring Relationship' in A. H. Bishop and J. R. Scudder, eds, *Caring, Curing, Coping: Nurse, Physician, Patient Relationships*, Birmingham, Alabama: University of Alabama Press 1985, 31–43.

Gadow, Sally, 'Whose Body? Whose Story? The Question About Narrative in Women's Health Care,' *Soundings* 77/3–4 (1994), 295–307.

Gadow, Sally, 'Restorative Nursing: Toward a Philosophy of Postmodern Punishment', *Nursing Philosophy* 4/2 (2003), 161–7.

Gilligan, Carol, *In a Different Voice: Psychological Theory and Women's Development*, Cambridge, Massachussets: Harvard University Press 1982.

Gilligan, Carol, 'Moral Orientation and Moral Development' in Eva Feder Kittay and Diana T. Meyers, eds, *Women and Moral Theory*, London: Rowman & Littlefield 1987, 19–33.

Gillon, Raanan, 'Medical Ethics: Four Principles Plus Attention to Scope', *British Medical Journal* 309 (1994), 184. Web address: *http://bmj.com/cgi/content/full/309/6948/184?maxtoshow* Accessed 1 May 2004.

Hanford, Linda, 'Nursing and the Concept of Care: An Appraisal of Noddings' Theory' in Geoffrey Hunt, ed., *Ethical Issues in Nursing*, London: Routledge 1994.

Holm, Søren, *Ethical Problems in Clinical Practice*, Manchester: Manchester University Press 1997.

Hudson Jones, A. 'Narrative in Medical Ethics' in T. Greenhalgh and B. Hurwitz, eds, *Narrative Based Medicine*, London: BMJ Books 1998.

Hunter, K. Montgomery, *Doctors' Stories: The Narrative Structure of Medical Knowledge*, Princeton: Princeton University Press 1992.

Hunter, K. Montgomery, 'Narrative' in T. R. Warren, ed., *Encyclopedia of Bioethics*, New York: Simon & Schuster Macmillan 1995, 1789–94.

Jonsen, Albert and Stephen Toulmin, *The Abuse of Casuistry: A History of Moral Reasoning*, Berkeley: University of California Press 1988.

Kohlberg, Lawrence, *The Philosophy of Moral Development*, San Francisco: Harper and Row 1981 (a).

Kohlberg, Lawrence, *The Meaning and Measurement of Moral Development*, Massachusetts: Clark University/Heinz Werner Institute 1981 (b).

Kuhse, Helga, *Caring: Nurses, Women and Ethics*, London: Blackwell 1997.

Kuczewski, M. G., 'Commentary, Narrative Views of Personal Identity and Substituted Judgement in Surrogate Decision Making', *Journal of Law, Medicine and Ethics* 27/1 (1999), 32–6.

Lipp, Allyson, 'An Enquiry into a Combined Approach for Nursing Ethics', *Nursing Ethics* 5/2 (1998), 122–38.

Little, Margaret Olivia, 'Why a Feminist Approach to Bioethics?' in James Lindemann Nelson and Hilde Lindemann Nelson, eds, *Meaning and Medicine*, New York: Routledge 1999, 199–209.

MacIntyre, Alasdair, *After Virtue: A Study in Moral Theory*, London: Duckworth 2000.

McPherson, Gladys, Patricia Rodney, Michael McDonald, Janet Storch, Bernadette Pauly and Michael Burgess, 'Working within the Landscape: Applications in Health Care Ethics' in Janet L. Storch, Patricia Rodney and Rosalie Starzomski, eds, *Toward a Moral Horizon*, Toronto: Pearson Education Canada 2004, 98–125.

Murphy, Sharon, Personal communication, 2004.

National Commission for the Protection of Human Subjects of Biomedical and Behavioral Research, *Belmont Report*, Washington DC: Government Printing Office 1979. Web address: *http://ohsr.od.nih.gov/mpa/belmont.php3* Accessed 1 May 2004.

MacKenzie, Catriona and Natalie Stoljar, *Relational Autonomy*, Oxford: Oxford University Press 2000.

Melia, K. M., 'Just Passing Through', *Nursing Times*, 18 May 1983, 16–27.

Nelson, Hilde Lindemann, ed., *Stories and Their Limits*, New York: Routledge 1997.

Nelson, Hilde Lindemann, *Damaged Identities: Narrative Repair*, New York: Cornell University Press 2001.

Noddings, Nel, *Caring: A Feminine Approach to Ethics and Moral Education*, Berkeley: University of California Press 1984.

Noddings, Nel, 'In Defense of Caring', *Journal of Clinical Ethics* 3 (1992), 15–18.

Nussbaum, Martha, *Love's Knowledge*, New York: Oxford University Press 1992.

Nussbaum, Martha, *Poetic Justice: The Literary Imagination and Public Life*, Boston: Beacon Press 1995.

Peter, Elizabeth and Joan Liaschenko, 'Whose Morality is it Anyway? Thoughts on the Work of Margaret Urban Walker', *Nursing Philosophy* 4/3 (2003), 259–62.

Peter, Elizabeth and Joan Liaschenko, 'Feminist Ethics is Not a Subject Matter', 8th International Philosophy of Nursing Conference, 7–9 September 2004.

Ricoeur, Paul, *Time and Narrative*, Vol. 3, trans. Kathleen Blamey and David Pellauer, Chicago: University of Chicago Press, 1988.

Rodney, Patricia, Bernadette Pauly and Michael Burgess, 'Our Theoretical Landscape: Complementary Approaches to Health Care Ethics' in Janet L. Storch, Patricia Rodney and Rosalie Starzomski, eds, *Toward a Moral Horizon*, Toronto: Pearson Education Canada 2004, 77–97.

Scott, P. Anne, 'Nursing, Narrative, and the Moral Imagination' in Trisha Greenhalgh and Brian Hurwitz, eds, *Narrative Based Medicine*, London: BMJ Books 1998, 149–158.

Sherwin, Susan, *No Longer Patient: Feminist Ethics and Health Care*, Philadelphia: Temple University Press 1992.

Sherwin, Susan, 'A Relational Approach to Autonomy in Health Care' in S. Sherwin and The Feminist Health Care Ethics Research Network, eds, *The Politics of Women's Health: Exploring Agency and Autonomy*, Philadelphia: Temple University Press 1998, 19–47.

Smith, Katharine V. and Nelda S. Godfrey, 'Being a Good Nurse and Doing the Right Thing: A Qualitative Study', *Nursing Ethics* 9/3 (2002), 301–10.

Tong, Rosemarie, *Feminist Approaches to Bioethics*, Colorado: Westview Press 1982.

Tong, Rosemarie, 'Just Caring about Maternal-Fetal Relations: The Case of Cocaine-Using Pregnant Women' in Anne Donchin and Laura M. Purdy, eds, *Embodying Bioethics*, Lanham, Maryland: Rowman & Littlefield 1999.

Veatch, Robert M., *A Theory of Medical Ethics*, New York: Basic Books 1981.

Walker, Margaret Urban, 'Picking up Pieces, Lives, Stories, and Integrity' in Diana Tietzens Meyers, ed., *Feminists Rethink the Self*, Boulder, Colorado: Westview Press 1997.

Walker, Margaret Urban, *Moral Understandings*, London: Routledge 1998.

Watson, Jean, *Nursing: Human Science and Human Care*, New York: NLN Press 1988.

Woods, Martin, 'A Nursing Ethic: The Moral Voice of Experienced Nurses', *Nursing Ethics* 6/5 (1999), 423–33.

Index